40 Years in
Family Medicine

JOSEPH E. SCHERGER, MD, MPH

DEDICATION

To my family who have supported me
in pursuing all my dreams.
My wife Carol and my sons, Adrian and Gabriel.

To my mentors, colleagues, dedicated staff,
residents, students and patients,
I have learned from all of you.

ACKNOWLEDGMENT

To Helen Searing, my assistant
at Eisenhower Medical Center, who worked
painstakingly to make this book come out so well.

CONTENTS

Part II: Maturing with Family Medicine, 1978-1984

Part III: Leadership 1985-92

Part IV: Managed Care and Family Medicine, 1992-98

Part V: The Internet Changes Almost Everything, 1999-2005

Part VI: New Models of Care, 2006-2014

PREFACE

40 Years in Family Medicine

I did not plan to go into family medicine. My demographics predicted it was likely. I grew up in a small town in Northwest Ohio, Delphos, where the only physicians were general practitioners. While I was talented in math and science, I was drawn to the social sciences and had a minor emphasis in philosophy while in college. While studying in the turbulent late 1960s, I said medicine would be my profession while philosophy would be my hobby.

I was a cerebral kid. I exercised my mind but had limited physical skills. I never fixed my bicycle, or anything I can remember. Internal medicine would be my specialty and maybe rheumatology since I was fascinated with unlocking the secrets of autoimmune disease. Then again, I was drawn to child psychiatry.

My conversion to family medicine happened during the third year of medical school at UCLA. I was on the emergency medicine rotation at a large county hospital. Each day the medical students were triaged to either the medical or surgical areas of the emergency room. On the surgical side I discovered I could fix things, such as sewing up lacerations, putting on splints and casts. I loved it! When I was triaged to the medicine side, the tedium had me not looking forward to going in. That rotation was followed by the joy of delivering babies in obstetrics and the joy of seeing children in pediatrics. I wanted it all and was drawn to the new specialty of family medicine.

I did not just choose family medicine, I had a conversion. It was 1974 and I read about the creation of the specialty from general practice in 1969. I joined the American Academy of Family Physicians as a student member and helped start the UCLA family medicine interest group. I read about how the Society of Teachers of Family Medicine was started by Lynn Carmichael. G. Gayle Stephens became my family medicine philosopher. I saw Tom Stern leave his family medicine residency program in Santa Monica, where he was the real Marcus Welby, and go to Kansas City to lead the development of more family medicine programs.

Helping other medical students choose family medicine became a passion. Preceptorships, where students would spend time in a practicing family physician's office, became popular. I saw that some of these experiences worked and some turned the students off. That topic became the focus of my first published article and early presentations. I shared insight into how preceptorships were effective and why they were not.

I was gifted in giving presentations since high school, and doing them was easy and fun. A mentor during medical school, Len Hughes Andrus from the University of California, Davis, expressed to me that the spoken word just evaporates but the written word is eternal.

I was not a natural writer. Growing up in Delphos, Ohio, English was taught by either nuns or athletic coaches. On my first college paper, my English teacher wrote, "Mr. Scherger, you have no semblance of logical organization". By mid-term my parents were warned that I might fail the class. Getting an A in freshman English was one of my hardest accomplishments. I learned that writing was an activity you had to exercise. I became committed to writing and this book is the result.

Collected here are the articles I am most proud of and I think made some contribution to family medicine at the time. The articles are not a complete look at the issues central to the growing specialty and academic discipline of family medicine during the 40 years between 1974 and 2014. They reflect those areas of my involvement, such as student interest in the specialty, especially during the 1970s and 1980s; family centered maternity care in the 1980s and 1990s; managed care in the 1990s; and the emergence of the internet and information technology resulting in new ways to provide family medicine in 2000 and beyond.

I hope these articles are useful not only from an historical perspective but also as a guide to the future. As Winston Churchill said, "The farther backward you can look, the farther forward you are likely to see". At a minimum, I hope in reading this you experience some of the joy in this career journey.

Joseph E. Scherger, MD, MPH
La Quinta, CA

June 2014

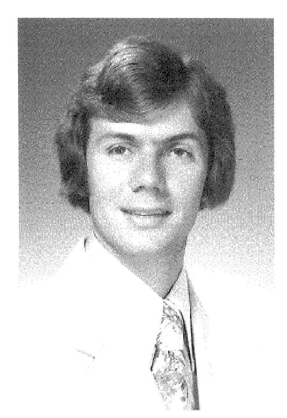

JOSEPH E. SCHERGER, MD
FAMILY MEDICINE RESIDENT, 1976

JOSEPH E. SCHERGER, MD, MPH

PART I: BEGINNINGS WITH FAMILY MEDICINE, 1974 TO 1978

Born in 1969, the new specialty of family medicine (then called family practice) was gaining attention during my medical school years, 1971-75. After I converted to family medicine in 1974 and helped start the FMIG at UCLA, preceptorships in practicing physicians' offices became popular. I observed that about half the time, the preceptorship experience actually turned off the student to family medicine. My first published article was an essay to would-be preceptors and those who ran these programs in order to make them most often positive experiences for the students. This article became the most copied of all articles I have ever published and was highlighted by John Geyman in Archives of Family Medicine, Volume I in 1980.

A Medical Student's Perspective on Preceptors in Family Practice

Journal Family Practice
1975;2(3):201-203

Reprinted (with Commentary)
Archives of Family Medicine
1980
John P. Geyman (Ed.). New York: Appleton-Century Crofts

Abstract: Preceptorships have become an important means by which medical students are exposed to family practice. In order for a preceptor to be successful in nurturing student interest in family practice, he must have a good understanding of certain characteristics of today's medical students. Important differences exist between preclinical and clinical students, and the preceptorship must be designed accordingly. Unless preceptors are carefully selected and trained, they may have a negative influence on student interest in family practice.

The preceptorship is an educational experience in which a medical student spends a period of time with a physician preceptor in a practice setting outside the academic center. Teaching of family practice may be somewhat limited within the academic center, and the preceptorship is an important means by which the student can see the family physicians as a role model and experience the scope and flavor of family practice. The student may be either positively or negatively reinforced in his interest in family practice, and the preceptor is very influential in the decision making process of a student considering a career in family practice.

Having experienced several preceptorships during my medical education and discussed many others with my peers, I have concluded that too often preceptors are unaware of the responsibilities of their position and the delicate nature of their interchange with students. If they are aware, too often they lack the insight or training to make the preceptorship experience effective. The existing literature on the subject of guidelines for preceptors[1] or student views of the preceptor role[2,3] is very limited. This paper attempts to provide preceptors with a better understanding of the students they will encounter in the hope that this will improve their teaching effectiveness.

It is most important for a preceptor in family practice to have a good understanding of the medical student preceptee: Who are today's medical students? What are their anticipations about family practice? What is the student's perspective on the practice of medicine at the present time in his training? Though the answers to these questions show some individual variation, there is considerable similarity among most students and this must be understood by family practice preceptors.

Many, if not most, students entering medical school today are interested in becoming some kind of primary care physician. Besides professional independence and financial security, the image of a first contact doctor-patient (and family) relationship is a strong motivational factor in students who enter the field of medicine. This image, however, is usually untested and far removed from the real practice of family medicine, and it must undergo a great evolutionary process during medical school if a student is to choose family practice residency training. There are many nurturing opportunities and stumbling blocks during this evolution, and the family practice preceptor may contribute to both.

A discussion of the preceptor-student relationship should distinguish between the student in his preclinical (usually first two years of medical school) and clinical periods of training. Students in these two periods are so different that if a preceptor is teaching both types without marked differences in the conduct of his preceptorship, he is certain to be ineffective with at least one of these groups.

The Preclinical Student

The student entering a preceptor's office early in his medical education is usually quite eager for any clinical experience. In some ways the preclinical student is the easiest and least intimidating preceptee because his lack of medical background makes him likely to find any medical treatment given by the preceptor acceptable without question. In other ways these students may be a burden to the preceptor because they require an explanation of the most basic aspects of clinical practice and generally cannot compensate for this extra time by seeing patients.

At this stage in their training, most preclinical students feel certain deficiencies in their education which a preceptor can counteract and, in the process; he can nurture student interest in family practice. Though students enter medical school with a strong desire to begin training in the clinical role of the physician, the curricula of most schools involve almost complete delayed gratification of this desire during the basic science years. Family practice can get the jump on the other clinical specialties by providing the student an opportunity to participate in a clinical environment.

3

Family physician preceptors should realize a unique quality of the preclinical student that is often forgotten in the medical school curriculum. The student in the early years of his transition to the doctor's role still identified himself more as patient than as doctor. The preclinical student is therefore keenly sensitive to the feelings of patients, probably more so that the practicing physician long entrenched in the role of provider. Though a preceptor may feel confident that he knows what his patients feel, he should allow the student to interview them as a patient or family advocate to test these conceptions. The preclinical student in a clinical setting has the opportunity to learn a tremendous amount about what patients feel, an opportunity that may be lost as he becomes enveloped by the content of medical science.

Though the preceptorship role for a preclinical student is largely that of observer with respect to patient management, the preceptor should provide the student with as much active participation as possible. For example, depending on the student's experience and what he has learned in the preceptor's office, the student should actively participate in history taking, physical examination, office laboratory procedures, and even in a discussion of diagnostic possibilities and therapeutics. The preclinical student should also assist the preceptor in such procedures as obstetric delivery and major or minor surgery.

Several stumbling blocks that preceptors can throw in the way of a preclinical student's interest in family practice should be mentioned. Any student with a realistic chance of entering medical school today has a strong background in the biomedical sciences together with a respect for the latest advances in science and an awareness that these advances may have a profound effect on the practice of medicine. If a student perceives a practice setting as being outdated and the preceptor as being unaware of modern advances in biomedical science, he will have a negative reaction to that kind of practice and physician. The family physician preceptor must convincingly demonstrate to the student that his knowledge and his practice are appropriate to the modern practice of medicine, and that the specialty of family practice has designed a mechanism for maintaining quality among its members through continuing education.

The preceptor should also realize that today's preclinical students are products of high school and undergraduate education during the late 1960's and early 1970's when a revolution in social values occurred among the younger generation. Many medical students are interested in family practice because of the humanistic values they acquired during that era. The family practice preceptor must, to a certain extent, share in these social values (not to be confused with political ideology) and stress the humanistic aspects of his practice. He should not stress the material benefits of his practice as he might to a resident (who he may see as a potential future partner) for these are not appropriate to the preclinical student's interests and may negatively affect his feeling toward family practice.

A third stumbling block to the preclinical student's interest in family practice relates to the preceptor's actual clinical practice. Though the preclinical student may not have the experience to evaluate the diagnostic and therapeutic activities of the preceptor, he may react negatively to the experience retrospectively after subsequent training. Hence, the preceptor must be certain that the student understands the reasoning behind the care given, even if it is somewhat beyond the student's present training.

Finally, the preceptor should realize that preclinical students maintain an image of themselves as future physicians which is based on idealized concepts rather than clinical experience. To be a successful role model, the preceptor must convey his personal philosophy of being a physician to the student in such a way that it is compatible with the student's image. The preclinical student with any interest in family practice has a physician image which is largely built around the art of medicine, i.e., the human element in the successful doctor-patient (and family) interaction, and the ability to provide continuing care relevant to the total well-being of the patient. Family practice is unique among the specialties in its strong emphasis on the art of medicine and the family practice preceptor should eagerly convey through conversation and action this artistry to the student. The preclinical student who has personally experienced, through a role model, the art of medicine in family practice will have a torch to carry which will guide the way through the remainder of his medical education. Only family physicians who practice a humanistic approach to patients and are concerned with their total well-being should be preceptors. Those family physicians who have abandoned that artistry for the sake of expediency or defensive medicine should never be preceptors.

The Clinical Student

The medical student during his clinical clerkship years is in an extremely rapid period of development. As if overnight, the student senses his acquisition of enough skills to relate to patients in the role of doctor. Many of his previous images of himself and medicine fade into oblivion during this rebirth and his world becomes largely confined to the walls of the hospital ward. If his academic mentors are successful, the mere words "headache" or "low back pain" will instantly trigger in the mind of the student a large differential diagnosis, and he embarks on a comprehensive work-up. Out of this environment the haggard student arrives, by requirement or elective, at the office of the family physician for a look at family practice.

The clinical student interested in an alternative to the secondary and tertiary care of the academic center will be taking a very close look at the family physician, his life-style, and his practice. Many physicians today are concerned about the advent of peer and government review of their practice, but the potential preceptor should realize that student review will be far more critical than these two. The clinical student from the academic center brings with him standards and a philosophy of medicine which the preceptor must be prepared to deal with. He should be able to put these in a proper perspective and present viable alternatives.

An optimal preceptorship environment for clinical students can easily be summarized. If a preceptor accepts a clinical student for anything more than a few hours, he should be prepared to allow the student a significant amount of participation in the practice. If limited to a role of observation, the student with clinical experience will quickly become bored and frustrated no matter how capable the preceptor nor how interesting the patients. Some physicians may be concerned about their private patients being examined alone by medical students, but if the student is appropriately introduced (or introduces himself) as a "doctor-in-training" working with Dr. X, and it is made clear that the patient may see Dr. X and will definitely have his consultation, patient dissatisfaction is generally not a problem. Many patients enjoy having a young mind from the academic center hear their problems, and their respect for the family physician is greatly increased when they realize he is involved with teaching medical students.

At the onset of the preceptorship program, the student should be oriented in the office setting as if he were a new physician member of the health care team. The student should then observe the preceptor seeing a few patients to get a feeling for his approach to patients. The preceptor may then want to observe the student in history taking and physical examination to evaluate his competence and offer suggestions. After this introductory period, which should last about half a day, the student should begin seeing patients. He should take whatever history and perform whatever physical examination he feels is appropriate, decide upon the most likely diagnostic possibilities, and consider a management plan. Then the student should present his findings and ideas to the preceptor for discussion and evaluation. The preceptor may want to review with the patient pertinent aspects of the history and physical examination for verification and for teaching purposes. When the final management plan is decided upon, often it will be a joint decision by the student and the preceptor.

At the end of a day in the office, the preceptor should spend at least 30 minutes discussing with the student the experiences of the day and relating these to a general view of the clinical practice of family medicine. During this period, the student should be able to both describe the positive features of the preceptorship experience and provide constructive criticism.

Other aspects of the preceptorship should include hospital rounds where the preceptor and student discuss the management of each patient. The student should also participate as much as his experience allows in surgical procedures and obstetrics, always under the close supervision and guidance of the preceptor.

In order to conduct a preceptorship as outlined above, the preceptor should realize that he must either decrease his patient volume or increase the amount of time spent in the office. The latter is usually the most acceptable and reflects the dedication of the physician to the preceptor's role of being both a doctor and teacher. No physician should be a preceptor who thinks he can increase his patient volume or time off by bringing in a student with clinical experience.

Beyond the content of the preceptorship itself, the experience will be successful only if the preceptor is a successful role model. The same comments made in the last paragraph in the section on the preclinical student concerning the role model apply to the clinical student. In order for the preceptorship to nurture the clinical student's interest in family practice, the preceptor must embody and convey the art of medicine in family practice.

Concluding Remarks

This paper is an attempt to give family physician preceptors some insight into the preceptorship experience from the perspective of a medical student. It is hoped that these comments will be considered by those involved in the development of preceptorship programs and the recruitment of preceptors. The guidelines presented here are essential to the achievement of a positive experience for most students.

It is my impression that a great number of the students presently choosing family practice are doing so by default, i.e., they are rejecting the role models of the academic center and opting for family practice. The students usually have had limited exposure to family physician role models and hence their career choice is largely conceptual. With the increasing emphasis on family practice in medical education, preceptorship opportunities are increasing such that the student will have more experience upon which to base his career choice. Unless preceptors are carefully selected (e.g., by aptitude testing and evaluation of the practice setting) and trained (e.g., in workshop training sessions) to provide a positive experience to most students, preceptorship education will have a negative influence on the number of students choosing family practice.

Acknowledgement

I would like to thank L. Robert Martin, MD for his review of this paper and helpful suggestions.

Commentary

Since writing this article as a senior medical student, I have completed a family practice residency and am now engaged in full time practice. I am a clinical faculty member in family practice at a nearby medical school, and serve as a role model in a variety of preceptorship electives. Reviewing my former perspective reminds me of critical issues in being an effective preceptor.

I believe that the content of this article is currently relevant. Although a revolutionary spirit is less noticeable, the medical student of 1980 appears similar in orientation to that of the early and middle 1970s. Certainly the greatest change during this period has been the highly visible establishment of family practice departments and the growth of preceptorship programs organized by medical schools.

As a medical student I demanded very high standards for the selection of preceptors in family practice. I suggested that anything less would be counterproductive in nurturing student interest in the field. Re-reading this article makes me pause and wonder if even I live up to these standards in practice. However, I maintain that I must live up to them to be an effective preceptor, and I do not soften my plea for a most careful selection and training of preceptors in family practice.

References

1. Preceptorships: Learn by teaching in your own office. Patient Care 8(16):182-197, 1974.
2. Heller RF, Heller CA: Studentships in general practice. Lancet 1: 745-746, 1968.
3. Rosenberg L: A student's view of the preceptorship program. J Med Educ 34:654-656, 1959.

Nurse practitioners and physician assistants emerged as primary care providers in the early 1970s. I studied their impact during a project on innovations in health care as a senior medical student. After starting residency training in 1975, a nurse practitioner, Sally Flaherty, was assigned to our resident team but not to the two others. We used Sally for continuity of care when we were not in clinic. I studied this impact in the following article. I believe this is the first article to describe a co-practice relationship between an NP and a family physician, a model I still prefer to independent practice.

A Nurse Practitioner in a Family Practice Residency: Role Description and Impact on Continuity of the Practitioner-Patient Relationship

Joseph E. Scherger, MD, Marshall H. Eaton, MD,
Sally Flaherty, RN, and Michael J. Gordon, PhD

The Journal of Family Practice
1977;5(5);791-794

The nurse practitioner and physician's assistant are new health practitioners providing primary health care. When teamed with family physicians, these new health practitioners can extend patient services. Family physicians should be trained to work with new health practitioners effectively. Presented is a model where a nurse practitioner and family practice residents work as co-practitioners in a family practice unit. A nurse practitioner in this role can improve the continuity of the relationship between patient and provider in a family practice residency.

The nurse practitioner (NP) and the physician's assistant (PA) have emerged as examples of new health practitioners (NHP) providing primary health care. It is generally agreed and legislated that the NP and PA should work under the supervision of physicians when providing medical care. Studies have shown that in certain settings these new health practitioners can provide care that is comparable to physicians,[1,4] that patient satisfaction is high,[2-6] and that economic viability is possible.[4,7-9]

In family practice, a NHP can bring specific expertise and medical manpower to the health care team. Advantages to the family physician in working with a NHP include assistance with: health maintenance, such as well-child care and physical examinations, common acute problems, such as upper respiratory tract infections and urinary tract infections, and the stable phase of common chronic problems, such as hypertension and diabetes. The nurse practitioner can also extend nursing skills into medical practice through counseling and identification of behavioral or social problems. If the NHP functions as a co-practitioner with a family physician for a given patient population, in the absence of either one, practitioner-patient continuity may be maintained.

It is being increasingly recognized that physicians need training in working effectively with new health practitioners.[4,5,17] This paper describes a model for the role of a nurse practitioner in a university-based family practice residency.

The continuity of the interpersonal relationship between practitioner and patient has been described as an "element"[10] or "dimension,"[11] of continuity of patient care, an essential of family practice. Geyman has described the many factors which work against continuity of care in a family practice residency program.[12] We felt it important to study and report on the manner in which the continuity is affected by a nurse practitioner in a residency program unit.

Nurse Practitioner Role Description

The University of Washington Family Medical Center (FMC), clinical teaching unit of the university-based family practice residency, employs a nurse practitioner. This NP functions on one of three teams (Team 1) in the FMC and serves as a co-practitioner in the practices of a limited number of family practice residents.

Each team in the FMC consists of six residents (two from each year), two faculty with limited practices, one nurse, a medical assistant, and a secretary. Each team is structurally identical except for the addition of the NP on Team 1. Each resident spends two or three half days each week in the FMC seeing patients.

Prior to beginning work in February 1976, the NP negotiated one of three working agreements with each of the Team 1 physicians:

Working Agreement A – MD and NP serve as co-practitioners for an entire practice.

Working Agreement B – NP serves as co-practitioner for a limited number of families in MDs' practice.

Working Agreement C – NP not primarily involved in physician's practice, but may provide coverage as a practitioner within the team.

The essential elements of the co-practitioner relationship are listed in Table 1.

Table 1

Physician and Nurse Practitioner as Co-Practitioners – Essential Elements of Practice

Both MD and NP must accept the philosophy of sharing patient care responsibility.

Exchange will be that of peer professionals. The physician will maintain a general supervisory role over medical care.

Faculty will maintain a supervisory role over Resident-NP practices.

NP will develop protocols or "patient care guidelines"[16] for the diagnosis and management of common conditions. These must be reviewed and accepted by any physician working as a co-practitioner.

Each co-practitioner, by mutual agreement, may emphasize certain patient problems, e.g., NP will emphasize patient problems for which she has a mutually agreeable protocol for diagnosis and management.

Patients will have the option to express preference for one of the practitioners.

Co-practitioners must agree to maintain open communication concerning all aspects of the practice. This requires regular meetings to discuss common patient concerns, review charts, create or modify protocols, and evaluate the co-practitioner roles.

The role of the co-practitioner in patient encounters will vary at the discretion of the practitioners or patients. A given patient may be seen by the co-practitioners together, by the MID or NP alone, or in another combination, for example, the patient is initially seen by the MD but the NP follows through with certain aspects of management. The frequency of each type of encounter should be recorded and evaluated (see Table 2).

When one of the co-practitioners is absent, the other will maintain primary responsibility for patient care. When the primary MD is absent, one or more MDs on Team 1 will provide back-up and supervisor for NP in medical aspects of practice.

Initially, by mutual agreement between the NP and each physician on Team 1, the NP had Working Agreement A with the two first and the two third-year residents, Working Agreement B with the two second-year residents, and Working Agreement C with the two faculty members. Because of administrative responsibilities not related to her NP role, the NP was forced to change the Working Agreement from A to B for the two third-year residents. The study in this report compares the two first-year residents on Team 1 with Working Agreement A, with the first-year residents on other teams not working with the NP.

As co-practitioners, the NP and resident work together seeing patients during the regularly scheduled two or three half days each week. The NP also sees patients in each practice in which she is a co-practitioner for acute visits when the resident is not present in the FMC (inpatient rotation, vacations), using an available Team 1 physician as back-up, if necessary.

All patient visits involving the NP are logged and characterized as shown in Table 2. As expected, during the first month the NP functioned, the frequency of parallel visits was low (eight percent of encounters) and the frequency of consulting visits to MD was high (64 percent). After five months the frequency of parallel visits rose to 52 percent, and the frequency of consulting visits to MD fell to 35 percent. The frequency of the other types of visits did not change significantly. Studies using the NP at other sites have shown that the frequency of patient visits seen by a NP not requiring immediate MD consultation stabilizes at 67 to 77 percent.[13]

Table 2	
Classification of Encounters	
All patient visits involved the NP are documented as follows:	
Parallel Visit	NP manages patient visit (per protocol). MD may acknowledge patient or sign prescription.
Shared Visit	MD and NP see patient together.
NP Initiated Visit MD Consults	NP sees patient initially and involves MD in consultation.
MD Initiated Visit NP Consults	MD sees patient initially and involves NP in consultation.

Continuity Study – Methods

The practices of the two first-year residents on Team 1 with the NP as a co-practitioner were compared with the practices of the first-year residents on Teams 2 and 3. Four hundred and twenty-eight patient records were randomly selected for study, with 198 being from the two resident-NP practices on Team 1, 127 records from 2, and 103 records from Team 3. Two time periods were selected: September 1975 to January 1976 (before the NP) and February 1976 to July 1976 (NP working on Team 1). All encounters listed in the progress notes as involving an MD or NP were analyzed. The frequency of patient encounters which involved a break in continuity with the primary practitioner(s) was calculated. A break in continuity was defined as a visit recorded in the progress notes by someone other than the patient's primary practitioner(s). A primary practitioner was defined as the first-year resident assigned to the patient, or the NP who worked as a co-practitioner during the second study period. Encounters involving a consultation requested by a primary practitioner were excluded, as well as those with the team nurse, social worker, pharmacist, or other non-physicians.

Because the University of Washington Family Practice Residency uses a resident pairing system,[14] all encounters involving a resident's partner were included in the analysis. These encounters were considered a break in continuity, the justification for which is supported by the data (see discussion).

The number of different practitioners seeing each patient during the study periods was also examined with the same exclusions.

	Team 1	Team 2	Team 3	Team 2 & 3
Table 3				
Comparison of Breaks of Continuity During Two Study Periods*				
Charts reviewed during period 9/75-1/76 (No NP)	198	127	103	230
Visits	235	127	119	246
Breaks in continuity	30	19	25	44
% Breaks in continuity	13	15	21	18
Differences from Team 1	--	NSt	NSt	NSt
Period 2/76-7/76 (NP on Team 1)				
Visits	365	191	217	408
Breaks in continuity	38	44	63	107
% Breaks in continuity	10	23	29	26
Differences from Team 1	--	$p<.0002$	$p<.0001$	$p<.0001$

*Comparison of the breaks in continuity in the study practices on each team during two five-month periods. The NP worked as co-practitioner with the residents on Team 1 during the period February 1976 thru July 1976.
tNS = Not Significant, $p>.05$.

Continuity Study – Results

The frequency of breaks in continuity in the three teams during the study periods is presented in Table 3. The most striking finding is the highly significant difference in breaks in continuity between Team 1 and the other teams during the second study period with the NP working on Team 1. There were no significant differences in the time any of the residents spent away from their practices during the study periods. The only known difference among the teams during the second period was the addition of the NP as a co-practitioner with the two residents on Team 1.

Also present in Table 3 is the noticeable but not statistically significant ($p > .05$) increase in breaks in continuity on Teams 2 and 3 during the second study period. This difference could not be accounted for by a change in time the residents spent away from their practices. One factor which may account for the increase in breaks in continuity is the increase in number of encounters in the selected population during this period. Since this increase in patient visits occurred for all three teams, we suggest that the frequency in breaks in continuity during the second period would have also occurred on Team 1 without the NP.

An analysis of the continuity of the practitioner-patient relationship is presented from the perspective of the patient in Figures 1 and 2. These figures analyze the number of physicians seen by patients who made two or more visits during each of the study periods. All of these patients were seen at least once by their primary practitioner(s). The patterns for the three teams during the first study period (without the NP) were similar. Between 30 and 45 percent of patients saw more than one practitioner. Of interest is that the resident's partner sees very few of the patients not seen by the primary resident, minimizing the partner's ability to maintain continuity. During the second period a greater percentage of patients was seen by more than one practitioner with the most striking changes on Team 1 and 3. However, on Team 1 most of the patients seeing a second practitioner were seen by the NP. Except for the NP on Team 1, there was no other consistent practitioner seeing patients when they were not seen by the patient's primary resident.

Discussion

New health practitioners such as the nurse practitioner and physician's assistant are already involved in delivering primary care, usually as members of health care teams.

If family physicians are to be effective members of health care teams with new health practitioner they must be trained.[4,5,17,18] A logical time and place for this to occur is during residency training in the family practice unit.

At the present time many family practice residencies do not have new health practitioners in their family practice units. In an informal survey by one author (JES), the reason most often stated by program directors for not having NHP's is that they would compete with residents for patients.

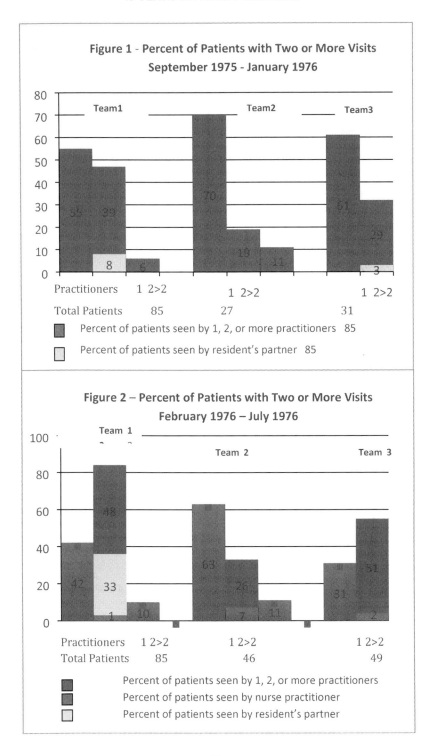

Figure 1 - Percent of Patients with Two or More Visits
September 1975 - January 1976

Figure 2 – Percent of Patients with Two or More Visits
February 1976 – July 1976

There are two aspects of the model presented here which reduce the possibility of competition between the resident and the nurse practitioner. First, the NP functions as a co-practitioner with the resident for a given practice; she does not have her own panel of patients. This shared involvement in patient care fosters more of a complementary rather than competitive relationship. Second, resident involvement with the NP occurs on an optional and negotiable basis. Those residents not interested in having NP involvement with their patients are not required to do so. All residents receive some exposure to the NP by observing her function in the family practice unit and because she occasionally sees their patients for acute visits under Working Agreement C. There would need to be a NP on each of the three teams in the unit (six residents per team) in order to allow each resident the option of working with the NP as co-practitioner for all or part of his or her practice.

Because family practice residents are by necessity part time providers in their practices, patients in these practices may have frequent breaks in continuity with their primary resident. In the study presented here, 10 to 29 percent of all patient visits involve a break in practitioner continuity. Of patients with more than one visit over five months, 30 to 60 percent see at least one practitioner other than their primary physician.

In discussing the lack of continuity in family practice residencies, Geyman presents several approaches to the problem.[12] These include: group practice with modular organization into resident teams, use of the problem-oriented record, use of the resident pairing system,[14] and use of full-time family practice rotation. All of these approaches are employed by the University of Washington family practice residency and are helpful in facilitating patient coverage by an organized group of residents. However, there remains a striking lack of continuity in the resident practices examined in this report.

As demonstrated by Starfield et al,[15] continuity of the flow of patient information relating to care is better when the practitioner providing follow-up care is the same from one visit to the next. Since family practice residents are not consistently available to their patients, there is a need for another primary practitioner on the team that is in close communication with the resident and is consistently available to the patient. Because a resident's partner in a pairing system is also inconsistently available and is concerned primarily with his or her own patients, the partner is limited in ability to maintain continuity in the model unit. As demonstrated here, a nurse practitioner working as a co-practitioner with residents is helpful in maintaining the practitioner-patient continuity.

Acknowledgement

This work was supported in part by HMEIA Interdisciplinary Team Training Grant No. MBD 000017 MBD 21 W. K. Kellogg Foundation Grant, UW Budget No. 63-2994. The assistance of Lynn Crowell and Jennifer Clough of the Interdisciplinary Health Care Team Project is gratefully acknowledged.

References

1. Sackett DL, Spitzer WO, Gent M, et al: The Burlington randomized trial of the nurse practitioner: Health outcomes of patients. Ann Intern Med 80:137-142, 1974.
2. Batchelor GM, Spitzer WO, Comley AE, et al: Nurse practitioners in primary care IV: Impact of an interdisciplinary team on attitudes of a rural population. Can Med Assoc J 112:1415-1420, 1975.
3. Flynn BC: The effectiveness of nurse clinicians service delivery. Am J Public Health 64:604-611, 1974.
4. Lewis CE, Resnick BA: Nurse clinics and progressive ambulatory patient care. N Engl J Med 277:1236-1241, 1976.
5. Merenstein JH, Wolfe H, Barker KM: The use of nurse practitioners in a general practice. Med Care 12:445-452, 1974.
6. Nelson, EC, Jacobs AR, Johnson KG: Patient's acceptance of physician's assistants. JAMA 228:63-67, 1974.
7. Estes EH Jr: The Duke physician assistant program: A progress report. Arch Environ Health 17:6901, 1968.
8. Spitzer WO, Russell, WAM, Hackett BC: Financial consequences of employing a nurse practitioner. Ont Med Rev 40:96-100, 1973.
9. Stetson LA, Draye MA: The nurse practitioner as an economic reality. Medical Group Management 22(5):24-27, 1975.
10. Hansen MF: Continuity of care in family practice: Measurement and evaluation of continuity of care. J Fam Pract

2:439-444, 1975.

11. Hennen BK: Continuity of care in family practice: Dimensions of continuity. J Fam Pract 2:371-372, 1975.

12. Geyman JP: Continuity of care in family practice: Implementing continuity in a family practice residency program. J Fam Pract 2:445-447, 1975.

13. Pickard CG: Family nurse practitioners: Preliminary answers and new issues. Ann Intern Med 80:267-268, 1974.

14. Lincoln JA: The three-year paired residency program: A solution to a teaching dilemma. J Fam Pract 1(2):31-33, 1974.

15. Starfield BH, Simborg DW, Horn SD, et al: Continuity and coordination in primary care: Their achievement and utility. Med Care 14:625-636, 1976.

16. Hoole AJ, Greenberg RA, Pickard CG: Patient Care Guidelines for Family Nurse Practitioners. Boston, Little, Brown and Co, 1976.

17. Alpert J, Charney E: The Education of Physicians for Primary Care. Bureau of Health Services Research, Rockville, MD, DHEW Pub No (HRA) 74-3113, 1973.

18. Kindig D: Primary health care teams: Issues for team delivery and interdisciplinary education. J Med Educ 50:97-110, 1975.

During residency I was given the opportunity to write the Residents' Viewpoint Column for Family Practice News. Bruce Bagley preceded me as the first resident columnist and recommended me to continue, a platform I enjoyed. I wrote 12 columns in 1977-78 on a wide variety of topics. Seven are reprinted here.

Residents' Viewpoint Column, *Family Practice News*:

Family Physician Role Eroded

Family Practice Views
Residents' Viewpoint Column
July 1977

Just what family physicians are able or allowed to do in the care of their patients is now in question. The role of the comprehensive, jack-of-all-trades family doctor is being eroded. As a neophyte family physician, I am wondering if many of the skills I am enthusiastically acquiring will be my privileges in future practice.

What is happening? First the specialties proliferated, and many procedures or medical problems once considered routine were rendered as suspect or forbidden for the family physician. Now the insurance industry is the villain, with skyrocketing malpractice premiums making many procedures prohibitive unless performed as frequently as a referral physician would perform them.

The days when the MD meant a license to do anything one dared in the care of the sick are fortunately gone. Only competent physicians should practice, but what is the measure of competence? Who decides?

The most active arena in the battle for privileges is the hospital. Here the credentials committees have the control, and they vary considerably among hospitals.

I recently had the opportunity of attending a credentials committee meeting of a community hospital; it was chaired by a family physician. Not by coincidence, there were still family physicians functioning in the operating rooms and coronary care unit. As the ratio of family physicians to other specialists continues to fall, particularly in urban areas, family physicians are being squeezed out of these units in many hospitals.

Coming to the rescue, the Joint Commission on Accreditation of Hospitals has stated that privileges should be granted on the basis of training, experience, and demonstrated ability. There should be no bias against any specialty. The American Academy of Family Physicians is preparing to defend this statement in court, if necessary, for family physicians who are denied privileges in areas in which they are competent.

If a family physician feels threatened in the hospital, he can no longer retreat to his private castle, the office. Here the malpractice premium, already taking its toll on hospital procedures performed by family physicians, is threatening the feasibility of many office procedures. As my uncle, a senior family physician in California, vividly said, to no longer be able to do for patients what he had done for years is having a devastating effect on his morale in practicing medicine.

Solving the malpractice problem is too complex to be generalized upon here. One aspect pertinent to family physicians is that the insurance industry must become more selective in its malpractice premiums. The price of my auto insurance is dependent not only on whether I drive but also how many miles. Likewise, malpractice insurance should reflect not only the nature of procedures but also the frequency with which they are performed.

Family practice residents are also feeling the squeeze on practice privileges. The cost of malpractice insurance for residents and faculty is threatening to limit the training opportunities in residency programs. The residency represents the future for the family physician, so it is essential that the breadth of experience is not jeopardized.

With regard to future hospital privileges, residents are beginning to realize the need for carefully documenting their training experience. Some residents, upon graduation, are being denied privileges they had as residents, even in the hospital in which they trained.

Whether in the hospital, the office, or in residency training, a major priority of organized family physicians must be the protection of our practice privileges. Family physicians must be ever present in the development of standards of competence. We must be the leaders in defining the limits of our competence as family physicians.

Within these limits, residencies must train for competence in all areas, and the residents' experience must be documented. Family physicians should maintain competence in practice through documented experience and continuing education. If given the chance, the demonstrated ability of the family physician will guarantee a comprehensive and satisfying practice.

Art of Medicine or Deception?

Family Practice Views
Residents' Viewpoint Column
July 1977

The practice of medicine can be divided into the scientific aspects of diagnosis and treatment and the nonscientific aspects of meeting patients' needs, the art of medicine.

In medical school I learned the science of medicine. There I diligently studied the basic sciences and gained a thorough understanding of the pathophysiology of disease. In the clinical years I learned to apply this knowledge to a wide variety of interesting patients who came to the academic center.

Yet, when I started my family practice residency, I lacked the ability to care for patients. Though I could take a through history, perform a complete physical examination, and diagnose and treat specific illnesses, I had little idea how to satisfy patients by meeting their needs.

The art of medicine is the nonscientific part of a successful doctor-patient interaction. For a doctor-patient interaction to be successful, not only must the illness be appropriately addressed, but both patient and physician must be satisfied.

In the university environment, the art of medicine often gets inadequate attention. Indeed, most academic physicians think that only scientific medicine exists and that patients should be satisfied with a sophisticated approach to their problems. Some patients are satisfied, but many are disgruntled. It is not unusual for a patient, after a $1,000 work-up, to go to a family physician or chiropractor for satisfaction.

I was eager to discover the art of medicine at its finest during my rotation away from the university in a rural community. During these 2 months I looked for the pearls of wisdom that allowed community physicians to be so successful. I found that a very explicit technique was used by some physicians to achieve not only satisfaction but adoration from their patients. Unfortunately, this technique is dishonest.

Early in my community experience I was impressed by how often patients told me a doctor had saved them. I heard such statements as "Doctor X saved my leg," or "Doctor X saved my life." I know that it does occur, but not as often as I was hearing it.

Investigating these statements I found such stories as, "One day I twisted my ankle very badly, and it became quite swollen. My doctor told me I could lose my leg from this but that he would take X-rays, put my leg in an Ace bandage, and give me crutches. In 3 days I was well. I am so thankful he saved my leg."

And, "One day I had a temperature of 104. All of my muscles ached, my head hurt, and I had a terrible sore throat and cough. My doctor told me I could die from this, but he gave me a medicine and made me stay home. I was sick for about 2 weeks, but I got better. He saved my life."

Is the art of medicine the art of deception? This horrifying thought actually came to me after hearing several such stories, but I learned that most of the physicians involved in such stories were not well respected by their colleagues.

I learned many honest techniques for successfully caring for patients. The several family physicians with whom I worked, all clinical instructors associated with my residency, were impeccably honest and taught me to combine compassion and efficiency.

Despite learning many positive techniques and having good role models, I left the community experience somewhat saddened by the lack of integrity that can exist in the profession. I was naïve in believing that all the nonscientific aspects of medicine that made patients happy must be good.

By experiencing deception, I learned why quackery continues to flourish despite the widespread availability of honest medical care. Most significantly, I learned the importance of a sometimes frustrating humility; my patients with sprained ankles and influenza will not believe I saved their lives.

Importance of Behavioral Skills

Family Practice Views
Residents' Viewpoint Column
September 15, 1977

What is so special about a family physician? Is it the breadth of knowledge that allows us to manage problems from the newborn to the aged? Is it that we are able to treat entire families, allowing us the privilege of observing family interactions in illness? Or is it that we approach our patients differently than the other specialties?

As a neophyte family physician, I would respond "Yes" to all of these questions.

There is a somewhat controversial aspect of family practice

training that attempts to develop many of these special qualities. For lack of a better term this aspect of our training has been called behavioral science.

Behavioral science deals with the psychological or sociologic aspects of patient problems, or the nonphysical aspects. It has been shown that up to two-thirds of patient problems presenting to a primary physician are either entirely nonphysical or have a significant nonphysical component.

Family physician teachers have tried to identify and provide behavioral science teaching to residents, usually with difficulty because of the lack of an organized approach to this area in their own training. Many family practice programs have hired behavioral specialists such as psychologists, psychiatrists, or sociologists to present behavioral science training. In certain programs behavioral science has become the dominant part of the training.

As family physician teachers are struggling to define and present behavioral science in our training, many of them are grumbling. "Do they really need this, whatever it is?" I am sure that many practicing physicians reading this column are thinking, "I didn't have any of that in my training and I am doing fine."

A large emphasis on behavioral science has made many family physicians uncomfortable. They fear a loss of identification with "blood and guts" medicine and an excessive identification of the family physician as counselor.

The editor of a local newspaper in a town with a family practice program emphasizing behavioral science expressed this same concern. He wrote about going to the family practice center with a shoulder complaint and reports that the resident asked a large number of psychological questions and never examined the shoulder.

If one assumes that the major reason for family practice residencies is to preserve the traditional model of the general practitioner, then one could argue against formal behavioral science training. Certainly the GP learned much about the behavior of patients and families by caring for them over a long period of time. However, a look at the diagnoses recorded by general practitioners reveals an almost exclusive recognition of physical ailments, with only occasional mention of psychosocial and family problems.

Many teachers and residents look on family practice as a reform movement as much as an attempt to preserve a traditional discipline.

Part of this reform is the inclusion of a solid background in the recognition and management of common behavioral problems as part of the comprehensive care provided by family physicians.

Simultaneous with the growth of family practice is a discussion about the need for a new medical model with a change in the way physicians approach patient problems.

George Engle, M.D., a medical philosopher and professor of medicine and psychiatry at the University of Rochester (N.Y.), has written that the traditional biomedical model is obsolete and calls for a biopsychosocial model for patient care in "The Need for a New Medical Model: A Challenge for Biomedicine" (Science, April 8, 1977).

Herrick Petersen, editor of Patient Care, agrees and states in his column of May 1, 1977 that family practice is the likely discipline to sponsor such a new model. Essentially, this model calls for an approach to patient care that combines and integrates the potential biologic, psychological, and social components of illness.

Our limited biomedical approach to patient care is illustrated in the traditional medical history. The review of systems asks for only physical complaints except for the occasional, "Have you ever been hospitalized for psychological reasons?" Many of us are learning to take sexual histories but find it awkward to include them in the present general history format.

The practice of medicine has always been a changing art, and an increasing emphasis on psychological and social problems is certain. The challenge for family practice to incorporate attention to behavioral problems into an efficient medical practice is enormous. Ireton and Cassata, two psychologists in the department of family practice at the University of Minnesota, have made an important contribution in this area by providing a concise "Psychological Systems Review" (J. Fam. Pract., April 1976).

Just because many teachers are uncomfortable with behavioral science is not a reason for avoiding it. The content of knowledge in family practice should become clearer as the academic life of the specialty matures. Certainly, an orientation to behavioral science should in no way erode the many physical "blood and guts" skills required of a family physician.

Incorporating behavioral skills in family practice is not to suggest that the family practice is not to suggest that the family physician becomes all things to all people. It is increasingly recognized that a comprehensive approach to patient care often requires a term effort that includes nurses, social workers, and others. The family physician is usually the first contact for patients, so he must be able to recognize physical, psychological, and social components of problems and manage or refer management appropriately.

We must not forget the patients' desires when deciding the scope of medical practice. The patient who only wants his shoulder examined should get just that. The patient who asks, "Why have I not been feeling well for some time?" deserves a biopsychosocial approach.

Including behavioral science in our training and using a biopsychosocial model when appropriate should preserve and advance those special qualities of family physician.

Gaining Ground in Academia

Family Practice Views
Residents' Viewpoint Column
November 15, 1977

Family practice has arrived at a crossroads. The intellectual arena of academic medicine has extended an invitation to family practice.

What is the evidence of this invitation into the scientific elite? Certainly the fact that most medical schools now have departments or divisions of family practice is impressive testimony. However, this could be more the result of incentives such as increased funding than intellectual acceptance: the most prestigious schools, such as Harvard, Yale, and Stanford, are holding out.

Very dramatic evidence, to me at least, is that the Pharos, the publication of the national medical honor society, Alpha Omega Alpha, recently had a cover article entitled, "The Intellectual Worthiness of Family Practice."

In this article Dr. Walter Spitzer, a Canadian family physician and epidemiologist, says that for some time entering family practice was considered "intellectual suicide." He then describes how family practice will earn intellectual worthiness by defining its patient care and through developing a scientific research base.

As a third-year resident who feels comfortable with his clinical skills. I have elected to spend a year having a look at the intellectual arena to see how it might apply to my concepts of family practice. By the intellectual arena, I am referring to the academic realm and to the elite who perform definitive research and govern medical education.

The academic department of any clinical field is usually divided into areas of patient care, education, and research. Patient care is so close to the heart of family practice that the academic departments are having little trouble standing out in this area. Family practice has assumed a leadership role in the important patient care issues such as comprehensive care, cost containment, providing primary care to underserved areas, team care, and in including behavioral and social problems in the medical model.

Family practice departments are also off to a good start in the educational component of the academic mission. Curriculums in family medicine are flourishing in those medical schools that make room for them. Standards for residency training have kept pace with the phenomenal growth of programs.

Research, however, receives the most attention for admission for admission into the intellectual arena. Certainly the invitation extended to family practice is contingent upon the development of a solid research base. It is in this area that I elected to work during my third year.

Quality clinical research requires basic skills in epidemiology and biostatistics. After completing course work in each of these areas, I undertook a reading of the medical literature in an area of interest: quality-of-care assessment. I hoped to identify an intellectually worthy research project applicable to family practice.

Reading the medical literature in this area raised in my mind the incongruity between the intellectual arena and the family practice movement.

Impracticality pervades most intellectual research; rather than useful methods of quality assessment. I found very elaborate research designs.

Family physicians are true pragmatists. We are generally interested only in what will help patients. The research efforts of family physicians should contain this same practical value. However, most research in the intellectual arena appears self-serving to a body of knowledge, with little attention to its usefulness. In the intellectual arena it appears that being tediously compulsive is admired but being practical is suspect.

My bias is that unless clinical research somehow affects the practice of medicine, either today or in the future, it is meaningless. By this standard, much of the research that fills the medical journals is not worth the funds and effort that supported it. This abundance of meaningless research must result from the publish or perish law that exists in the academic realm.

Family physicians will be inclined to do research if it affects or validates their practice.

I despair at the thought of the wasted effort if family physicians are pressured to perform research for its own sake to obtain intellectual worthiness.

Family practice has been a reform movement in patient care and education. Family practice should have a research base to validate itself and advance. Unless research in family practice is both practical and meaningful, however, a town and gown separation will certainly develop. The invitation from the intellectual arena should be accepted with caution.

Reluctance to Leave Academia

Family Practice News
Residents' Viewpoint
February 15, 1978

It is self-evident that the main purpose of medical school and residency training is to prepare physicians for the practice of medicine. However, as I reach the end of this long training process, I feel more hesitant than prepared to enter practice.

It has become apparent to me that medical education, like many other academic areas, tends to serve itself rather than the public.

I have often felt it both amusing and tragic that large numbers of graduate students in many fields are reluctant to leave the university environment. They become "professional students."

To my chagrin, I am witnessing among other residents, and to a certain extent feeling myself, a reluctance to leave the university environment and a desire to become "professional residents." The servitude of the residency experience can be lessened by becoming a fellow or junior faculty, while the familiar and sheltering surroundings of the university are retained.

Is the reluctance to leave the university for the outside world simply a normal human response to a major change or is it instilled during the process of medical education? I believe that to a certain extent the latter is true.

Medical education fails in that it does not give attention to socializing physicians for practice in the community. Instead, medical students and residents become socialized to the academic environment and have to break this tie to start practicing in the outside world.

This misdirected socialization occurs for several reasons:

First, medical education occurs almost exclusively in the peculiar environment of university hospitals; the outside world of community practice remains a mysterious unknown.

Second, the vast majority of role models in medical education are academicians who have very little, if any, community practice experience. Consequently, students are residents are continuously surrounded by mentors who relate only to the academic environment.

Third, and probably most significant, is that medical education stresses only medical competence. Indeed, combined with the two reasons above, senior residents develop a general impression that their medical competence exceeds that of most community-based physicians. Other skills that are important to the practice of medicine in the community, such as practice management and coordination of patient care in the context of a community (community medicine), are largely ignored.

The university represents both a haven for medical competence and a shelter from the unknown.

Family practice, as a new venture in medical education, has an opportunity to avoid this misdirected socialization process and actually stimulate students and residents to enter community-based practice. This can be done by giving attention to and avoiding the problems mentioned above.

A significant part of family practice education should occur in community settings. For the medical student this would mean carefully selected preceptorships and community-based clerkships in settings that would nurture interest in community practice. For the university-based resident this would mean community-based rotations in similar settings.

The majority of educators in family practice should either be actively in practice or remain very close to the environment of community-based practice. As role models, these educators can bring an outside-world perspective into the university setting.

Medical competence should be stressed but put in the perspective of quality standards for practice in the community. Tertiary-care work-ups should be regarded as such, and realistic primary and secondary care should be taught. Experiential training in other important skills such as practice management and community medicine should be stressed.

By the end of formal training, the resident should feel ripened and eager for the total experience of community-based practice if that was his purpose in acquiring a medical education.

For family practice residency programs that are based in community hospitals, the problems discussed here regarding medical education are virtually nonexistent. If the community hospitals have the resources and the commitment for teaching, I would be surprised should many graduates of these programs be hesitant about entering practice.

My own hesitance and that of some of my colleagues must be related to our socialization in the university environment. Our residency program is a good one and does make some effort to avoid the traps mentioned above. Graduates of our program seem to be entering community-based practices at a greater rate than from other residency programs within the university system.

However, the self-serving overall process of medical education in the university affects us.

I would never suggest that family practice residency training should not occur in the university environment. But a worthy reform function of our new academic discipline would be to redirect the process of medical education in the university.

The Future of Solo Practice

Family Practice News
Residents' Viewpoint
April 15, 1978

What is the future for solo practice? Do many residents still consider this time-honored form of medical practice a viable alternative?

Solo practice has been and remains the most common form of medical practice. A survey by the American Medical Association (1975) estimated that 20% of all active private physicians are in groups of three or more, an estimated 15% are in partnership practice, and over 60% of private physicians are in solo practice.

With little factual information in the medical literature, but ample intuitive reasoning, solo practice has fallen into disfavor in many circles. The environment of most training programs, including family practice, is such that most graduates express a preference for group or partnership practice.

Experts in health services, who seem to have a liking for larger organizations and an aversion to professional independence, consistently express a preference for group practice. Even the AMA has expressed a preference of group practice in its practice management manual, "The Business Side of Medical Practice."

Data from the AMA ("Socioeconomic Issues in Health, 1976") show that group practice has grown in popularity since 1932, when less than 1% of all private physicians worked in groups. The most rapid rate of growth of group practice occurred between 1959 and 1965 with an increase in number of groups of 18.5% per year. Since 1969, the rate of growth of group practice has decreased. This suggests that solo practice is not rapidly headed for obsolescence.

The most common form of solo practice is that of sole proprietorship with a fee-for-service method of payment. However, solo practice can still occur without the physician's ownership and with other payment mechanisms.

Traditionally, American solo physicians have practiced with extreme independence and autonomy. Whenever possible, they would provide coverage 24 hours a day, 7 days a week. It would not be unusual for a small town with seven solo physicians to have all seven covering their own patients every night and weekend. In this traditional arrangement, solo physicians tend to view other physicians as competitors and strive to keep all aspects of their medical practice as private and separate.

This traditional form of solo practice seems to be very unattractive to residents and is likely to become rate.

However, in parallel with the growth of group practice, changes have been adopted by many in solo practice that make it more attractive. These physicians have arranged to enjoy some of the advantages of group practice while maintaining their independence.

These arrangements include sharing after-hours coverage with other physicians to increase personal free time and sharing office space and major medical equipment to reduce professional expenses and provide more technical services. In larger communities, solo physicians have aggregated in medical office buildings, which facilitates sharing arrangements and also establishes informally organized referral arrangements.

These sharing arrangements may be resulting in more collegial and less competitive relationship among solo physicians.

Even with these organizational changes, the chief factor in a decision to enter solo practice is still the professional personality of the physician. The strong-minded physician who wishes to control his working environment and make individual decisions will certainly prefer solo practice.

The long-term survival of solo practice depends on this choice of practice by a certain number of graduating residents. Data from the division of education of the American Academy of Family Physicians indicate that 13.6% of residents graduating in 1976 entered solo practice. In 1977, this percentage increased slightly to 14.5%. The number of graduating residents who enter group or partnership practice and later change to solo practice is unknown, but there is some suggestion by the AAFP that this number may be sizable, particularly with the new sharing arrangements.

The decision by residents to enter solo practice may be largely influenced by the training environment. Most family practice residencies are centered around a family practice center with a group-practice model. These residents are trained to share patient coverage in a team arrangement. However, in one family practice program in which the program director is strongly oriented to solo practice, virtually all of its graduates choose solo practice.

There will always be some physicians who make that choice. Certain physicians have personalities that necessitate their working alone, and the special independence of the doctor-patient relationship in solo practice appeals to many patients and some physicians.

Given the present 60% of physicians in solo practice, and this limited data on graduating residents, it would be reasonable to estimate that the prevalence of solo practice will drop to a plateau of around 15-20% of private physicians. This percentage may be higher if solo physicians make their model of practice more visible.

Collision Over Childbirth

Family Practice News
Residents' Viewpoint
June 15, 1978

Childbirth is receiving a great deal of attention today because of a collision that is occurring between two large and growing movements.

The first is the continued medicalization of childbirth through the use of advanced technology, with the purpose of maximizing safety. The second movement is to make childbirth as natural as possible to maximize the personal qualities of the event.

The collision is most acutely manifested in the controversy over home birth. Historically, childbirth had been predominantly a home event, even in this country up until the past three decades. Without modern living conditions, prenatal care, and skilled personnel, infant and maternal morbidity and mortality were quite high.

The first hospital delivery services were designed to give the destitute a place to give birth. For many years, particularly before antibiotics came into use, the rate of complications was much higher in hospital deliveries than in those attended at home.

The growth of modern obstetric practice over the past three decades had led to a routine and nearly universal form of hospital-based labor and delivery. The hospital routine developed around an emphasis on two factors: the convenience of the staff and the safety of the mother and infant.

Academic obstetric practice added another emphasis, a prevailing attitude that labor and delivery are potentially pathologic events that require aggressive monitoring and intervention.

Unfortunately, an emphasis on the personal experience of childbirth was largely left out.

The trend toward home births is the continuation of a public movement that began with putting fathers in the delivery room and challenging the routine use of obstetric analgesia. This movement is a manifestation of a growing feeling that the experience of childbirth has been coopted by the hospital-based system. Physicians who have observed the great advances in obstetric care are usually puzzled as to why a sensible couple would want their baby to be born at home. Given the present state of hospital deliveries, the reasons are:

- Decreased fear and pain associated with a familiar environment.
- Unrestricted presence of family members.
- Greater opportunity for control and involvement in decision making.
- Avoidance of routine and sometimes needless hospital procedures (those that derive from the emphasis on staff convenience).
- The greater opportunity for minimal or no anesthesia, which maximizes the mother's participation, particularly in the second state of labor.
- No separation of mother and infant to foster bonding and breast feeding.
- Decreased cost.
- The desire to view childbirth as a natural event rather than a pathologic process.
- The avoidance of iatrogenic complications from improperly applied technology. (To many couples, avoiding this risk more than offsets whatever increased risk they perceive from home birth.)

The home-birth question became more than academic for me when the wife informed me during her recent pregnancy that she wanted to give birth at home. She is a registered nurse and felt deeply that the hospital experience she observed during her training and at work was not what she wanted in the delivery of our first child.

Facing this question personally, I set out to review the world's literature on the safety of home birth. I did this through a computer library search and by consulting a physician friend who has extensively studied this subject. I was unable to draw any firm conclusions regarding the overall safety of home birth.

From my review, it is apparent that all births should be attended by skilled personnel. Low-risk patients who successfully give birth at home appear to be at least as safe from complications as those in the hospital. Those who begin the process at home but must be transferred to a hospital because of certain complications represent a special risk group with the risks dependent on the time delay in transfer.

One very disturbing finding was that most of the data presented against home birth was more political than scientific.

For example, the American College of Obstetricians and Gynecologists is widely publicizing uncontrolled state health department figures as evidence against home birth (Family Practice News, March 1, 1978, page 1). The problem with these figures is that although all hospital births are reported, many normal home births are not, and there is a bias toward reporting those that are complicated.

It is also disturbing that a large case-control study of home and hospital births in California that showed no differences could not get published in a scientific obstetric journal (figures reported in the same issue of Family Practice News, page 49).

Like many other physicians who are open minded and sympathetic toward this public movement, I am too uncertain to be an advocate for or against home birth. I am attracted by the concept of home-styled birth centers that would combine a home-like environment with medical facilities. I wish that hospitals or medical groups were moving faster in this area.

I do advocate that serious attention be given to each of the nine reasons cited earlier for home birth to maximize the personal experience of childbirth. I will reiterate with slight modification the three principles espoused by Dr. Richard Beard, chairman of the department of obstetrics at St. Mary's Hospital in London, and featured in Patient Care (Nov. 15, 1977):

1. Ask the parents what the priorities are in the experience of childbirth and accommodate them as much as possible.

2. Intervene in natural labor and delivery only if the mother's or baby's health is threatened.

3. Keep the experience of childbirth within the context of the family. Let the mother decide who should be present, and facilitate the relationship by getting the parents immediately involved in the infant's care. The impact of this principle on later child rearing is only beginning to be realized.

The alarming rate of unattended home births indicates that the medical profession should act quickly on these principles. Traditional physicians and hospitals that refuse to change should realize that they are the greatest contributors to growth of the home-birth movement.

During residency two strong practice interests emerged, childbirth and end-of-life care. They were to remain strong interests throughout my career, although I provided maternity care for just 18 years. The following essay was written while a resident in Seattle on the increasing problem of supporting a natural death with the new technologies of modern medicine.

Death and Modern Medicine

The Bulletin
King County Medical Society
1978;57(2):25-26

I attended a seminar recently in which the speaker presented the merits of the influenza vaccine. Now that influenza can be prevented, these deaths have been rendered unacceptable by the standards of modern medicine.

Life-threatening illnesses fall into two categories; those that are preventable or treatable, and those that presently cannot be prevented or successfully treated. As physicians, we have been indoctrinated to feel in general that death by a preventable or treatable illness is a mistake, but a death that cannot be prevented or treated is unfortunate but acceptable.

As manifested in death certificates, we have been trained to think that every death has a specific cause, and "old age" is no longer acceptable. The task of modern medicine has been to attack every cause of death and render it preventable or treatable. Medical care is evaluated by longevity and mortality rates. Our profession is waging a war against death, despite its inevitability. As we advance in our understanding and treatment of disease, the fallacies in this orientation toward death become more apparent.

As physicians, we tend to label patients as dying only when they have a disease that is beyond successful treatment. In the past, such patients commonly had advanced tuberculosis or tertiary syphilis. Today, those with end-stage cancer or intractable heart failure are more common. I would never criticize the discovery of antibiotics or research into cancer treatment. My concern is that, when all causes of death become readily treatable, it will be very difficult to die in a medical-care setting.

Very few physicians would disagree that relieving human suffering is more important than preventing death. To cure sometimes but comfort always is as accepted as motherhood and apple pie. However, I have found the application of these principles the exception rather than the rule in the practice of modern medicine. Many times I have heard that aspiration pneumonia can be "the old man's friend." As a student and resident, I have never been allowed to let a patient die of aspiration pneumonia. Why? Because it is easily treated.

When a patient's meaningful life has ended, and suffering becomes pervasive, why do we continue to treat? The reasons are many. I will describe two. First, human suffering is more difficult to recognize and quantify than other manifestations of disease. Particularly when a patient loses his orientation to time and place, a separation between us and the patient dampens our perception of suffering, while the pneumonia remains obvious. The second reason has to do with our basic orientation as physicians. After recognizing a treatable condition, it is virtually impossible for us not to treat. Even when the appropriateness of death is obvious to the patient and family, we often hospitalize and provide intravenous hydration, tube feedings and antibiotics, while hoping for some unrecognized malady to end the life.

It is unlikely that we will change in our basic nature toward treating disease. In order for us to limit or eliminate the suffering of the dying patient, we must develop a new orientation toward death. We must learn the management of the death itself, not just the causes of death.

We all agree that death is inevitable, and whether we believe it is an end or a transition, we agree that it is a phase of our existence. As a phase, death could be compared to birth. Optimally it should be a positive experience without suffering.

In our zealous effort to prevent and treat disease, we have expropriated the management of birth and death from the public. While both formerly occurred at home, the status quo is that they now occur in hospitals under technological monitoring and intervention. In our fight against disease, it is apparent that we often ignore the quality of these experiences.

Through public concern and the influence of Lamaze[1] and Leboyer,[2] the quality of the birth process has gotten renewed attention. The same phenomenon is occurring with death in a more gradual manner.

A detailed discussion of the management of the dying patient is beyond the scope of this article. I will only present a few general concepts. There is an expanding literature on the care of the dying to which I hope to motivate interest.

A prerequisite to helping patients with the dying phase is an acceptance of our own and our patients' mortality. This acceptance must be more than an intellectual acknowledgement of death; it must be an acceptance through introspection which affects our world view and lifestyle. The physician who lives in a delusion of immortality is unlikely to accept the death of his patients.

The key element in the management of the dying phase is preparedness. To manage a dying patient without preparation is similar to managing a delivery without prenatal care. Though a discussion of death is appropriate at any time in life, it becomes very important when a patient enters a time when his lifetime appears more limited than the general population, e.g., advanced age, onset of congestive heart failure, or at the discovery of a malignancy. Virtually all patients give thought to their death at these times, and the greatest barrier to a discussion is a reluctance of the physician.

Preparing a patient for dying has many elements and a checklist may be helpful. These elements include business affairs (e.g., will), family affairs, desired location for dying (home vs. hospital), and symptom management (e.g., pain). A living will[3] and resulting discussion among patient, family and physician before the terminal phase can be very helpful in decision-making after a patient becomes irrational or loses consciousness.

Kubler-Ross has described various stages a patient and family may go through in the dying process.[4] Though the sequence and number of stages vary, the goal is to help the patient and hopefully the family reach a stage of acceptance, the manifestation of a positive death experience. If the physician accepts the death of his patient, he can help the patient reach this important stage. If the physician denies the dying process and gives the patient and family false hope for continued life, he may obstruct the patient's development and compromise the death experience.

When a patient has reached the stage of acceptance of death, and meaningful life has been replaced by suffering or a vegetative state, the physician can avoid his compulsion to treat inappropriately by avoiding diagnostic efforts. It is easier not to order a chest x-ray than it is to withhold antibiotics when a pneumonia has been diagnosed. Diagnostic efforts can be replaced by supportive attention and the patient will not feel abandoned.

The act of dying itself deserves comment. The evidence is overwhelming that the death of an ill person is a painless relief. This is literally described by Tolstoy in *The Death of Ivan Ilych*.[5]

Moody has provided clinical evidence from interviews of over 100 people who experienced physical death and recalled the process after being resuscitated.[6] Whether "death" occurred from sudden trauma or a chronic illness, these accounts of the death experience are remarkably similar and provide a provocative insight into the fate of our consciousness after physical death.

Death resulting from a preventable or treatable illness may not only be acceptable, but appropriate. The management of the dying phase is an essential part of complete patient care, to some high-risk persons, the influenza vaccine is inappropriate. Our standards of modern medical care must include the management of dying patients and a scrutiny of treatment that affects the quality of the death experience.

References

1. Lamaze F. *Painless Childbirth: The Lamaze Method.* Chicago: Henry Regnery Co., 1970.
2. Leboyer F. *Birth Without Violence.* New York: Knopf, 1975.
3. Bok, S. "Personal Directions for Care at the End of Life." *New England Journal of Medicine*, 295:367-9, 1976.
4. Kubler-Ross E. *On Death and Dying.* New York, MacMillan Co., 1969.
5. Tolstoy L. *The Death of Ivan Ilych* (1886). New York: The New American Library, 1960.
6. Moody RA. *Life After Life.* Couiagton (Georgia): Mockingbird Books, 1975.

During my third year of residency I used my elective time to get a Master of Public Health (M.P.H.) in health services at the University of Washington. My thesis research project was to study the differences in diagnostic methods used by family medicine and internal medicine, in this case senior residents from each field. This article contributed to the literature that distinguished family physicians from internists in the care of adults. Each specialty has its own culture, and family physicians are therapeutic pragmatists while internists are more compulsive diagnosticians. This article was written during my residency but published in 1980 after I started practice.

Comparison of Diagnostic Methods of Family Practice and Internal Medicine Residents

Joseph E. Scherger, MD, MPH, Michael J. Gordon, PhD, Theodore J. Phillips, MD, and James P. LoGerfo, MD, MPH

Journal of Family Practice
1980;10(1):95-101

The diagnostic methods of third year residents in internal medicine (N=23) and family practice (N=22) were compared with respect to common ambulatory patient problems. Five written simulated patients were presented and the dependent variables were: initial and revised diagnostic hypotheses, physical examination items, and laboratory charges. The two groups considered the same number and type of diagnostic hypotheses. There were large differences in the selection of physical examination items ($P<.001$), with the family practice group selecting fewer items. Laboratory charges were significantly greater for the internal medicine group with two patients ($P<.05$), and the charges were nearly identical with two patients. A high degree of patient-specific behavior was demonstrated by both groups. These findings have implications for the future training of primary care physicians.

Recent studies indicate that different types of physicians may use different diagnostic strategies in the same clinical situations. In the primary care setting in the United States, where different specialties care for similar clinical problems, the use of different diagnostic strategies among these specialties may have important implications for graduate medical education in primary care, and for cost and quality of medical care.

Although the issues of primary care training, costs, and quality give a timely curiosity to the study reported here, the motivation for this study lies at a more basic level of specialty description. So little is known about physician behaviors at the end of specialty training, that to generalize about specialty types is risky at best. As Donabedian concluded in a classic paper,[1] "....before one can make judgments about quality, one needs to understand how patients and physicians interact and how physicians function in the process of providing care." This study is simply a descriptive look at the diagnostic behaviors of senior residents from two specialty groups, family practice and internal medicine. The effect of training is suggested, the issue of cost is mentioned relating to laboratory use, and the issue of quality is deferred.

The clinical method generally taught in medical school is to collect exhaustive data by a thorough history and physical examination before formulating diagnostic hypotheses. The work of Elstein and Shulman[2,3] and Barrows[4] has demonstrated that practicing physicians rarely, if ever, use this exhaustive diagnostic process. Rather, physicians consistently begin to generate diagnostic hypotheses very early in a clinical encounter, and the diagnostic process is largely one of testing, reformulating, and verifying these hypotheses.

There have been very few studies comparing the clinical strategies used by family physicians and internists. Smith and McWhinney[5] used a live simulated patient with three separate complaints (fatigue, sore throat, and headaches) and compared the diagnostic methods of nine family physicians and nine internists who were members of a university faculty. Their study emphasized history taking and found that the family physicians asked significantly fewer questions. They also found that the family physicians requested fewer items of physical examination and fewer laboratory tests.

Feightner, Norman, et al,[6] as part of a larger study of clinical methods at McMaster University,[7] reported a comparison of 20 family physicians and 20 general internists, all randomly selected from practice. They used four live simulated patients with diagnostic problems more complex than in the study cited above. With an emphasis on the diagnostic process, they found that the two groups conformed similarly to the model of early hypothesis generation and verification as described by Elstein and Shulman.[2,3] They found no differences in the number of type of diagnostic hypotheses generated throughout the encounter. They did find that the family physicians asked significantly fewer history questions and performed less physical examination resulting in a greater efficiency score.

It is important to mention that both of these studies were done in Canada where internists are limited to a consultant practice. Also, the family physicians in these studies generally predated family practice residency training.

The study reported here concerns family practice and internal medicine residents at the end of their training in the United States. The focus is on the formation of diagnostic hypotheses and objective data collection (physical examination and laboratory tests). The study was set up to test the following hypotheses: that the family physicians would consider fewer diagnostic hypotheses; that the family physicians would select fewer items of physical examination; and that the family physicians would order fewer laboratory tests resulting in smaller laboratory charges.

Methods

The two study groups were all of the third year residents in internal medicine at the University of Washington and all of the third year residents in family practice in five University of Washington affiliated programs (University Hospital, Providence Hospital, The Doctors Hospital, Group Health Cooperative of Puget Sound, and Family Medicine Spokane). All of these programs are well established and competitive in being able to select from many highly qualified applicants. The data were collected during March 1978, when all of the residents were in the last four months of their training program.

Five written simulated patients were used in this study. In brief, these were:

1. A 43 year old male laborer with a six-week history of low back pain. There is no history of trauma. He is married, the father of

three children, and has not missed work.

2. A 34 year old woman with a one-month history of recurrent epigastric pain. She is having a concurrent marital problem.

3. An active widowed 76 year old woman with a two-year history of occasional palpitations. The remainder of her cardiac history is negative.

4. A 64 year old retired man with a six-month history of fatigue and weight loss. He is a chronic smoker, drinks alcohol regularly, and has symptoms in several organ systems.

5. A 48 year old salesman with a six-to eight- month history of intermittent, cramping, middle and lower abdominal pain. He has had an increased frequency of loose stools without melena, and rectal bleeding. He is thin and his weight is stable. He is single and his future career is uncertain.

The five patients were selected using three criteria: (1) The presenting problems are common in ambulatory practice for both internists and family physicians, being in the top 20 most common presenting problems in the National Ambulatory Medical Care Survey for 1975[8]; (2) Each patient does not have an obvious diagnosis, but rather has symptoms which suggest a number of diagnostic possibilities; (3) The evaluation of the presenting problems has not been well established by a protocol. The specific details of the patients were adapted from actual patients in the practice experience of the author (J.E.S.)

The five patients were presented in a standardized printed format, resembling the Patient Management Problems developed at the University of Illinois,[9] and the Diagnostic Management Problems developed by Helfer and Slater.[10] The instructions with the study instrument explicitly stated that problems were episodic visits in which the physicians should address the presenting problems only.

A brief but complete history was given for each patient. After each history, the residents were asked to write a prioritized list of the diagnostic hypotheses they would consider in this patient. Items of physical examination were then selected using a checklist in which the physical examination was arbitrarily divided into 52 items. The same checklist was used for each patient. The resident was given the option of selecting specific physical examination items, or selecting "General Physical Examination" which included all the items. On the page following the physical examination checklist, the resident was given information on the positive findings of the physical examination. All the patients has physical findings which were limited to the area of symptoms in order to avoid directing the unsuspecting resident to go back and check other areas of the examination. After the information on the physical examination was given, the residents were asked to write a revised prioritized list of diagnostic hypotheses. In the final step with each patient problem, the residents were asked to select whatever laboratory tests they would order. A rather thorough checklist was given in order to resemble the laboratory request sheets usually used and to avoid cueing the subjects. The same checklist was used for each patient and included tests in the following categories: x-ray, hematology, urine studies, chemistry, endocrine, immunology, and coagulation. Certain special studies and procedures were also listed which varied with the patient problem, and blank lines were provided for writing in additional lists.

The instrument was administered in the following manner: Each resident was contacted by telephone and urged to participate in the study. The purpose of the study and the make-up of the study groups were not shared in order to avoid biasing the responses. The residents were informed that the study would be done anonymously, that there were no right or wrong responses, and that the study simply wanted to look at how residents approach common ambulatory problems. Each resident who agreed to participate and returned a completed instrument was given $10. The materials were sent to the residents' homes with a stamped return envelope, and a three-week limit was put on the study. Those residents not responding after two weeks were again contacted by telephone and urged to complete the instrument. Of the 28 residents in internal medicine, 27 could be contacted and received a questionnaire, and 23 responded (85 percent). Of the 25 residents in family practice, 22 responded (88 percent).

Four dependent variables were analyzed for differences among the patient problems and between the two study groups using a repeated measures analysis of variance. These variables were: (1) initial diagnostic hypotheses (following the standardized history); (2) revised diagnostic hypotheses (following the selection of physical examination items and the standardized results); (3) items of physical examination; and (4) laboratory charges. The laboratory charges were calculated using the charges for each test at the University of Washington Hospital at the time of the study. The repeated measures analysis of variance permits comparisons among the five problems irrespective of specialty training, comparisons between the two specialty groups on the series of problems considered as a whole, and interaction effects (i.e., differential performance between groups on particular problems). This allows an analysis of the individual problems and the series of five problems as a whole while taking into consideration the correlation in performance by a single resident with the five problems.

The selection of specific items of physical examination and specific laboratory studies were compared using a chi-square analysis. Fisher's exact test was used when the number of observations of any item was less than five.

Results

The study groups were compared with respect to age, sex, medical school and year of graduation, previous postgraduate training other than present residency, and previous clinical experience other than present residency. No differences existed in the two groups except that 8 of 22 family practice residents had attended the University of Washington School of Medicine, compared to 1 of 23 internal medicine residents. No distinct pattern of responses was apparent for graduates of the University of Washington. Other postgraduate or clinical experience was negligible in the two groups.

A comparison of the study groups was made with respect to future practice intentions. Expressed in mean percent of professional time, the internal medicine residents indicated a mean 40.5 percent in primary care practice compared to 87.0 percent for the family practice residents. Intended time in primary care among the internal medicine group ranged from zero to 100 percent. The internal medicine residents with greater or lesser intentions for primary care practice were kept together in the analysis, because an analysis of them separately (divided into two groups by the median) showed no significant differences in their responses to any of the variables.

The results with respect to the four variables are presented separately.

Diagnostic Hypotheses

The initial and revised diagnostic hypotheses were analyzed by looking at the total number of diagnoses listed. The mean number of initial and revised diagnoses in both groups varied between three and six for the five problems. The differences were significantly related to the particular patient problem (P<.01), but not to the two study groups. Although the family practice residents tended to list slightly fewer diagnoses, none of the differences approached statistical significance.

Table 1 Number of Physical Examination (PE) Items Selected by Two Study Groups							
Patients							
		1	2	3	4	5	All
Internal Medicine	(N=23)						
Mean Total Charges		35.4	28.8	33.0	49.7	36.0	36.5
Family Medicine	(N=22)						
Mean PE Items		16.3*	11.1*	22.5**	45.9^{NS}	17.6*	22.7*
*P<.001							
**P<.05							
NS = Not significant							
Total possible number of items = 52							

Physical Examination

The greatest differences between the two groups occurred in the selection of the physical examination. Table 1 lists the mean total physical examination items selected for the five patients. Significant difference (P<.001) occurred for patients 1, 2, and 5, and for patient 3 (P<.05), with the family practice residents selecting many fewer items.

In patient 4, with non-localized symptoms, the differences between the two groups largely disappeared.

The most striking finding comparing the two groups was the tendency for the internal medicine residents to select a general physical examination. Eight (35 percent) or more of the internal medicine residents selected a general physical examination on each patient. These were not always the same residents with each patient. Overall, the internal medicine group selected a general physical examination with a 50 percent frequency compared to 23 percent for family practice (P<.001). The family practice residents tended to limit the examination to items which corresponded to the presenting symptoms. In a patient with non-localizing symptoms (patient 4), the differences between the groups largely disappeared, with both groups selecting the general physical examination.

Even discounting those residents who selected the general physical examination, and looking at only those residents who selected a "limited physical examination," the internal medicine residents selected more items than the family practice residents (P<.01). Particular items which had significant differences in this analysis were the lymph nodes and certain areas of the neurologic examination (mental status, cranial nerves, coordination, and upper extremity sensory, motor strength, and reflexes). An attempt was made to see if more frequent selection of these items corresponded with hematologic and neurologic diagnostic hypotheses, but these relationships were not present.

A high degree of patient-specific behavior was again demonstrated by the number of physical examination items selected by the residents in both groups (P<.001). This was more striking for family practice than internal medicine because the latter group consistently selected the general physical examination.

Table 2 Total Laboratory Charges Incurred in the Selection of Laboratory Tests by the Two Study Groups							
Patients							
		1	2	3	4	5	All
Internal Medicine	(N=23)						
Mean Total Charges		$43.71	56.34	157.59	158.84	193.38	121.97
Family Medicine	(N=22)						
Mean PE Items		$23.59*	39.99	141.13	175.20	144.82*	104.91**
*P<.05 **P<.114							

Laboratory Tests

The dependent variable chosen to represent laboratory tests selected by the residents was total charges for the tests. Total charges were chosen in order to give a meaningful weighting to the laboratory test data.

Table 2 displays the total charges generated by the study groups for the five patients. Significant differences (P<.05) occurred for patients 1 and 5, with the family practice group incurring lower laboratory charges. For patients 3 and 4, the behavior of the two groups with respect to laboratory charges was nearly the same. The difference in laboratory charges between the two groups for all five patients together was not significant.

The patient-specific behavior of the residents in both groups is apparent (P<.001) by repeated measures analysis of variance. An analysis of the residents individually showed a high degree of variability in laboratory charges among the five patients.

Some significant differences occurred between the study groups with certain tests in certain patients, but with the large number of tested differences the significant findings may be spurious. Whenever significant differences did occur, the internal medicine group selected the test more often. With these patients, the greatest differences occurred in the selection of chemistry batteries (patients 1 and 5), and chest x-ray films in patients without symptoms referable to the chest (patients 1, 2, and 5).

Discussion

This study, which indicates differences in the clinical strategies used by residents from two specialty groups, has three limitations which must be considered in interpreting the results. These limitations arise from the selection of the study groups, the method, and the selection of patient problems.

The approach used in this study was to identify the clinical strategies used by residents in the two specialties at the end of their training. This selection of study group focuses on the effect of graduate medical training while not considering the effect of practice experience after training. Residents during the final months of their training probably use different clinical strategies than practicing physicians with years of primary care experience. Also, the internal medicine group was in a traditional residency curriculum with less than half the primary care activities experienced by the family practice group. Although a career interest in primary care among the internal medicine residents did not affect the data, simply a different amount of time in primary care training may explain some of the differences in this study. Finally, other personal characteristics of the residents selected into the respective programs under study, which were not considered in this study, may account for some of the differences in clinical strategy.

The format of simulated patient problems may be a limitation in studying the strategies that are used with actual patients. The validity of written simulated patients with formats similar to that used there has been considered reasonable.[3,9,10] This study contained a measure of internal validity by the patient-specific responses that were obtained with nearly all the residents. An evaluation of the study instruments by the residents in both groups indicated a nearly unanimous response that the five simulated clinical situations were realistic representations of common ambulatory patients. The use of a standardized history, which gave all the residents the same core of information on each patient, may have limited the study of diagnostic hypotheses and objective data collection in the two groups. This factor would tend to make the strategies more alike than if the histories were solicited by the residents. However, certain differences were demonstrated despite this limitation.

The third limitation lies in the specific patient problems that were chosen. The patient problems in the study reported here were chosen to give a sampling of common ambulatory problems in order to find consistencies within the two groups. The great variation in responses to different patient problems indicates that the selection of patient problems is a major determinant of the results in a study such as this. This conclusion was also reached in the studies of Elstein et al.[3] If patients 3 and 4 had not been a part of this study, the authors might have been led, as in a previous study,[5] into making more general statements about the clinical strategies in family practice and internal medicine. This study suggests that, depending on the patients, the clinical strategies of family practice residents and internal medicine residents may be the same or quite different.

Keeping these limitations in mind, some statements can be made from this study. The finding of no significant differences in the number of diagnostic hypotheses during the encounter agrees with the findings of Feightner et al[6] using live simulated patients. Contrary to the prestudy hypothesis, it appears that residents in the two specialties tend to generate similar lists of diagnostic hypotheses with ambulatory patients when provided with the same information. Both studies support the work of Elstein[3] that the number of hypotheses considered at any one time is limited and usually does not exceed five.

The difference in physical examination strategies used by the two groups is the most impressive finding. This difference is supported by the two previous studies.[5,6] The finding that with four of five patients, the family practice group consistently limited their physical examination to selected areas, while the internal medicine group tended to depend on a more general physical examination, suggests that there are major differences in the way the two groups used this diagnostic method. Internal medicine residents appear to use the thorough and exhaustive clinical method that generally is taught in medical school. The justification for this method is the traditional high priority given to the compulsive avoidance of making errors of omission.[11] Family practice residents, on the other hand, appear more inclined to limit the physical examination to those areas which would directly relate to the list of diagnostic hypotheses. This approach would more closely correspond to the hypotheses testing described by Elstein.[3] In more complex patients with non-localized symptoms, family practice residents may use the same strategy as the internists by changing to a general physical examination.

The behavior of the two groups with respect to laboratory tests and charges were less consistent than with the physical examination, and more patient specific. Previous studies of internists in ambulatory settings have shown great variations among physicians in the use of laboratory tests,[12,13] and no association with quality of care.[13] Great variation occurred with both groups in this study, not only among physicians, but among the patient problems for a given physician. The significantly lower use of laboratory tests and lower charges by the family practice group in two patients agrees with the study by Smith and McWhinney[8] which showed lower laboratory testing by family physicians in two of three patients. However, the nearly same laboratory testing behavior of the two groups with two patients indicates that a more selective strategy of laboratory testing in family practice, resulting in lower laboratory costs, may be true for only certain ambulatory patients.

These findings, which suggest similar conceptualizations of diagnostic hypotheses yet different strategies of objective data collection in certain ambulatory patients, have implications for the future training of primary care physicians. The field of family practice is seeking to define itself in academic terms. The strategies described here, used by senior family practice residents, are quite similar to the strategies advocated by early scholars in general practice.[14,15] Selective clinical strategies based on hypotheses testing, which differ from the traditionally taught clinical method, are currently being validated as an approach to patients.[3]

The field of internal medicine is seeking to define its role in primary care.[16] New curricula are being developed for the training of internists specifically for primary care. Whether these curricula will result in different strategies of objective data collection than those reported here is conjectural.

Current options include a continuation of the present system with different specialties training physicians in parallel programs to deliver primary care to overlapping groups of patients, often using different diagnostic methods. Another option is a merging of primary care training in which more consistent diagnostic methods are developed.

Either way, it is likely that both family practice and internal medicine training programs will affect each other's strategies in the continuing development of primary care physicians.

Acknowledgement

This study was supported in part by a grant from the W.K. Kellogg Foundation No. 63-2994, administered through the Department of Family Medicine, University of Washington.

References

1. Donabedian A: Evaluating the quality of medical care. Mibank Mem Fund Q 44:193, 1966.
2. Elstein AS, Kagan N, Shulman LS, et al: Methods and theory in the study of medical inquiry. J Med Educ 47:85, 1972.
3. Elstein AS, Shulman LS, Sprafka SA: Medical Problem Solving: An Analysis of Clinical Reasoning. Cambridge, Mass, Harvard University Press, 1978.
4. Barrows HS, Bennett K: The diagnostic (problem-solving) skill of the neurologist. Arch Neurol 26:273, 1972.
5. Smith DH, McWhinney IR: Comparison of the diagnostic methods of family physicians and internists. J Med Educ 50:264, 1975.
6. Feightner JW, Norman GR, Barrows HS, et al: A comparison of the clinical methods of primary and secondary care physicians. In Proceedings of the Thirteenth Research in Medical Education Conference (RIME). Washington, DC, Association of American Medical Colleges, 1974.
7. Barrows HS, Freightner JWS, Neufeld VR, et al: Analysis of clinical methods of medical students and physicians. Hamilton, Ontario, McMaster University, 1978.
8. National ambulatory medical care survey: Ambulatory medical care rendered in physicians' offices, United States, 1975. In National Center for Health Statistics (Hyattsville, Md): Advance Data from Vital and Health Statistics, No. 12, October 1977. DHEW publication No. (HRA) 77-1250. Government Printing Office, 1977.
9. Williamson JW: Assessing clinical judgment. J Med Educ

40:180, 1965.

10. Heifer RE, Slater CH: Measuring the process of solving clinical diagnostic problems. Br J Med Educ 5:48, 1971.

11. Ledley RS, Lusted LB: Reasoning foundations of medical diagnosis. Science 130:9, 1959.

12. Schroeder SA, Kenders K, Cooper JK, et al: Use of laboratory tests and pharmaceuticals. JAMA 225:969, 1973.

13. Daniels M, Schroeder SA: Variation among physicians in use of laboratory tests: Part 2: Relation to clinical productivity and outcomes of care. Med Care 15:482, 1977.

14. Crombie BL: General practice today and tomorrow: Diagnostic method. Practitioner 191:539, 1963.

15. Hull FM: diagnostic pathways in general practice. J R Coll Gen Pract 22:241, 1972.

16. Petersdorf RG: Internal medicine and family practice: Controversies, conflict, and compromise. N Engl J Med 293:326, 1975.

PART II: MATURING WITH FAMILY MEDICINE, 1978-1984

I started my practice career after residency in 1978 by volunteering with the National Health Service Corps. I became a migrant health physician in Dixon, California and lived 8 miles away in the college town of Davis. I stayed 14 years, starting a private solo practice in 1980 that grew to 5 physicians as Family Practice Associates of Dixon.

Family Practice News asked me to write a commentary to my Residents' Viewpoint columns two years after starting practice. I have a strong preference for residency graduates going into a community practice to actualize all the skills acquired during residency.

Reflections on Leaving Academia

Family Practice News
Perspective & Commentary
January 1, 1979

During the past 2 years, while writing the Residents' Viewpoint column for *Family Practice News*, I was a resident trying to express my perspective on issues related to family practice education and patient care. When I wrote about patient care, I would usually receive letters from a few practicing physicians questioning some of my statements because I had never been in practice. At least one physician doubted whether I would ever enter practice.

I am proud to state that I am now actively in practice, and I offer some reflections on getting started.

After a 4-month search for the "right" place and setting, I chose to practice in an agricultural town with a population of 6,000 in north-central California. The town has a severe shortage of physicians, with only one other family physician, who no longer has hospital privileges or takes night calls.

My practice setting has a few peculiar features: I am being subsidized for 2 years by the National Health Service Corps; there is a community advisory board; and we have a federal grant to subsidize care for a large population of migrant farm workers. Otherwise, the practice is similar to that of any other fee-for-service private office.

I have been in solo practice with a nurse-practitioner for the first month, and we will be joined by another residency-trained family physician. We are using two hospitals in nearby towns, and our practice includes coronary care and obstetrics.

In the Feb. 15, 1978 column ("Reluctance to Leave Academia"), I expressed concern that my medical education had failed to socialize me for entering a community-based practice. Having taken the step into practice, I continue to feel this way with certain exceptions. My fund of medical knowledge and abilities are highly adequate, and I believe my patients are receiving a level of care they had not had previously.

Two experiences during my residency were most valuable in preparing me to enter practice. These were a community-based rotation and a course in practice management.

The two-month rotation in a rural teaching practice was exceedingly important as a model for my present practice, and it afforded me insight and experience in relating to a small community hospital. My recollection of this rotation from 18 months ago was vivid as I admitted my first patient.

Practical material in office practice management has not received academic credibility except in family practice.

With a new residency director during my third year, I was

fortunate to receive such a course even though it was quickly thrown together and presented in the evening. I didn't realize how much I had learned or the importance of this material until starting practice.

Most practicing physicians are aware that the most important task of a new physician in public relations. Becoming known and selling yourself must occur with both the general community and the medical community.

The message that the general community wants above all others is a promise of availability. The comfort of knowing that a personal physician is available at a time of need seems to take great precedence over the amount of training or the level of care provided.

Curiously, this promise of availability seems to bear little relation to the actual number of after-hours calls.

Realizing this overriding community need, I have kept a low profile in maintaining personal time away from the practice.

Public relations with the medical community have been more delicate and time-consuming, particularly because I have ties with the federal government. I am impressed by the fine line that exists between gracious acceptance and open resentment from other physicians. Taking the time to make personal contacts and expressing an eagerness to work with the medical community in the area makes referrals and hospital care much more pleasant.

Starting practice has been a transition that I approached with at least as much anxiety as I felt in starting medical school and internship.

Thus far it has been as difficult but much more enjoyable and satisfying. I look forward to a career in family practice with an optimism that I do not believe exists among other specialties.

I was a full scope of practice semi-rural family physician in Dixon and was brimming with youthful confidence and some self-deception. Delivering babies was my favorite activity closely followed by seeing elderly and preterminal patients at home. Early in practice I boldly removed a newborn from an academic health center so I could care for my patient in a community hospital. This essay tells that story.

Doctor as Patient Advocate

The New Physician
1983;32:35-36

Family physicians will occasionally face the dilemma of questioning or even terminating the diagnostic work-up initiated by another specialist in order to protect the patient from potential harm. The following case report describes my role with a premature infant in a university medical center neonatal care unit.

While I was out-of-town on a Saturday, a 27 year old primigravidas female, paraplegic due to a spinal cord injury five years previously, went into labor at 33 weeks gestation. The family physician covering for me decided to send her to the regional university medical center for delivery, anticipating a premature infant. That Saturday afternoon, the patient delivered a 5 lb., 1 oz. boy. The infant was delivered by outlet forceps due to the mother's paralysis and inability to push in the second stage.

The newborn examination was normal except for an abnormal origin of the left fifth finger and possible undescended testes. I was notified of the baby's excellent status Sunday afternoon, 24 hours after birth.

With Monday morning rounds, new diagnostic and management considerations began. The total bilirubin was high at 9.5 MG% at 36 hours of age. In response, the child was placed under phototherapy. The infant's head circumference at birth was 34 centimeters, placing it at the 90th percentage for 33 weeks. The weight was at the 75th percentile. Questioning the appearance of the head, the attending neonatologist determined that potential macrocephaly should be investigated. A computerized tomography (CT) scan gave equivocal results. A suggestion of hygromas was observed laterally in the subdural areas. A second CT scan using a different body scanner was obtained the next day, which again showed uncertain signs in the subdural areas.

Bilirubin values were obtained three to four times daily on Monday and Tuesday with the child remaining under the lights. All values were between 9 and 10 MG% with a bilirubin binding alarm level of 16 MG%.

Monday afternoon I received a phone call from the mother suggesting that I come to the medical center to evaluate her baby and consider a transfer to our local hospital. She questioned why the physician would not leave her baby alone.

On Tuesday, while still under the bilirubin lights, the infant had showed a weight loss of seven ounces and required periodic lavage feedings. A neurologic exam showed sluggish Moro and sucking reflexes and below normal head control. Neurologic and neurosurgical consultations were obtained and a septic work-up was done.

On Tuesday afternoon, I saw the infant and discussed the management with the attending physician and the staff. The attending neonatologist felt that the child was neurologically deteriorating, that the findings on the CT scan could not be ignored, and that treatment with bilirubin lights was still required. I questioned whether the infant's sluggishness might be due to the continuous phototherapy. I suggested that the child be observed out of the lights and with regular feedings, but got a negative response.

On Tuesday night at 10:30 pm, the attending neonatologist reported to me that the child had an elevated blood ammonia level. He stated that this might suggest enzyme defects, indicating the infant's inability to digest protein. He suggested that the child might be sluggish as a result of the infant formula that he was taking.

The attending physician discouraged any transfer from the medical center and indicated that a further work-up for metabolic abnormalities was essential. He also informed me that the infant now had overlapping suturae in the skull which might suggest brain atrophy. Furthermore, a hearing test of the child suggested that he could not hear.

On Wednesday morning, I returned to the medical center. The

parents at this time were very distraught and were hopeful that I could remove their baby, whom they felt was normal, from the medical center. The child showed an improved neurologic examination after 12 hours of simply feeding and sleeping. His improved status would be short-lived, however. The elevated venous ammonia level of the night before was to be investigated. All protein formula feedings were discontinued and the child was placed on a glucose-electrolyte solution.

Arterial punctures were required to accurately determine the ammonia levels. One was obtained early in the morning and was normal, but the attending and neonatology fellow were unsure of its significance because of its timing from the last feeding. With a normal value they were now curious about an arterial-venous differential in the ammonia levels.

A follow-up arterial ammonia level was obtained with difficulty from an artery in the neck on the right side after failure to obtain an adequate specimen from both brachial arteries and the left side of the neck.

By noon on Wednesday, still under the bilirubin lights and after these procedures, the child was again thought to be neurologically depressed. The suturae had a greater degree of overlap and the child quickly fell asleep.

By this time, I wanted strongly to transfer the child to the intermediate care nursery at the community hospital. To my dismay, there would be no space available for the infant until the following morning.

On Thursday morning, at four and one-half days of life, the infant was transferred. The attended neonatologist expressed his serious concern regarding the prognosis of this child. The long list of abnormalities suggested a syndrome, he insisted. He stated that I was inappropriately interrupting the diagnostic work-up and that a small nursery would not have the resources to benefit this child. Urologic, genetic, and orthopedic consultations were indicated but had not yet been obtained. Neurologic and neurosurgical evaluations had not been completed.

My plan at the community hospital was simply to nurture the child and observe him. The bilirubin lights were stopped and no value was ordered until the following morning. In a consultation, a general pediatrician agreed with me that the infant was probably normal with a crooked finger.

Over 36 hours, the infant thrived. With rehydration, the overlapping suturae retreated. The infant became vigorous and alert with a completely normal neurologic examination. Only one laboratory test was done in the hospital, a bilirubin level which by the next day dropped to 8 MG%.

The parents, who had been frightened into the possibility of a markedly abnormal child, were now very encouraged. The child was discharged to home at one week of life having regained five ounces of weight in two days. At six months, the child was thriving with normal growth and development, including normal hearing. The testes were descended into the scrotum by two months. The crooked finger is functioning and awaits an orthopedic evaluation.

Discussion

This case report illustrates the potential morbidity of an extensive diagnostic evaluation and continuous phototherapy in a premature infant. It also illustrates the "Catch 22" of diagnostic evaluation.

This infant's "abnormalities" could readily be explained by rather obvious circumstances. The delivery by forceps could explain the "fuzziness" on the CT scans in the subdural areas. An aggressive management of hyperbilirubinemia using phototherapy appeared to depress this child, resulting in the sluggish neurologic exam and overlapping suturae. The general pediatrician at the community hospital stated that he frequently sees such findings in premature infants undergoing continuous phototherapy and resulting dehydration.

The effects of insufficient nurturing of the infant were also apparent. With different personnel doing the various consultations and testing, little regard was given to the infant's sleeping and feeding schedule. He seemed to do well only during the night when left along except for nursing care.

This case typifies how apparently healthy premature infants may become victims of a tertiary care center. Undeniably, severely ill infants can survive only as a result of the care provided in such centers. However, extensive diagnostic and therapeutic interventions can be harmful; particularly to fragile premature infants can survive only as a result of the care provided in such centers. However, extensive diagnostic and therapeutic interventions can be harmful, particularly to fragile premature infants, and of course expensive. (The cost for this child's four and one-half days in the medical center was nearly $4,000.)

This case also underscores the importance of the family physician remaining involved while a patient and family are under care in a tertiary center. The family physician is in the unique position of having an understanding and perspective on the medical center while being knowledgeable and understanding of the family.

Group practice was taking off in the 1980s and Medical Economics ran an article stating that small practices were not likely to survive. As managing partner of our small practice in Dixon I took offense and wrote this essay that they were kind to publish. This generated lots of supportive comments from small practice FPs around the country.

Small Practices Won't Survive? Don't You Believe it!

Medical Economics
1984;61:33-36

"I believe we're witnessing the beginning of the end of small medical practices….. I'm telling my clients that bigger is now better," management consultant Leif C. Beck wrote in *Medical Economics* earlier this year.

I strongly disagree.

Speakers at the last annual meeting of the Society of Teachers of Family Medicine echoed Beck's theme. The keynoter lamented the not-too-distant time when we'll all be practicing in medical "supermarkets." And at a seminar, faculty members were urged to prepare their family practice residents for careers as mega-group employees, rather than small-office entrepreneurs.

I also disagree with the chairman of the department of family practice of the University of California School of Medicine at Davis –

where I teach part time. He, too, predicts the demise of small offices and advises residents to look to large HMOs for their future economic security.

According to critics of solo and small partnership practice, current economic trends give a big advantage to large multispecialty medical groups. They say such organizations have a competitive edge because of their broader range of services, greater efficiency, and marketing clout.

Well, I find such claims more theoretical than proven. They're at odds with my own experience and that of other small office practitioners I know. In fact, I'm convinced that the future of neighborhood practices with four or fewer doctors is brighter than that of the large groups. Here are my reasons:

Patients prefer the personalized service they get in small offices. Six years ago, after my residency, I joined a two-man family practice partnership located in a semirural community in northern California. I'm still with it. Although even then there was no shortage of primary care MDs locally, my practice developed so fast that by the third year I had to limit the number of new patients. Many people transferred to us from a prestigious, 65 doctor multispecialty clinic. Their chief reason for switching was frustration at being unable to see the same physician for all their medical problems.

Since the demand for our services continues to grow, we've recently taken on a fourth partner. Some of our patients are now concerned that we may get too big to provide the kind of personalized care that attracted them. They can relax, though; we're determined not to add any more doctors. Our patients can count on seeing the physician of their choice except in an emergency. We handle more than 90 percent of their problems without referral, and we're always available to assist at surgery. With the aid of consultants, we provide comprehensive medical services 24 hours a day, seven days a week. As a result, patients almost never leave us for a larger group.

Small practices are more efficient. They are still the choice of most private practitioners – and with good reason. A 1984 survey by *Medical Economics* shows that 76 percent of all office-based MDs practice either solo or in partnership with no more than two other doctors. Where partnerships of six or more exist, I believe it's mainly to give physicians built-in coverage, rather than to serve patients better.

A group that grows to that size tends to become unwieldy and inefficient – a victim of its own success. It's more difficult to manage, and its ratio of expenses to income often gets out of hand. Theoretically, the partners should be able to keep control by hiring a full-time clinic manger, but it usually doesn't work that way. On the other hand, as managing partner of my small group, I've been able to hold our overhead to 50 percent of gross receipts in each of the past four years.

That may seem high to physicians in some parts of the country, but I checked nearly 40 other solo and small partnership practices in our area and found that their expense ratios are about the same as ours. In contrast, every group of five or more doctors I've queried reports a much higher ratio, often well over 60 percent. Why? Because the larger groups generally employ more personnel less efficiently and have more costly billing systems.

Small offices save patients money, too. Contrary to the belief of many employers and other health care purchasers, small offices are more efficient to lowering costs for patients and their insurers. Because I already know most of the patients I see, and because I rely more on interviewing than on using expensive diagnostic tests, I can manage cases much more economically than a primary care physician in a large multispecialty clinic. And unlike me, the big group doctor has a financial incentive to utilize in-house ancillary services and to refer within the group.

One of my recent cases clearly illustrates the relative economy and effectiveness of small-office practice: A middle-aged man went to the big clinic I mentioned before, complaining of periodic dizziness. After a $950 workup, he was sent home with nothing but the suggestion that he eliminate before-dinner cocktails.

Dissatisfied, the patient then consulted me. After examining and interviewing him thoroughly, I concluded that his dizziness was due to psychological stress and improper diet rather than alcohol. I did recommend limiting his pre-prandial drinks to two, but I also advised him on diet and how to cope with stress. After two visits with me his problem was solved – at a total charge of $60. He'll be returning for follow-up visits every three months, but he'll wind up spending less with me in a year than he did in one visit to the clinic.

It's much the same story with periodic adult health exams. The local multispecialty clinic gets $350 or more, depending on lab fees. In contrast, the three small-office internists in town each charge $175, not counting outside lab fees, while our office charges $125. We also include urinalysis, an ECG, and a pulmonary-function test, all done in our office. So our patients normally pay a total of only $140, including outside lab work.

The difficulty large multispecialty groups have in controlling costs was dramatically demonstrated not long ago when a huge IPA-type prepaid health insurance program in northern California, Washington State, and Utah folded. Introduced in 1975 by the Safeco Insurance Co. of Seattle, United Healthcare grew rapidly through 1980, then closed down in 1982 with estimated losses of about $5 million.

The decision to use the "gatekeeper" approach – paying primary care physicians a capitation allowance and letting them control the utilization of all health care services for enrollees – was probably wise. So, I believe, was its policy of making the gatekeepers share the financial risk. However, the rewards and penalties for participating physicians were too small to inspire changes in practice patterns, so costs kept exceeding the premiums.

In our immediate area, United Healthcare began by contracting exclusively with the local multispecialty clinic. Around 1978, the plan's managers woke up to the fact that the big clinic doctors couldn't hold down costs. Attempts were then made to recruit small offices, whose care they'd found to be less expensive. But apparently it was too late.

Small practices can successfully compete for large blocks of patients. Increasingly, corporate employers and government agencies are looking to large groups to help fight the escalating cost of medical care. More and more HMOs and PPOs are being formed to vie for this business. One might assume that volume health care purchasers can save by arranging preferred-provider contracts with big groups, and at present that's often the case. But the situation is changing.

Medical care is much more a personal service than a commodity. That's why comparisons to supermarkets and discount drug chains are invalid. I shop in supermarkets, but medicines in discount drugstores, and buy clothes in large department stores. However, my financial adviser, accountant, and attorney are in small offices, and I trust only my neighborhood auto mechanic.

Given a choice, patients prefer to be treated in small primary care offices. And more of them whose bills are paid by employers or government agencies will get that choice as small-scale practices everywhere become more competitive.

Most of us in solo or small partnership practice know how to deliver good medical care economically, but individually we're in no position to compete for large scale contracts. The answer, of course, is for more of us to organize network-type IPAs, each with a negotiator well-qualified to make preferred-provider deals.

This movement has already begun in some areas, including my own. Foundation Health Plan, the IPA to which my partners and I belong, contracts only with small medical offices. It was organized some years ago to compete with the Kaiser Foundation Health Plan of Northern California. Our IPA now has 80,000 enrollees, half of whom switched over from Kaiser. It uses the gatekeeper system, requiring patients to see a primary care practitioner before they can be treated by anyone else. It also saves money by requiring that all diagnostic studies be done in low-cost, independent labs, rather than in the physicians' offices.

Health insurance, unfortunately, is so expensive these days that self-employed people with families can no longer afford it. I hope to see that problem disappear as more and more small-office, IPA-type PPOs spring up.

When people really matter, small is beautiful.

In 1981 I became the main advisor to medical students interested in family medicine at the University of California, Davis. The 1980s was a decade of rapidly escalating health care costs and the incomes of procedural specialists rose dramatically. It became an economic sacrifice to enter family medicine. We appealed to the values of the medical students and were successful in getting many to become family physicians. One evening a medical student wrote down about 15 challenging questions about family medicine as a career. These questions become the basis for an article that would be published and revised over two decades. Turns out John Beasley at Wisconsin was writing the same article so we combined our efforts and included Stephen Brunton at AAFP. The first article in this series follows.

Responses to Questions Frequently Asked by Medical Students About Family Practice

Joseph E. Scherger, MD, John W. Beasley, MD, Stephen A. Brunton,
MD, T. Warner Hudson, MD, Gary J. Mishkin, Kenneth W. Patric,
MD, and Steven H. Olson
Davis, California; Madison, Wisconsin; and Kansas City, Missouri

The Journal of Family Practice
1983;17(6):1047-1052

During their medical school years medical students are frequently exposed to misinformation about family practice from faculty members in other specialties. Responses to 26 questions frequently asked by medical students about family practice are presented with a review of recent literature. These responses may assist medical students and their advisors when considering careers in family practice.

Medical students frequently have questions about the specialty of family practice. Exposed to academic tertiary care specialists throughout most of their clinical rotations, many students are given misinformation about family practice. There are common misconceptions or myths perpetuated in the academic environment that can be destructive to a student's interest in family practice as a career choice.

The following is a list of questions gathered by medical students at the University of California, Davis, and the University of Wisconsin-Madison. Responses were compiled by residency-trained family physicians from their experiences and a review of recent literature. These responses may be useful to medical students and their advisors as a supplement to a predoctoral program for developing careers in family practice.

Question 1: What is a family physician, and how does this role differ from that of a traditional general practitioner?

Response: By definition the family physician is "educated and trained to develop and bring to bear in practice unique attitudes and skills which qualify him or her to provide continuing, comprehensive health maintenance and medical care to the entire family regardless of sex, age, or type of problem, be it biological, behavioral, or social. This physician serves as the patient's or family's advocate in all health-related matters, including the appropriate use of consultants and community resources."[1]

Family practice residencies were developed in response to a need perceived by the public, the medical profession, and government for the development of a well-trained generalist. The general practitioner of the past usually began practice after an internship or brief residency largely consisting of inpatient rotations. After World War II came an age of specialization during which very few graduates selected general practice. To fill the need left by the decline in general practice, family practice became a specialty in 1969, the twentieth specialty recognized by the American Board of Medical Specialties. Family practice follows the general practice tradition, but has some major differences. Before entering practice, in addition to a broad inpatient training, family physicians receive extensive training in outpatient medicine for all ages. As a specialty, family practice has stringent requirements for continuing education and board certification. Family practice combines the content of general practice and other clinical disciplines, including the behavioral sciences and preventive medicine, and integrates them into a single specialty with a focus on patient care in the context of the family and community.[2]

Question 2: Is it possible to be a competent family physician? How can one know enough about the many clinical areas in medicine?

Response: The amount of knowledge necessary to be a good family physician is not greater than the amount of knowledge necessary to be any other specialist such as a pediatrician or a neurologist.[3] The difference is that the body of knowledge in family practice spreads across many disciplines without the need for an esoteric depth in any discipline. Seventy percent of all the problems seen by a family physician fit into 30 diagnoses.[4,5] It is not extraordinarily difficult to acquire and maintain high-quality clinical skills to manage the great majority of common problems that patients bring to physicians in a primary care setting.

Question 3: Do family physicians refer many of their patients to other specialists?

Response: Family physicians manage exclusively over 90 percent of problems they encounter with the confidence that they are handling these problems as well as or better than any other specialist. A consultation is requested for about 7 percent of problems, and the family physician continues to manage the patient. When a referral is made (0.9 percent to 3 percent of problems), the family physician remains active in the care of the patient.[6-8]

Question 4: What will be the role of the family physician in the future, when there is a surplus of other specialists?

Response: The public, third-party payers, and government health officials recognize that family physicians are the appropriate providers to manage most health problems. Because of the efficiency and cost effectiveness of having a family physician as the entry into the health care system, the role of the family physician seems secure.[9] Current trends in government and other third-party reimbursement systems suggest that family physicians will maintain and probably will enlarge their role in the health care system.

Question 5: Will family physicians be able to maintain hospital privileges, particularly in obstetrics?

Response: With well-documented residency training, it is not likely that family physicians will be denied hospital privileges. The American Academy of Family Physicians has established the maintenance of hospital privileges for family physicians as a top priority.[10,11] Criteria have been negotiated with other specialty organizations for the approval of hospital privileges for family practice residency graduates. These criteria have been tested in court, and generally the family physician has won.[12] A recent survey of family practice residency graduates has shown that over 96 percent have all the hospital privileges they requested, with 89 percent having privileges in intensive care units and 64 percent of graduates doing obstetrics.[13,14] As long as the profession of family practice in this country considers hospital privileges to be an important priority, it is unlikely there will be any significant change in the hospital-based role of the family physician.

Question 6: Is family practice a satisfying career choice, or does it become monotonous?

Response: Surveys of family practice residency graduates in practice indicate high levels of personal and professional satisfaction.[13,15] Only 4 percent of recent graduates find boredom to be a problem.[15] The variety of medical problems is such that no day in the office is the same. In an average month, a family physician may see patients with up to 400 different diagnoses.[16]

The family physician receives the greatest satisfaction, however, from the intense involvement in the changing lives of his or her patients rather than from the treatment of the health problems with which they present. Being a family physician is a fascinating and privileged role that increases with time as the physician gains a deeper understanding of the people in a community.

Question 7: Do family physicians take care of patients with serious illnesses?

Response: Patient visits to family physicians include not only preventive care and health promotion, but also the management of acute and chronic illnesses, be they minor or serious. A large survey of patient visits to family physicians indicated that about one third of visits were for serious or potentially serious problems (for example, cardiovascular disease and abdominal pain).[16]

Question 8: Are family physicians adequately trained for their job?

Response: Residency training in family practice is designed specifically to prepare family physicians for their job. Surveys indicate that recent graduates feel well prepared for their work as a result of their residency training.[13,15] Only 1 to 2 percent of recent graduates indicate having to care for medical or surgical problems beyond their training as a serious problem.[15]

Question 9: Do family physicians see too many patients to do a good job?

Response: In the 1980 the average number of patient contacts per week for family physicians was 172, compared with 160 for pediatricians and 112 for internists.[17] More recent figures from other sources show that family practice residency graduates have an average of 141 patient contacts per week.[4] The range is great, since physicians may set their own pace. The data suggest that family physicians may spend somewhat less time with patients at each visit but see them more often.[4] Only 8 percent of residency graduates rate having too many patients to see as a serious problem.[15]

Question 10: What is life like for a family physician: Is there time for a good personal and family life?

Response: The typical family physician works 50 to 60 hours per week in direct patient care.[13,14] About 80 percent of residency graduates practice in partnerships or group practices that have call-sharing arrangements.[13,18] Family physicians in solo practice may also share calls with a group. Coverage arrangements can be made so that the physician may work part-time and be on call only when desired and still maintain a continuous involvement with patient care. Most family practice residencies train their graduates to work with colleagues so that they will have ample time for personal and family priorities. A survey by the Robert Wood Johnson Foundation has shown that family physicians spend more time with personal and civic activities than do general internists, most medical specialists, obstetrician-gynecologists, and some surgical specialists.[19]

Question 11: What about malpractice insurance; could the high cost prevent family physicians from doing obstetrics and other procedures?

Response: Family physicians enjoy special malpractice rates formulated for their specialty. A family physician can do basic obstetrics, surgical assisting, vasectomies, dilation and curettage, and office surgeries in an intermediate category with very affordable insurance rates. The mean malpractice insurance costs for family physicians in the United States in 1981 was about $2,000 per year, with considerable geographic variation. This compares with mean malpractice insurance costs for obstetrician-gynecologists and other surgical specialists of over $10,000 per year.[20, 21]

Question 12: What practice opportunities will be available in the future for family physicians?

Response: Although the United States is heading for a potential physician surplus by 1990, a continuing need for primary care physicians, including family physicians, has been projected.[22] Many areas of the country are greatly underserved and need family physicians. Family practice openings are numerous in urban, suburban, and rural locations. A recent *Physician Placement Bulletin* of practice opportunities in California listed more family practice positions than internal medicine, pediatrics, and obstetrics and gynecology combined.[23]

Family practice has an advantage over other specialties in that a population of 2,000 is adequate to keep a family physician busy. It takes an unserved population of over 10,000 to accommodate most other specialists.[24] Hence, growing communities frequently need more family physicians.

Question 13: Is family practice only for rural communities, or is this specialty appropriate for urban areas?

Response: There is a great public demand for family physicians in all locations. While it is true that communities with fewer than 10,000 people are best served by family physicians almost exclusively, family physicians also enjoy nearly the same role in urban areas, where there are many other types of specialists.[10,11,16] Surveys of recent graduates of family practice residencies have shown that although about 50 percent practice in communities of less than 25,000 people, 25 to 30 percent practice in cities with more than 100,000 people.[25,26]

The presence of many subspecialists does not preclude the need for family physicians. The family practice model is so embraced by the public that family physicians have little difficulty competing with other specialists for primary care.

Question 14: How do family physicians keep up with medical advances?

Response: Continuing education occurs in a variety of ways, including dialogue with colleagues, learning from consultants, reading medical journals, and attending sources and medical meetings. The number of major advances each year altering patient care on a primary care level is not great.

The American Board of Family Practice was the first specialty board to require recertification for ongoing membership. Recertification involves a cognitive examination and an audit of a selected number of the physician's office practice records. No other specialty requires a comparable degree of continual updating of medical knowledge and skills.

Question 15: Can I specialize in a field such as general surgery or obstetrics and gynecology and still do family practice?

Response: Although there is nothing to restrict any licensed physician from doing general practice, physicians in practice readily acknowledge their lack of expertise in handling problems outside their specialty area. The ability to manage confidently a wide variety of problems from sick infants to orthopedic problems to chronic disease in the elderly requires years of generalist training beyond medical school. There has been a documented rapid decline in broad clinical knowledge during the first year of residency training in specialties other than family practice.[27] Furthermore, board certification in family practice requires residency training in family practice.

Question 16: Can a family physician be an expert in anything?

Response: The family physician is an expert in the evaluation and management of common health problems, with an understanding of the whole person in the context of a family and community, and with an emphasis on disease prevention and health promotion.

Along with this expertise, many family physicians develop a special interest in certain areas. For example, family physicians commonly have a special interest and expertise in sports medicine and fitness, preventive medicine, care of the elderly, and hospice care for the dying. The variety in family practice allows the physician to have expertise and be active as a community leader in diverse areas.

Question 17: After family practice residency training, what career options are available, for example, in emergency rooms, health maintenance organizations, student health centers, public health, or international medicine?

Response: A family practice residency provides a broad and liberal training that gives the graduate many options besides a traditional practice. Many family practice residency graduates work in community hospital emergency rooms, student health centers, and health maintenance organizations. Often the family physician is in a management role in these locations. The great variety of opportunities is illustrated by the offerings in the *Physician Placement Bulletin*[23] or the classified advertisements of many medical journals.

Family practice residency training also prepares a physician to pursue a role in public health and international medicine. The World Health Organization is becoming increasingly aware of the value of family practice training, and the residency format in this country is spreading throughout the world.

Question 18: How do physicians' assistants, nurse practitioners, and midwives fit in with the role of the family physician in the future? Will they replace the need for family physicians?

Response: Physicians' assistants, nurse practitioners, and midwives developed as new members of the health care team, particularly in response to the need for providers in medically underserved areas. They were never intended, nor are they trained, to replace family physicians. These practitioners can extend the breadth and quality of family practice, particularly though health promotion, screening, and patient education; however, the family physician is an essential provider of comprehensive and continuing care for families. In addition, as a substantial physician surplus is developing, the number of training positions for physicians' assistants and nurse practitioners is decreasing.

Question 19: What is a family practice residency, and how does it vary in structure around the country?

Response: In the United States all family practice residencies are three years and provide a relatively standard curriculum. About 70 percent of family practice residencies are located in community hospitals that usually do not have other residency programs. About 30 percent of family practice residencies are in academic teaching centers. Most community hospital programs are affiliated with a medical school.[28]

The most striking characteristic of all family practice residencies is an outpatient experience in a family practice center that allows the resident to assume the role of a family physician for a limited number of individuals and families throughout the three years of residency. The amount of time spent in the family practice center increases with each year in the residency.

The hospital experience during the first year of residency is similar to that of a rotating internship. During the second year, the resident assumes greater responsibility for hospitalized patients and usually has some elective time. In the third year the resident commonly has more outpatient rotations, electives, and inpatient rotations with greater responsibility.

Important aspects of family practice residency training include behavioral science, counseling skills, practice management, and an approach to health maintenance and preventive medicine. All of these are integrated to develop a physician with an orientation to the whole person and to families. Flexibility is usually built into the curriculum to allow the resident to pursue such diverse interests as high-risk obstetrics, clinical hypnosis, and research. In other words, the third-year resident will usually select training experiences that fit a future practice interest.

Question 20: How difficult is it to get into a good family practice residency?

Response: There are currently 387 family practice residencies in the United States.[28] A Residency Review Committee, (with representation from the American Medical Association, the American Academy of Family Physicians, and the American Board of Family Practice), carefully evaluates these programs to maintain an overall quality. While considerable competition exists for the most popular programs, it is not difficult for a student of at least average academic standing to match into a good family practice residency.

Question 21: Is it possible to do a flexible internship and then enter a family practice residency?

Response: Although this option is possible, it is more difficult than entering a family practice residency the first year. The attrition rate for family practice residencies is very low. For those limited number of available positions in the second year, there is generally great competition. Residents completing a flexible internship would have to compete with physicians having practice experience who would want to complete a family practice residency.

Question 22: What are the academic qualifications of students entering family practice?

Response: In one study, the average Part II National Board Examination scores for students entering family practice residencies was 541. The average of the entire group of students entering all specialties was 539. For Part III, the score was 549 for family physicians and 526 for all specialties.[27] Another study done in 1982 indicated that the premedical academic qualifications of students selecting family practice (as measured by undergraduate GPA and MCAT scores) are comparable to those of students selecting other specialties.[29] In general, students entering family practice have the same qualifications as those entering other specialties.

Question 23: What is the average income of a family physician, and how does this compare with other specialists?

Response: Family physicians enjoy an income that compares favorably with other specialists in primary care. A recent survey in *Medical Economics* indicated that the average net income for family physicians in 1981 was about $70,000 per year.[30] This amount was slightly greater than that for pediatricians and general practitioners and slightly less than for psychiatrists and internists.

Question 24: What are the opportunities for teaching in family practice?

Response: Since family practice is a relatively new academic discipline that has grown rapidly, there are many unfilled teaching positions. Family physicians teach full-time or part-time in both medical schools and community hospital programs. There is also a great need for family physicians to teach medical students and residents in their office settings. Sixty percent of recent family practice residency graduates are currently involved in some form of teaching.[18]

Question 25: What are the opportunities for research in family practice?

Response: The opportunities for research in family practice are varied and are receiving increasing support. The spectrum for family medicine research includes the natural history of disease and illness behavior in individuals and families, clinical studies of diagnostic and treatment methods, the organization of health services, and public policy.[31,32] The developing collaborative networks among practicing physicians will provide a rich base for future research.[33] The American Academy of Family Physicians (AAFP) and the Society of Teachers of Family Medicine (STFM) have active research committees that work to improve research skills and stimulate projects. The Family Health Foundation of America (FHFA), the philanthropic arm of family practice, provides increasing support to research activities. The National Institutes of Health (NIH) recently held a symposium on family medicine research.

Question 26: Is family practice a growing specialty?

Response: The number of board-certified family physicians has risen from 0 in 1969 to nearly 30,000 in 1982. In the same period, the number of residencies has gone from 0 to 387. The number of residents in training has increased yearly, exceeding 7,200 in 1982. The AAFP, with over 55,000 members, is the largest specialty organization in the world. There is a projected growth of 10 percent in the number of family physicians between 1980 and 1990.[22] The numbers reflect a discipline that is well established, growing, and here to stay.

Comment

These responses reflect the wisdom of several recent residency graduates who are enthusiastic about the specialty of family practice. There is room for further elaboration and varying opinions. Most students with an interest in or a healthy skepticism about family practice will have other questions not listed above. While many academic specialists in other fields will readily give their opinions about family practice, it is hoped students will obtain counsel from family physicians. Departments of family practice in medical schools should have a group of family practice advisors who are readily accessible and who frequently meet with students to discuss these questions.

References

1. American Academy of Family Physicians: Official definition of family practice and family physicians, reprint 303.AAFP Reporter 2:10, 1975
2. Perkoff GT: Family practice: Potential for a key role in medical care. Arch Intern Med 141:979, 1981
3. Spitzer WO: The intellectual worthiness of family medicine. Pharos 40:2, 1977
4. Rosenblatt RA, Cherkin DC, Schneeweiss R, et al: The structure and content of family practice: Current status and future trends. J Fam Pract 15:681, 1982
5. Marsland DW, Wood M, Mayo F: A data bank for patient care, curriculum, and research in family practice: 526,196 patient problems. J Fam Pract 3:25, 1976
6. Geyman JP, Brown TC, Rivers K: Referrals in family practice: A comparative study by geographic region and practice setting. J Fam Pract 3: 163, 1976
7. Brock C: Consultation and referral patterns of family physicians. J Fam Pract 4:1129, 1977
8. Taylor RB: Categories of care in family medicine. Fam Med 13(4):7, 1981
9. Farrell DL, Worth RM, Mishina K: Utilization and cost effectiveness of a family practice center. J Fam Pract 15:957, 1982
10. Clinton C, Schmittling G, Stern T, et al: Hospital privileges for family physicians: A national study of office based members of the American Academy of Family Physicians. J Fam Pract

13:361, 1981

11. Stern T, Schmittling G, Clinton C, Black RR: Hospital privileges for graduates of family practice residency programs. J Fam Pract 13:1013, 1981

12. Lavin JH: FPs: No longer shortchanged on hospital privileges. Med Econ 58:97, 1980

13. Geyman JP: The emerging profile of the residency trained family physician. J Fam Pract 11:717, 1980

14. American Academy of Family Physicians: Academy survey profiles office-based family practice. AAFP Reporter 7(7):1, 1980

15. McCranie EW, Hornsby JL, Calvert JC: Practice and career satisfaction among residency trained family physicians: A national study. J Fam Pract 14:1107, 1982

16. Marsland DW, Wood M, Mayo F: Content of family practice: Part 1. Rank order of diagnoses by frequency. Part 2. Diagnoses by disease category and age/sex distribution. J Fam Pract 3:37, 1976

17. Owens A: Doctor surplus: Where things stand now. Med Econ 57:63, 1980

18. Black RR, Schmittling G, Stern TL: Characteristics and practice patterns of family practice residency graduates in the United States. J Fam Pract 11:767, 1980

19. Medical Practice in the United States: A Special Report. Princeton, NJ, The Robert Wood Johnson Foundation, 1981, pp 32-47

20. Recent trends in physician liability claims and insurance expenses. SMS Rep 1(7):1, 1982

21. White JS: Practice expenses: Has all the fat been trimmed? Med Econ 59:130, 1982

22. Report of the Graduate Medical Education National Advisory Committee to the Secretary, Department of Health and Human Services, vol 1: GMENAC Summary Report. Health Resources Administration (Hyattsville, Md). DHHS publication No. 81-651. Government Printing Office, 1980

23. Physician Placement Bulletin: California Opportunities. San Francisco, Physician Placement Service, California Medical Association, November-December, 1982

24. Review of Health Manpower Population Requirements

Standards. Health Resources Administration (Hyattsville, Md). DHEW publication No. (HRA) 77-22. Government Printing Office, 1976

25. Geyman JP, Ciriacy EW, Mayo F, et al: Geographic distribution of family practice residency graduates: The experience of three statewide networks. J Fam Pract 11:761, 1980

26. Report on Survey of 1982 Graduating Family Practice Residents, reprint 155-H. Kansas City, Mo, American Academy of Family Physicians, 1982

27. Gonella JS: The impact of early specialization on the clinical competence of residents. N Engl J Med 306:275, 1982

28. Three Hundred Eighty-seven Accredited Family Practice Residencies, July 1982, reprint 150-D. Kansas City, Mo, American Academy of Family Physicians, 1982

29. Burkett GL, Gelula MH: Characteristics of students preferring family practice/primary care careers. J Fam Pract 15:505, 1982

30. Owens A: Earnings: Where do you fit in? Med Econ 59:246, 1982

31. Phillips TJ: Research considerations for the family physician. J Fam Pract 7:121, 1978

32. Culpepper L, Franks P: Family medicine research: Status at the end of the first decade. JAMA 249:63, 1983

33. Nelson EC, Kirk JW, Bise BW, et al: The cooperative information project: Part 1. A sentinel practice network for service and research in primary care. J Fam Pract 13:641, 1981

Without any curriculum time, we were successful at UC Davis in recruiting many students to family medicine. Our strategy became a model of career development and the following article was the basis for presentations at STFM predoctoral conferences.

A Predoctoral Strategy for Promoting Careers in Family Practice

Joseph E. Scherger, MD; Jeanne Woolsey, MSPH; Candelaria Perez-Davison, MSW

Family Medicine
1984;16 (1):19-23

Abstract: An important but often neglected part of medical school education is career development. While 30% to 40% of entering medical students have personal interests and characteristics for family practice, only 13% to 15% of students enter family practice training. Given the need for more students to choose a career in family practice, predoctoral programs should place a high priority on maintaining student interest in family practice.

Career decision making by medical students is a longitudinal process. To be successful in promoting careers in family practice, predoctoral programs should develop a strategy consisting of extracurricular activities and curricular offerings during the preclinical and clinical years. Using such a strategic approach, the University of California at Davis Predoctoral Program is successful in promoting family practice careers, even with limited departmental resources and limited curricular time.

Introduction

Medical school education has two overriding purposes: to provide a broad, basic medical education and to prepare the student for choosing a career in medicine. Most medical school curricula are designed to accomplish the first educational purpose, with little attention given to the second – career development. The most important decision a medical student will make is what type of physician to become. Unfortunately, most students make this decision in relative isolation with little help from their medical schools.

Although the medical school curriculum may not be designed to aid in a wise career decision based on a broad understanding of medical specialties, student experiences in medical school particularly during the clinical years, have a major impact on the choice of specialty.[1-4] While 50% to 70% of students entering medical school have an interest in some primary care field, less than half of graduates become primary care physicians.[5] Most students make their firm career decision during the third year or early in the fourth year, prior to or at the time of residency selection.[1,6] That students are exposed almost exclusively to academic subspecialty attendings during this time may account for the disproportionate number of students choosing specialties other than primary care.

Thirty percent to 40% of entering medical students have personal interests and characteristics appropriate for family practice.[5] The American Academy of Family Physicians has set a goal that 25% of medical students should enter family practice to maintain balance in the health care system.[7] Currently, only 13% to 15% of U.S. students enter family practice training. This figure has been stable since 1978.[8,9] The percentage of graduates selecting family practice varies from less than 5% to over 50% among medical schools.[10] Factors which have been correlated with a larger number of students selecting family practice include admission policies, institutional commitment (department status and faculty size), and extensive curricular time.[10-12]

Given the need for more students to select family practice careers, predoctoral programs should place a high priority on maintaining student interest in family practice. Whatever the admission policies, administrative status, and curricular time, family practice predoctoral programs can design a strategy of curricular offerings and extracurricular activities to promote family practice careers. The overall goal of such a strategy would be to give the students as broad a perspective of family practice as possible so that appropriate students will select this specialty.

This article describes the predoctoral strategy at the University of

California, Davis (U.C. Davis). This strategy, in a school with limited departmental resources and extremely limited curricular time, appears to be highly successful in promoting family practice careers. Currently, 20% to 30% of graduating students enter family practice residency training. This compares to an initial career interest in family practice of about 35% to 40%. Other schools report a similar initial interest in family practice with a much greater attrition by the fourth year.[2,5,13,14]

TABLE 1

A STRATEGY FOR PROMOTING FAMILY PRACTICE CAREERS

PRECLINICAL	CLINICAL
• *Identify* students interested in F.P.	• *Promote* a career decision in F.P.
• *Maintain* this interest	• *Guide* the residency selection process

Strategy

The predoctoral strategy at Davis is divided into the preclinical (first and second) and clinical (third and fourth) years. The principles of the strategy are presented in Table 1.

Identifying students interested in family practice is very important. Studies have shown that most students who select family practice have this interest when they enter medical schoo.[15] Identifying these students allows the program to begin a process of communication with, and a monitoring of, these students during the four years. At Davis, these students are identified in the first week of the first year by a questionnaire and by enrollment into a voluntary family practice pathway program described below. The predoctoral program continues to direct its activities toward all students in a class, since some of those not indicating an initial interest may later select family practice.

Once these students interested in family practice have been identified, the second objective for the preclinical years is to maintain their interest. Exposure to family practice role models appears to be the key method of maintaining this interest.[1]

During the clinical years of medical education most students either change their career decision or reaffirm their earlier decisions.[1,3,16] The first objective for this period is to promote a decision for family practice. Exposed to academic tertiary care subspecialists during most of their clinical rotations, many students are given misinformation about family practice. An ongoing program of student advising and carefully selected family practice experiences provide the key to promoting family practice career decisions.

The final objective in the strategy is to guide students who have chosen family practice with their residency applications. Students should be assisted as much as possible with the important process of selecting and matching with residency programs.

Family Practice Pathway

The Family Practice Pathway Program at U.C. Davis is an informal and voluntary mechanism through which the predoctoral strategy is implemented. The Program consists largely of extracurricular activities and electives which students can contribute to, or participate in, in any way that is of interest to them. The Pathway Programs are administered by the predoctoral faculty and staff, and are broader in scope than a family practice club or interest group. A student interest group may form within the Pathway, depending upon the level of student motivation.

TABLE 2

THE U.C. DAVIS PREDOCTORAL PROGRAM IN FAMILY MEDICINE: THE PRECLINICAL YEARS

FIRST YEAR	SECOND YEAR
• Introduction to Clinical Medicine (Required)	• No Required or Elective Curricular Time
• Family Practice Pathway Orientation	• Family Practice Pathway Community Physician Advisor
Community Physician Advisor	Communications
Counseling	Forum
Introductory Preceptorship (Elective)	Community Clinics

The first phase of the Pathway Program is directed toward the first- and second-year students (Table 2). During the first year of medical school,
students are introduced to the concept of the Family Practice Pathway through a department-sponsored introductory course in clinical medicine. Interested students are given a descriptive brochure outlining the philosophy of the Pathway and family practice activities and courses. A sign-up sheet is included for students to note the aspects of the Pathway they want to be involved in.

Major activities during the first two years of medical school include:

Orientation:

An orientation social is held at the beginning of the first year to introduce students to department faculty and staff members, community advisors, and upper classmates who share an interest in family medicine.

Community Physician Advisor Program:

Each Pathway student is paired with one of five locally practicing family physicians who serve as role models and general advisors to the students throughout medical school. These physicians provide students with a different perspective than they may receive from their traditional academic advisors. Most students initiate contact with their community physician advisors by spending a day in their offices.

Counseling/Information:

A full-time Pathway coordinator serves as a general counselor to the students and aids student involvement in family practice-related activities, including electives, research opportunities, site visits to preceptors' practices, and student forums.

Communications/Forums:

Articles and notices of upcoming activities are distributed to Pathway students to keep them informed of developments in family practice. An inhouse library is maintained for student use. Noon seminars and meetings serve as forums for the exchange of ideas and information. Student membership in the American Academy of Family Physicians is encouraged, as is student involvement in local and national academy activities.

Electives:

The first two years of the medical school curriculum offer little time for elective courses. At the end of the first year, there is a six-week block for students to make up deficiencies, take time off, or pursue educational areas of interest. During this time, an Introductory Preceptorship in Family Practice is offered. This is an extension of the first-year required course. The preceptors are family physicians located throughout California. In 1982, 20% of the class elected to participate in this preceptorship.

Two community clinics, a "free clinic" and one which serves an urban Spanish-speaking population, are available to second-year students for electives. Involvement with these clinics is longitudinal, and the students find time to work in them outside their required curricular time.

Elective opportunities for students to work with faculty members on research projects are also available.

TABLE 3

THE U.C. DAVIS PREDOCTORAL PROGRAM IN FAMILY MEDICINE: THE CLINICAL YEARS

<u>THIRD YEAR</u>	<u>FOURTH YEAR</u>
• No Required or Elective Curricular Time	• Family Practice Track Curriculum
• Family Practice Pathway Group Discussions Community Clinics	• Preceptorships/Clerkships
	• Residency Selection Workshops
• Fourth-Year Track Curriculum Planning	• Individual Counseling/Advising
	• Residency Applications/Letters
	• Match Day

The second phase of the Pathway Program is directed toward the third- and fourth-year students (Table 3). The third year of medical school contains no elective time and no curricular contact with the Department of Family Practice. Required rotations are largely inpatient and include medicine, surgery, obstetrics and gynecology, pediatrics, and psychiatry. Contact is maintained with students through Family Practice Pathway Track curriculum activities (described below) and through planning for the fourth-year curriculum.

The fourth-year curriculum is organized around a track system where students designate one of four track preferences: medical specialties, surgical specialties, family practice/behavioral specialties, and research. Students who choose the family practice track meet with the family physician track coordinator during the third year to design their fourth-year curricula.

The major activities of the Family Practice Pathway during the third and fourth years of medical school include:

Group Discussions:

During the third year, informal noon and evening meetings are held with students to discuss family practice as a career option and to answer students' questions regarding the field. Toward the end of the third year and through the early part of the fourth year, the Pathway discussions focus on family practice residency programs and the application process. Students are provided with a workbook to guide them with their residency applications and selections.

Preceptorships/Clerkships:

Students selecting the Fourth-Year Track Curriculum in Family Practice are encouraged to do a four-week preceptorship with a family physician early in the year. Preceptorships give students a community-based experience in family practice that may solidify or cause them to reconsider their career interests. Students are also encouraged to do a family practice clerkship in a residency program they are strongly considering as a training site.

Electives:

Special study electives are offered by the predoctoral program. These may involve reading, site visits and analysis of models of primary care, and research covering various facets of family practice. Many students continue their involvement in the community clinics during their clinical years. Some students continue their involvement in the community clinics during their clinical years. Some students take on leadership roles, becoming involved in directing the expansion of the clinic resources, recruiting students, and overseeing the general operation.

In summary, the Family Pathway is an informal mechanism by which the predoctoral program coordinates its activities and keeps in touch with students interested in family practice. Most students sign up the first year and remain on the Pathway roster for their class unless they specifically request to be moved. Some students enter the Pathway in later years as they develop an interest in family practice.

Resources

The predoctoral program at U.C. Davis has no full-time faculty. A local participating physician spends 30% to 40% time coordinating the overall strategy. One member of the Department of Family Practice faculty coordinates the required introduction to clinical medicine course for first-year students. Other departmental faculty members participate in student teaching upon request. Four local practicing physicians are paid 10% time to advise and teach students as part of the Pathway Program. Approximately 70 volunteer clinical faculty members participate each year as preceptors through the required course and preceptorship electives. Staff support consists of one full-time Pathway coordinator; two secretaries, and a half-time evaluator.

The program is supported largely by a training grant from the Department of Health and Human Services. The amount of this grant is comparable to other predoctoral programs. Along with limited departmental funding, some support is received from the regional Area Health Education Center in cooperation with U.C. Davis.

Discussion

Career decision making by medical students is a longitudinal process. Most studies of this process focus on the time at which students indicate making their decision. A closer look reveals that most, if not all, students reevaluate their career interests prior to, and throughout, medical school, with a large number changing their career interests during the clinical years.[1,3,16] This instability of career choice holds true for many students indicating an early interest in family practice.[13]

Attrition from family practice commonly occurs during the clinical years.[2,5,13,14] This may be because students who were initially naïve about their career interests later discover a more mature desire to become another kind of specialist. For many, however, there may be another explanation. During the clinical years, career decision making becomes greatly dependent upon experiences in medical school, particularly interaction with role models. Since students must make a career decision by the beginning of the fourth year in order to participate with their class in the residency selection process, the third year is the key clinical year for career decision making. In most schools, the third year consists almost exclusively of core clerkships in the specialties of internal medicine, surgery, pediatrics, obstetrics and gynecology, and psychiatry based in inpatient tertiary care centers with subspecialists as role model attendings. Negative opinions about family practice are commonly heard in these settings, and family practice predoctoral programs may have to expend considerable effort counteracting these influences.

A predoctoral strategy for promoting family practice careers should be longitudinal and address this attrition of interest. The goal should be to give students as broad a perspective as possible about family practice to allow appropriate students to select this specialty.

While there is evidence that having a family practice preceptorship in the third year may be associated with maintaining student interest in family practice,[17] several studies have shown that a single family practice rotation does not affect medical career choice.[15,18,19] In order to affect career choice, a multifaceted program or strategy that combines family practice experiences with advising seems necessary. Programs consisting of a longitudinal family practice track for the clinical years have been successful in promoting family practice career decisions.[20,21]

The predoctoral program at U.C. Davis has been successful in promoting family practice careers with limited resources and required curricular time only in the first year. Elective curricular time is limited to the summer after the first year and in the fourth year. By necessity, the program has had to emphasize extracurricular activities such as the community physician advisor program and a series of group discussions. One advantage of these extra-curricular activities is that they are longitudinal. A student interested in family practice may participate in one of these activities throughout the four years of medical school.

The predoctoral program is continuously evaluated with a goal of better understanding the career decision process and what influences have impact. Coker and colleagues have suggested that in a discipline which has lesser prestige in the medical school, the influence of role models and faculty advisors becomes especially important.[22] Brearley and associates have reported that the role model provided a major influence on students selecting family practice.[1] It appears that, at least for family practice, an ongoing advisor program supplemented with preclinical and clinical experiences is important.

Keeping in close contact with medical students throughout their four years can be a fascinating and rewarding experience. Students respond well to those who show interest in their futures. With a strategic approach, a predoctoral program in family medicine, even one with limited resources, may be able to help those students who should go into family practice to do so.

References

1. Brearley WD, Simpson W, Baker, R. Family practice as a specialty choice: effect of premedical and medical education. J Med Educ 1982; 57:449-54.

2. Sacha I. Medical specialty choice: replication and extensions. Proceedings of the 16th Annual Conference on Research in Medical Education. Washington, D.C.: American Association of Medical Colleges, 1977; 215-20.

3. Held ML, Zimet CN. A longitudinal study of medical specialty choice and certainty level. J Med Educ 1975; 50:1044-51.

4. Snyder DS. The relationship of students' experience before and during medical school to their conceptions of professional responsibility. J Med Educ 1967; 42:213-18.

5. Attitudes of medical students and recent graduates. Triennial Survey, 1981. Bureau of Research and Planning. Division of Research and Socioeconomics. San Francisco: California Medical Association, 1982.

6. Eagelson BK, Tobolic T. A survey of students who chose family practice residencies. J Fam Pract 1978; 6:111-18.

7. American Academy of Family Physicians. 1973 Congress of Delegates. Kansas City: AAFP Transactions; 1973; 45.

8. Goldsmith G. Medical student interest in family practice: how is it changing? Fam Med 1982; 14:13-16.

9. Geyman JP. Student selection of family practice residencies: a ten-year view. J Fam Pract 1981; 13:971-72.

10. Goldsmith G. Factors influencing family practice residency selection: a national survey. J Fam Pract 1982; 15:121-24.

11. Beck JD, Stewart WI, Graham R, Stern TI. The effect of the organization and status of family practice undergraduate programs on residency selection. J Fam Pract 1977; 4:663-68.

12. Boulger JG. Family practice in the predoctoral curriculum: a model for success. J Fam Pract 1980; 10:453-58.

13. Cauthen DB, Adams RI, De La Rosa F, Meyer GG, Holcomb J. Medical students and family practice: a prospective study. Texas Medicine 1980; 76:57-60.

14. Parmeter JT, Haf J, Scheifley V, Boger M. The cooperative Michigan longitudinal study of medical student career choices: research design and preliminary results. Proceedings of the 17th Annual Conference and Research in Medical Education, Washington, D.C.; American Association of Medical Colleges, 1978; 145-50.

15. Harris DL, Bluhm HP. An evaluation of primary care preceptorships. J Fam Pract 1977; 5:577-79.

16. Donovan JC, Salzman LF, Allen PZ. Studies in medical education: career choice consistency of medical students. Amer J Obstet Gynecol 1972; 112:519-23.

17. Influence of preceptorship and other factors on the education and career choices of physicians. DHEW Publication No. (HRA) 78-84. Washington, D. C.: Government Printing Office, 1978.

18. Rosenblatt RA, Alpert JJ. The effect of a course in family medicine on future career choice: a long-range follow-up of a controlled experiment in medical education. J Fam Pract 1979; 8:87-91.

19. Hale FA, McConnochie KM, Chapman RJ, Whiting RD. The impact of a required preceptorship on senior medical students. J Med Educ 1979; 54:396-401.

20. Phillips TJ, Gordon MJ, Leversee JH, Smith CK. Family

physician pathway and medical student career choice. JAMA 1978; 240:1736-41.

21. Harris DL, Coleman M, Mallea M. Impact of participation on a family practice track program on student career decisions. J Med Educ 1982; 57:609-14.

22. Coker RE, Back KW, Donnelly TG, Miller N. Patterns of influence: medical school faculty members and the values and specialty interests of medical students. J Med Educ 1960; 35:518-27.

PART III: LEADERSHIP 1985-92

I was fortunate to serve as the first resident member of the STFM board of directors in 1977-78. After starting practice in Dixon, I returned to the STFM board as the Chair of the Communications Committee. That was an exciting time, as Family Medicine Teacher became Family Medicine and the founder of STFM, Lynn Carmichael, agreed to serve as Family Medicine's Editor. Joel Merenstein formed a group of us with progressive leanings and used a Delphi method to produce a report, Training Residents for the Future (1986;18:29-37). The following is an editorial I wrote to accompany this report:

An Agenda for Change

Family Medicine
1986;18:39

The 21st century will be a time of easy access to information. Much of the information traditionally held by physicians will be readily accessible to the public. Much of the information traditionally held by subspecialists will be readily accessible to the generalists. Health care in the future will require good judgment by physicians and patients relating to an expansive array of technologies. The future will be an important time for the personal family physician.

The report by Merenstein et al. on training residents for the future describes the opportunities and priorities for family practice education. The brilliance of the report is that the agenda for the future is developed out of a fulfillment of the past. The recommendations of the Millis and Willard reports have been only partly realized, and by completing their mission we will be training residents for the future. The Merenstein recommendations begin by emphasizing the enduring qualities of the family physician. What is changeless about family practice is primary to what is changing. Meeting the health care needs in a "high tech" information society does not require a metamorphosis into some new type of provider. What needs to change most dramatically is the education structure by which we train family physicians.

Without reiterating the Merenstein report, I will list some priorities for the Society of Teachers of Family Medicine and other organizations of our specialty to begin addressing these timely recommendations.

1. Medical students need to be given much clearer information about the society in which they will be practicing. An understanding of the evolving roles of primary care and other specialties in the new systems of health care are essential in making an informed career choice.

2. If family practice is to be the main gatekeeper specialty in health care, far more students need to choose family practice and more residency positions are needed.

3. The structure of family practice residency education needs to be thoroughly reconsidered. The talents emphasized by Merenstein, such as gatekeeping within the ethics of medicine, use of the office as a clinical laboratory, and practicing community orientated primary care, have little place in most residencies. Rather, most residencies are structured around hospital care, and the traditional internship and second year often blunt the ideals and enthusiasm toward family practice which residents have when they enter programs. Hopefully, the Merenstein report will stimulate greater experimentation in residency education.

From a practical view, residency education can change when the funding base of programs shifts from hospitals to health systems with a strong primary care component.

The optimism expressed by Merenstein et al. was most refreshing. As a young specialty, family practice has much less inertia and should be able to meet the challenges of the future. A group of leaders generated the energy to establish the specialty of family practice. Similar leadership is necessary to develop appropriate training programs for the future. Merenstein and his task force have provided a direction for change.

By 1985, I had served as the Chair of both the Communication and Education committees of STFM and had more board experience than anyone else serving at the time. At age 35 I was elected president. The following is my first president column based on my speech upon taking office in 1986.

Where is Family Medicine in Medical Education?

Family Medicine
1986;18: 193-194,236-237

Usual presidential protocol would have me give a presentation about the state of STFM as an organization, or to cover the hot topics of today, such as corporate medicine, malpractice, or the funding problems of our programs. I am too restless as an educator to do that. Rather I will take some risks and give you a rather personal commentary on medical education, and the role of family medicine. Much of what I will present is familiar to most of you, but is not being discussed much at the present time.

My role as an educator, and the reason I am in education, is a concern for the career development of medical students and residents. What they learn in medical school and residency is important, but my priority is what happens to them in the process. I believe that the process of medical education is at least as important as the content; so, my remarks will focus on this process which has become a tradition over the last 75 years.

Let us begin at the very beginning – the orientation to medical school. Currently about 40% of students who enter medical school in this county want to become primary care physicians in a community. Ten years ago this figure was sixty percent,[1] but the fact remains there is still a tremendous reserve of interest in and potential for family medicine.

We all know the first two years of medical school rather well. I can summarize preclinical medical education and some of the problems with a quote from John Gardner's *Easy Victories*: "Much education today is monumentally ineffective. All too often we are giving students cut flowers when we should be teaching them to growth their own plants. We are stuffing their heads with the products of innovation rather than teaching them to innovate. We think of the mind as a storehouse to be filled, rather than as an instrument to be used."[2]

For many students, enthusiasm changes into anger and frustration. Many medical schools gear the first two years for good results on Part I of the National Boards. The irony of this is that virtually all practicing physicians, and most clinician faculty in any medical school, including the deans, could not pass Part I of the National Boards tomorrow. Although most students get by this hurdle of basic science memorization rather well, there are some casualties. Many minority students, or students who come to medical school with diverse rather than heavy science backgrounds, get discouraged or even depressed during the pre-clinical years and may drop out.

The third year of medical school begins formal clinical education by exposing students to the most difficult and the sickest of patients, all in a tertiary care academic setting. The irony is that at the end of this year we expect students to know what they want to do in medicine. No wonder there is an enormous attrition of that early interest in primary care or family medicine. The 40% potential for family medicine among students goes down to an average of 12% to 13%. The tragedy of this goes beyond the mere loss of interest in family medicine. Large numbers of students during their third year feel they do not like patient care, even though they had ideas earlier about becoming personal physicians. The fact is that the process and environment they are exposed to at this time is one they find tedious, not enjoyable, and many students retreat into non-patient care specialties. This loss of the desire to become a personal physician in a community, the loss of ideals which brought the student into medical school is one of the big tragedies that occur in medical education.

The fourth year of medical school is often a time of recovery, an opportunity for liberal education. It is a time when students gather their spirits back, and commencement is a joyous occasion. I am struck by the contrast between the pleasure of graduation week, with its sense of relief, and the beginning of internship and residency.

Before discussing the traditional academic internship and residency, I would like to comment on community based residencies which absorb many of our students. As a predoctoral director, my role is to work closely with all students in my medical school who go into family medicine. I get very close to about 25 students every year. They keep in touch through their residencies, and let me know how they are doing and how they grow. This has given me insight into the spectrum of residencies and the contrast between community and university programs. Residents in the finer community hospital programs relate an excitement, enthusiasm, and enjoyment for their residency education which I do not find in most university programs. I will go so far to state that some of the finer community hospital residencies in family medicine represent the best graduate education occurring in America today, regardless of specialty. These programs are not going to get any awards at the annual meeting of the Association of American Medical Colleges, but it is time we in family medicine recognize the excellence that occurs in graduate education in many of our fine community programs.

Getting back to the traditional academic process, I am curious about the current literature and what is being said about internships. This first year of graduate medical education is time honored as a general education. The *Journal of General Internal Medicine*,[3] and the most recent issue of *Pharos*,[4] each had an article from medicine residents who after their internships wrote to say that the year was hell but worth it.

I do not buy that. I say this because of what I see happen destructively during internship. I had a personal experience with one of my classmates in medical school – a very sensitive, caring person – who committed suicide during her internship. I also had the experience of two other colleagues who, as a result of the very common depression which occurs in over 50% of house staff in many teaching centers, committed suicide during internship. These suicides are just the tip of the iceberg of the destructive nature of what occurs during internship. Even more destructive are the many house staff that burnout on patient care and retreat from the healing role of doctor into a survival mode.

This is something I have not fully understood, but I think I have a clue. Eric Cassell, an internist and teach interested in ethics and the process of medical education, wrote recently:

"For at least two generations, academic medicine, as practiced on the medical wards of many teaching hospitals, has been ahead of – setting the example for – good medical practice by even the best of practitioners outside the hospital....Medicine was said to be academic to indicate that is was good medicine. An important aspect of the current problem is that academic medicine has fallen behind the practice of good medical care. Between the shift of technology to outside the hospital and the sophisticated demands and requirements of modern patients, the world of good patient care has changed drastically during the past ten years, and academic departments of medicine have failed to keep up with the change."[5]

Cassell goes on to describe three internal conflicts in many house officers today which result in negative feelings and which often compromise the development of healers learning to provide good medical care. He says that when students enter medicine, the idea of "the doctor" is someone who takes care of sick patients. This idealized belief of what medical care is supposed to be, and what doctors are supposed to do, comes into conflict with the requirements of internship and residency and the technology intensive and technology exclusive medicine most often practiced on academic wards. Functioning and survival on academic wards now often requires putting aside one's feelings for the patient in order to perform the duties of house officer – which often means the inflicting of pain. Second, Cassell describes the creative pathophysiologic thinking that was common among house officers in the past, and which is now largely absent on our teaching wards because most patients have their pathophysiologic thinking done before they arrive in the hospital. Third, Cassell describes a sentiment in academic teaching wards which favors knowledge, such as the quoting of articles, and may actually denigrate the experience of attendings in the care of patients.

The remainder of residency varies a great deal among location and specialty. Family medicine may lead the way in allowing a recovery of spirit and rediscovery of the human aspects of patient care. But there is still a great imbalance even in our specialty. Our third-year family medicine residents, for example, know far more about the parental therapy of malignant hypertension that they know about the non-pharmacologic therapy of patients with high blood pressure.

The tragedy of residency training is that so many residents, after more than twenty years of education and preparation for a professional career; feel burned out rather than having an enthusiasm to apply what they have been trained to do. They would rather not be on call because they know what being on call is like during residency. Many want to retreat from patient care and look for a comfortable alternative for an indefinite period of time.

Where is family medicine in medical education? I agree with Gayle Stephens that family medicine has a reform function in traditional medical education.[6] A more recent quote from Don Ransom summarizes the current situation:

"If family medicine can sustain its commitment and its unconventional approach for a bit longer, it may well assume leadership for all of medicine, both intellectually and in meeting patient needs. This is not so because family practice seeks to correct a gross imbalance in the kinds of medical services available, or because family physicians are more humanistic than their technology-minded subspecialty counterparts. It is because family medicine will prove to be more effective at what people go to physicians for: help to get well, to feel well, or suffer as little as necessary."[7] What Ransom is referring to is that healing may again become a priority in medicine.

The elements of change are before us. Institutions in medical education will not change because change makes sense. As Paul Starr stated, "The dream of reason did not take power into account."[8] But power in medicine is shifting from those who deliver health services to those who pay for them. The same is true for medical education. There is much to suggest that medical education may fundamentally change before the end of this century. It is up to us in family medicine, through whatever leadership we have, to be a part of that change.

Earlier in this conference, James Potchen mentioned the revolution in medical education which occurred in the earlier part of this century, bringing science into medicine. I have enormous respect for medical science. Medical science saves lives and has changed the course of history. However, medical science indiscriminately applied is not good medicine. The next major reform in medical education may be bringing the humanities fully back into medicine. Without the humanities, doctors cannot be effective healers, for this requires the integration of art and science in medicine.

Family medicine is laying the seeds for this change. We are doing much of the work which some day will be in the forefront of medicine if we hold out a bit longer.

We must seize the current opportunities for change and assume a leadership role. For example, in predoctoral education the GPEP report has tacitly endorsed problem based learning and greater ambulatory and community based clerkships. As teachers of family medicine, we have experience and are gaining expertise in these areas, and we can use the GPEP recommendations to be leaders in our medical schools. On the residency level, the curricular structure is being reexamined to provide residents with appropriate training for future practice. In the early days of our specialty, there was an ethic of sending residents to medicine and surgery wards to show that our residents were just as good as they were. That mentality needs to change. We need to ask how do we train the best family physicians? How can we train family physicians who are sophisticated in what family physicians do? Certainly there needs to be inpatient training, but the balance needs to shift in order to make room for training in family systems, community oriented primary care, health promotion and disease prevention, geriatrics, and cost-effectiveness. These are areas to which many of you are devoting your careers as teachers, yet our senior residents know little about them.

One of the strengths of STFM in effecting change in medical education is our multidisciplinary membership. The movement of bringing the humanities more into medicine is not arising primarily from physicians, but from scholars in other disciplines who have dedicated themselves to medical education and to medicine as a healing profession. STFM can be on the cutting edge of change because we are rich with such teachers and scholars.

Leadership has been a common theme at this conference, and my presentation is essentially a call for leadership in medical education because there are symptoms of a lack of leadership in family medicine. For example, our nominations committee struggles every year to come up with a slate to run for office, and there are numerous open department chairman positions. Is there less leadership in family medicine now than 15-20 years ago, and if so why? John Gardner raised a concern about leadership which I think applies to the current situation. He states:

"We are immunizing a high proportion of our most gifted young people against any tendencies to leadership. The process is initiated by society itself. The conditions of life in a modern complex society are not conducive to the emergence of leaders. . . . .

"Most of our intellectually gifted young people go from college directly into graduate school, or into one of the older or more prestigious professional schools. They are introduced to – or; more correctly, powerfully indoctrinated in – a set of attitudes appropriate to scholars, scientists, and professional men. This is all to the good. The students learn to identify themselves strongly with their calling and its ideals. They acquire a conception of what a good scholar; scientist or professional man is like.

"As things stand now, however, that conception leaves little room for leadership in the normal sense; the only kind of leadership encouraged is that which follows from the performing of purely professional tasks in a superior manner. Entry into what most of us would regard as leadership roles in society at large is discouraged.

"In the early stages of a career there is good reason for this: becoming a first-class scholar, scientist, or professional requires single-minded dedication. Unfortunately, by the time the individual is sufficiently far along in his career to afford a broadening of interest, he often finds himself irrevocably set in a narrow mold."[5]

Gardener is referring to leadership in society, but medical education can be considered in this broad context. Our fellowship programs have been considered as training grounds for future leaders. I raise a word of caution that our fellowships may be furthering the narrowness of our future teachers rather than developing leaders for medical education.

In closing I would like to give a prescription for leadership. As a practicing doctor I like to give prescriptions, and as I do with many of my patients, I will prescribe reading. Don Ransom's Random Notes series in *Family System Medicine*, is a powerful call for leadership in family medicine. The proceedings of the Keystone conference published in *Family Medicine* should be read not only for historical interest, but as a background to the leadership required to create the specialty, and the leadership necessary to bring family medicine farther along.[9] The GPEP report, in its complete form, gives a mandate with guidelines for change in predoctoral education.[10] A family medicine perspective on the GPEP report will be forthcoming in *Family Medicine*. The recent report, "Training Residents for the Future" in *Family Medicine* is pointing us toward new competencies for resident education.[11]

We must all work together as leaders for the education of medical students and residents. We must be leaders in our own institutions. Change will not trickle down from some national level. I learned this year that the Association of American Medical Colleges, in trying to implement the GPEP Report, is somewhat powerless in bringing about change in medical education; most of the power exists in local academic centers. We need to be leaders in that setting. In my medical school I was just given the role of chairing the curriculum committee. I was given the task partly because I am one of a handful of faculty among hundreds in the medical school who really cares about the whole curriculum enough to be a leader. I urge all of you to seek out such roles. If we work together as leaders, we will bring family medicine to a higher level, and medical education to a new era.

References

1. California Medical Association. Attitudes of medical students and recent graduates. Triennial survey, 1984. San Francisco: California Medical Association. 1985.
2. Gardner JW. No Easy Victories. New York: Harper and Row, Inc., 1968; 68. 127-9.
3. Schiedermayer DL. Internship – a personal cost-benefit analysis. *Gen Intern Med* 1986; 1:37.
4. Flynn TC. What makes internship so bad – and so good. *Pharos* 1986; Spring: 7.
5. Cassell EJ. Practice versus theory in academic medicine: the conflict between house officers and attending physicians. Bull

NY *Acad Med* 1984; 60:297.

6. Stephens GG. The intellectual basis of family practice. Tucson: Winter Publishing Co., Inc., 1982.

7. Ransom DC. Random notes: the unconventional future of family medicine. *Fam Syst Med* 1985; 3:120.

8. Starr P. The social transformation of American medicine. New York: Basis Books, Inc., 1982.

9. Proceedings from the Keystone Conference. *Fam Med* 198; 17:185-230.

10. Association of American Medical Colleges. Physicians for the twenty-first century: *J Med Educ* 1984; 59:1-208.

11. STFM Task Force on Training Residents for the Future. Training residents for the future: final draft report. *Fam Med* 1986; 18:29-37.

As past-president of STFM in 1987, the role of the family physician in maternity care was being seriously questioned. Technology was taking hold and impacting the process of natural labor resulting in rapidly escalating rates of Cesarean section. Ironically a group of men, such as Walt Larimore, Dale Moquist, Bruce Bagley, Bill Rodney, and myself, rose up to start the Family Centered Maternity Care initiatives in STFM and AAFP. Fortunately we were quickly followed by many women leaders. The following are two articles I published during this effort.

Family Physicians Strive to Continue Obstetrics

Joseph Scherger, MD, and Jeffrey Tanji, MD

California Family Physician
1987;38(July/August):12-13

Over half of the family physicians who were delivering babies in California during 1985 stopped doing so during 1986. The precipitating cause for this drop was the dramatic rise in the cost of professional liability insurance. Now that The Doctors' Company (the major insurer of California family physicians who do OB) is eliminating the low risk obstetrical category for family physicians, even more FPs will drop OB this year, rather than absorb a 35% increase in their premiums. The family physician who delivers babies has become an endangered species. For this reason, and to demonstrate that family physicians can be low risk providers of obstetrical care, the Family Practice Professional Liability Project was started.

The major goal of the project is to study whether medical malpractice risk can be managed through careful underwriting and an intensive risk management program. We have attempted to mobilize a study group of FPs who deliver babies and who would be willing to participate in the risk management program. From an original group of 529 physicians who were performing deliveries in 1985, 90 have applied to participate in the project (we estimate that this is about 40% of California FPs in private practice who are currently doing OB).

The most difficult part of this effort has been negotiating an affordable premium for family physicians participating in this project. As of this writing, The Doctors' Company has decided not to participate. NORCAL Mutual is studying the project and will consider a discount for participating family physicians. An insurance broker has been contacted to explore other options. In order to succeed with the study, there must be a means of controlling the rising costs of insurance to keep it affordable for family physicians.

Methods

A prospective study sample will be evaluated using underwriting criteria developed both by the research project group (UC-Davis) and participating insurance companies. At this time, the underwriting criteria proposed by the research group are: board certification in family practice; a willingness to present perinatal medical records, educational materials, and protocols to the study group for review; and a past claims experience which suggests low risk (e.g., a history of one or less claims for three years of practice).

Further underwriting criteria will be defined after consultation with the department of the sponsoring insurance company. All participating physicians must be found acceptable to both the study group and the sponsoring insurance company.

Once accepted into the intervention study group, the following risk management program will be presented (all participants must attend or participate in all aspects of the program):

- **Part A:** A prospective review of perinatal office and hospital records used in the care of obstetrical patients. Educational materials will also be presented and reviewed, including appropriate current genetic counseling and screening.

The project team will have standard recommended materials for medical records, perinatal risk assessment, genetic screening and counseling, and patient education. If the physicians' procedures do not meet these standards, the physicians must agree to modify their care accordingly. All participating family physicians will agree to abide to these criteria or be excluded from the project.

- **Part B:** Attendance at an annual risk management education conference sponsored by the research project, the sponsoring insurance company, and the CAFP.

Currently, a day-and-a-half program is being planned in conjunction with the CAFP's annual meeting in November 1988. This initial program would include: general risk management, focusing on failure to diagnose common cancers, proper interpretation of common laboratory tests, and techniques in medical record and data management in the office; fetal monitor interpretation; and other aspects of obstetrical risk management. All participating physicians will be required to attend. If a group of family physicians is participating in the project, and it is not feasible for all of the physicians to attend the conference, adequate representation from the group must be present with commitment to inform the entire group on the information given.

- **Part C:** Ongoing monitoring and evaluation of the participating physicians' practice.

A quality assurance committee of the project will review quarterly reports from each of the practicing physicians regarding outcomes in obstetrical practice, including number of new diagnoses of pregnancy, appropriate perinatal risk assessment, appropriate consultation and referral, and appropriate prenatal and labor and delivery management. All participating physicians must be willing to subject all aspects of obstetrical care to peer review by this committee. Ongoing intervention will be made as necessary to the physician's practice. Failure to comply with these interventions at any time may disqualify the physician from participating in the project.

Analysis

The professional liability claims and losses will be measured for the study sample over five years. These will be compared to a comparable group of physicians not receiving the interventions. A comparison will also be made with the study sample physicians during the years prior to the intervention. Appropriate tests of significance will be used to analyze the data.

The concept of affordability of professional liability insurance will also be analyzed during the study. Correlations will be made between the amount and type of obstetrical exposure and frequency of claims. It is anticipated that some physicians will drop out of the study and discontinue obstetrics because of a perceived unaffordability of the premium.

The AAFP has taken an interest in this project, and has referred it to their committee on professional liability for consideration as a national project, or for use in other states.

Other States

There have been changes in two states this year, which give some hope for relief in the cost in insuring obstetrical care. In Virginia, the legislature has approved a no-fault compensation fund for neurologically damaged infants. The fund is actually an insurance pool paid for by participating physicians and hospitals, and will replace the tort system in providing for these cases. Compensation for damaged infants and their families will be adequate and not exorbitant and it is hoped that, as a result, the cost of insurance will go down. In Maryland, the major professional liability carrier has announced an insurance plan with a set premium per delivery regardless of exposure rather than a yearly premium. This will help family physicians who have a relatively low number of deliveries compared to obstetricians.

Controlling professional liability for obstetrical care is an enormously complex and difficult task. If family physicians are to remain active in this area, we will need to educate the public, support tort reform, control our own risk through a high standard of care, and negotiate fair treatment by the insurance industry. This project is just one attempt to control the problem. Any physician interested in participating or wanting more information should contact us at the Department of Family Practice, 2221 Stockton Blvd., Sacramento, CA 95816.

Family-Centered Childbirth
A Philosophy Well Suited to Family Practice

Family Practice Recertification
1989;11(1): 23-26

The concept of family-centered childbirth, or family-centered maternity care, is well suited to family practice, because it focuses on how the birth of a child affects the entire family. A woman who gives birth forms new relationships with those close to her, and all family members take on new responsibilities to each other, the baby, and the community. (Children become brothers and sisters, mothers become grandmothers, and so forth.) Family-centered childbirth recognizes the importance of these new relationships and responsibilities, and has as its goal the best possible health outcome for all family members. Family-centered childbirth is an attitude rather than a specific program. It recognizes that birth is a vital life event rather than a medical procedure, and acknowledges the importance of childbirth to the woman and to those close to her. It respects the woman's individuality and need for autonomy, and accepts that she may not base her decisions solely on the advice of physicians or other medical professionals. It requires that a woman be guided, but not directed – that she be provided with all relevant information, but allowed to make her own decisions in accordance with her own goals. (This definition was developed at McMaster University in Canada, and has since been endorsed by The American Academy of Family Physicians and the American College of Obstetricians and Gynecologists.) The philosophy is applicable regardless of what medical professionals, birth place, and type of care a woman chooses.[1]

This approach to maternity care also emphasizes natural childbirth and avoiding routine use of unnecessary technology. Worldwide, scientific evidence supports the benefits of a natural approach to childbirth for most women.[2-6] The findings suggest that allowing women in labor to move about freely and to sit up in bed enhances the likelihood of spontaneous labor. For some patients whose labor is arrested, ambulation has been shown to be as effective as oxytocin.[7-11]

Other findings suggest that the use of continuous fetal monitoring should be avoided when risk is low.[12] Continuous monitoring has never been shown to improve perinatal outcome when compared with standard intermittent listening for fetal heart tones. On the contrary, false-positive findings have tripled diagnoses of fetal distress, and doubled rates of cesarean section.[13] In addition, continuous monitoring interferes with spontaneous positioning of the mother during labor.[8,12,13]

During the second stage of labor, the woman should be allowed to breathe and push down spontaneously, without being made to hold her breath or perform prolonged Valsalva maneuvers. Spontaneous pushing and breathing are more effective, and can avoid the increased risk of fetal oxygen deprivation associated with Valsalva maneuvers.[5,6] The pushing is often more effective when the patient is in an upright position, such as a squat, which improves intrauterine pressure and pelvic outlet diameter.[5,6,8,14-17] Other findings suggest that episiotomy is often unnecessary, and may result in more third-and fourth-degree lacerations.[18,19] When an incision is made in the perineum before the stress of birth, the chance of extensive tearing is much greater. No scientific evidence supports any benefit of episiotomy for the mother.[18,19]

Proponents of natural childbirth believe that keeping the family together both during and after labor enhances the experience for all family members. Each member (including siblings, depending on their ages) can participate in the birth by remaining in the room, or by staying at the hospital throughout. During this period, families can form a lasting bond that may be beneficial later on. Often mothers and infants can be discharged soon after delivery and followed up at home.[20-23]

Family practice bridges the gap between science and tradition. Working either alone or with a team of obstetricians and midwives, family physicians can bring to the delivery room excellent training in both the scientific and the humanistic aspects of maternity care. They have been shown to provide obstetrical care as safely as obstetricians;[24-25] and the maternity units of small rural hospitals have been shown to be as safe as those of larger hospitals.[26] Family physicians have been trained to be flexible in their approach to obstetrics, and to avoid the strategy of maximum use of technology that is promoted at high-risk obstetrical centers.[27]

Routine obstetrical care need not be offered solely by subspecialists; family physicians should also be well trained to deliver babies. Family-centered childbirth can also be advantageous for family physicians, because it will help to keep young and more complete families in their practices.[28] Family physicians should seek to define a role for themselves in the field of obstetrics, and should take the lead in investigating new, optimal methods of care.

References

1. International Childbirth Education Association adopts definition of family-centered maternity care. *Int J Childbirth Educ* 2(1):4, 1987.
2. Klein M, Reynolds JL, Boucher F, et al: Obstetrical practice and training in Canadian family medicine: conserving an endangered species. *Can Fam Physician* 30:2093, 1984.
3. Klein M: the Canadian family practice accoucheur. *Can Fam Physician* 32:533, 1986.
4. Odent M: *Birth Reborn.* New York, Pantheon Books, 1984.
5. Caleyro-Barcia R: The influence of maternal bearing-down efforts during second stage on fetal well-being. *Birth Fam J* 6:7, 1979.
6. Caldeyro-Barcia R, Giussi G, Storch E, et al: The bearing-down effects on fetal heart rate, oxygenation, and acid-base

balance. *J Perinatal Med* 9(1):63, 1981.

7. Fenwick L: birthing: techniques for management of physiologic and psychosocial aspects of childbirth. *Perinatal-Neonatal* 8(3):51-62, 1984.

8. McKay S, Mahan CS: Maternal position and movement during labor and birth. *Contemp Obstet Gynecol* 24:90-119, 1984.

9. Read JA, Miller FC, Paul RH: Randomized trial of ambulation versus oxtocin for labor enhancement: a preliminary report. *Am J Obstet Gynecol* 139:669, 1981.

10. Roberts J, Mendez-Bauer C: A perspective of maternal position during labor. *J Perinatal Med* 8:255, 1980.

11. Roberts J, Mendez-Bauer C, Wodell D: The effects of maternal position on uterine contractility and efficiency. *Birth* 10:243, 1983.

12. Simkin P: Is anyone listening? The lack of clinical impact of randomized controlled trials of electronic fetal monitoring. *Birth* 13:219-220, 1986.

13. Leveno KJ, Cunningham G, Nelson S, et al: A prospective comparison of selective and universal electronic fetal monitoring in 34,995 pregnancies. *N Engl J Med* 315:615-619, 1986.

14. Drahne A, Prang E, Werner C: The various positions for delivery. *J Perinatal Med* 10(suppl 2):72, 1982.

15. Russell J: the rationale of primitive delivery positions. *Br J Obstet Gynecol* 89:712, 1982.

16. McKay S, Roberts J: Second stage labor: what is normal? *J Obstet Gynecol Neonatal Nurs* 14(2):101-106, 1985.

17. Mahan CS, McKay S: Are we overmanaging second-stage labor? *Contemp Obstet Gynecol* 24:37, 1984.

18. Banta HD, Thacker SB: Benefits and risks of episiotomy, an interpretive review of the English-language literature, 1860-1980. *Obstet Gynecol Surv* 38:322, 1983.

19. Silverman S: Episiotomy – to cut or not to cut? If there really a question? *Cybele Rep* 6(1):2-4, 1985.

20. Klaus M, Jerauld P, Kreger N, et al: Maternal attachment. Importance of the first postpartum days. *N Engl J Med* 286:460-463, 1972.

21. De Chateau P, Winbert B: Long-term effect on mother/infant behavior of extra contact during the first hour postpartum. I.

First observations at 36 hours. *Acta Pediatr Scand* 66:137-143, 1977.

22. Siegel E, Bauman K, Schaefer E, et al: Hospital and home support during infancy: impact on maternal attachment, child abuse and neglect, and health care utilization. *Pediatrics* 66:183-190, 1980.

23. Larson C: Efficacy of prenatal and postpartum home visits on child health and development. *Pediatrics* 66:191-197, 1980.

24. Mengel MB, Phillips WE: The quality of obstetric care in family practice. Are family physicians as safe as obstetricians? *J Fam Pract* 24:159-164, 1987.

25. Franks P, Eisinger S: Adverse perinatal outcomes: Is physician specialty a risk factor? *J Fam Pract* 24:152-156, 1987.

26. Rosenblatt RA, Reinken J, Shoemack P: Is obstetrics safe in small hospitals? Evidence from New Zealand's regionalized perinatal system. *Lancet* 2:429, 1985.

27. Brody H, Thompson JR: The Maximin strategy in modern obstetrics. *J Fam Pract* 12:977-985, 1981.

28. Mehl LE, Bruce C, Renner JH: Importance of obstetrics in a comprehensive family practice. *J Fam Pract* 3:385-389, 1976.

In 1989, medical student interest in family medicine was in decline and three powerful leaders in family medicine, John Geyman, Jack Colwill, and Gerry Percoff, called for a merger into a single primary care specialty. Holding on to the belief that each specialty had its distinct culture, and diversity was better than consolidation in primary care, I wrote an opposing view of this effort:

Should There be a Merger to a Single Primary Care Specialty for the 21st Century? An Opposing View

The Journal of Family Practice
1989;29:185-190

This is a difficult time for primary care physicians. Medical student interest in the primary care specialties of family practice, general internal medicine, and pediatrics has declined. Reimbursement inequities have made the procedure-oriented specialties quite lucrative, whereas primary care is at the bottom of the earnings ladder.[1] While there is a growing surplus of non-primary care specialists, there is a shortage of primary care physicians in many areas. New managed care systems hold promise of a greater need for primary care physicians as gatekeepers or case managers, but often with increased financial risk and greater patient responsibility and without improved stature or economic reward.

These problems have led Geyman,[2] Colwill,[3] and now Peroff[4] to propose a merger of family practice, general internal medicine, and pediatrics into a single primary care specialty. They use a strength-by-consolidation argument. They cite the growing similarities of training and practice among the primary care specialties and suggest that the American people would be better served by having a single type of generalist physician.

While this merger and unification idea for primary care has some conceptual appeal, its reality now or in the future in American medicine is unlikely and undesirable. Do Americans really want a single choice of primary care physician? In our pluralistic society, I think now. While many Americans embrace the concept and practice of family medicine, others clearly want to be cared by an internist or an obstetrician-gynecologist and have their children cared for by a pediatrician. Many choose these specialists, not for their similarity to family physicians, but because of the distinct differences in focused expertise. Limiting the choice to some generic amalgamation of these specialists may not increase the power of primary care, as Geyman suggests; instead, it would likely have the opposite effect of restricting the potential power of primary care in the medical marketplace. The formation of a single primary care specialty would probably enhance the "hidden system" in primary care performed by other physician specialists and be a boon to other primary care health providers such as chiropractors and naturopaths. Americans like having choices are likely to exercise that freedom whenever possible.

Does a merger of family practice, pediatrics and internal medicine make sense from the perspective of these specialties? Most pediatricians have chosen that specialty because they want to focus their career on the care of children. Asking them to become primary care physicians for all ages is likely to result in widespread dissatisfaction. Are family practice and internal medicine enough alike to suggest a merger? Numerous studies have documented that family physicians and internists have markedly different practice styles with the same patient paroblems.[5-9]

Phillips[9,10] suggests that family practice and internal medicine have derived from very different medical traditions dating back to 18th century Europe (apothecaries vs physicians) and possibly even ancient Greece (Coan vs the Cnidian views of medicine). I suggest that in modern medical culture the internal medicine physician with a compulsive thirst for differential diagnosis remains quite different from the family physician with a focus toward pragmatic therapeutics. Attempting to merge these two specialties might make for interesting dialogue but is likely to cause considerable tension in practice styles.

Even if the American people would be better served by having a single primary care physician, and even if conceptionally an amalgamation of these specialties made sense, is such a merger organizationally or politically possible? In responding to the single primary care specialty ideas of Geyman and Colwill, Friedman,[11] an academic internist, states that merging internal medicine and family practice is impractical and unnecessary. Departments of internal medicine in academic institutions would never give up the general internal medicine component to an independent department. Departments of family practice, having struggled successfully for almost 20 years to gain an academic identity, would have to dissolve or transfer to some new primary care identity. In organized medicine, the single primary care physician concept has been virtually condemned by the American Academy of Family Physicians.[12]

A merger of the primary care specialties is unnecessary because most of the goals indicated by Geyman and Colwill can be achieved through greater interspecialty cooperation. Geyman suggests that competition is the alternative to a generic approach to primary care. While some interspecialty competition is inevitable and even desirable, a cooperation model is highly plausible for primary care.

Internal medicine and pediatrics do not generally compete, as the care is defined according to age. Family practice can compete with both and has, but more can be achieved by all three primary care specialties through cooperation. Friedman[11] describes five areas in which family practice and internal medicine are ready to cooperative: enhancing primary care training, developing primary care research, promoting academic viability of faculty, funding primary care programs and departments, and lobbying in the political arena. There are more than enough patient care needs to keep all primary care physicians busy. Working together, primary care physicians can promote reimbursement reform and improved professional status, which will make these fields more desirable to medical students. The American Academy of Family Physicians[12] has endorsed the idea of cooperation with other primary care fields. The concept of specialty merger or a generic physician seems counterproductive to improved relations among these specialties.

In summary, a merger of family practice, internal medicine, and pediatrics into a single primary care specialty is not appropriate, necessary, or practical. The American people like having choices, and having a single type of primary care physician is not likely to broaden public acceptance of primary care. The specialties of family practice and internal medicine have such different traditions, resulting in different practice styles, that a merger is probably impossible. Politically and organizationally a merger of these specialties would require compromises far too great to ever happen. Cooperation among the specialties is highly plausible and can achieve improved professional status and public acceptance for primary care. Let us stop this talk of merger and a common primary care specialty before such talk gets in the way of family physicians, general internists, and pediatricians working together to serve the American people; instead, let us promote academic achievement in primary care.

References

1. Owens A: How much did your earnings grow last year? Med Econ 1988; 65:159-180

2. Geyman JP: Training primary care physicians for the 21st 3century: Alternative scenarios for the competitive vs generic approaches. JAMA 1986; 2631-2635

3. Colwill JM: Education of the primary physician: A time for reconsideration? JAMA 1986; 255:2643-2644

4. Perkoff GT: Should there be a merger to a single primary care specialty for the 21st century? An affirmative review. J Fam Pract 1989; 29:185-188

5. Scherger JE, Gordon MJ, Phillips TJ, LoGerfo JP: Comparison of diagnostic methods of family practice and internal medicine residents. J Fam Pract 1980; 10:95-101

6. Merenstein JH: A comparison of residency trained family physicians and internists. Fam Med 1984; 16:165-170

7. Bertakis KD, Robbins JA: Gatekeeping in primary care: A comparison of internal medicine and family practice. J Fam Pract 1987; 24:305-309

8. Cherkin DC, Rosenblatt RA, Hart LG, et al: The use of medical resources by residency-trained family physicians and general internists: Is there a difference? Med Care 1987; 25:455-469

9. Phillips TJ: The intellectual roots of family practice. Pharos 1981; 44:26-311

10. Phillips TJ: Disciplines, specialties, and paradigms. J Fam Pract 1988; 27:139-141

11. Friedman RH: Family practice and general internal medicine: What kind of cooperation makes sense? JAMA 1986; 255:2644-2646

12. Spalding J: FP-IM merger is debated at FP educators' workshop. AAFP Rep 1988; 15(8):1-2

My uncle was a general practitioner and said while I was in medical student that low income patients would be the most appreciative of your help. In Dixon we cared for the entire community with one standard of care and I wrote the following essay as an expression of this service.

My Favorite Patients Are on Medicaid

The Western Journal of Medicine
1990;152(1):92

Two of my favorite patients died this past week. Sharon was truly inspiring. Crippled when an infant with spinal muscular atrophy, she lived 44 years with profound muscle weakness. Ten years ago she asked me to become her physician. With Harrington rods in her back and chronically infected staghorn calculi in her kidneys, she was a complex patient with many management problems. These were more than offset by her cheerful manner and the sight of the flowers she placed on the post of her electric wheelchair.

Seven years ago she announced her marriage to Michael, a young man with Marfan syndrome who also became my regular patient. Six years ago she caused me great alarm by becoming pregnant. Near term, Sharon developed respiration failure and required an emergency cesarean section that produced a normal little girl called Sara.

Subsequently, Sharon developed breast cancer in both breasts a year apart. Her chronic urinary infections and occasional sepsis led to an attempted lithotripsy for multiple renal stones. All of this kept Sharon and me close over the last five years. She died peacefully with congestive heart failure and metastatic cancer, and now I look forward to the future with Michael and Sara.

Evelyn, at the age of 80, moved from the city to live with her daughter in our small town. Weighing more than 200 pounds, and with blood sugar levels over 250 despite lots of insulin, she became my first patient every third Tuesday morning. During our first seven years together, she required only one hospital stay despite developing congestive heart failure and recurring arrhythmias. A year ago Evelyn had a major stroke that confined her to bed for the rest of her life. What her daughter Lola and I expected to be a few more months of life turned out to be a year of regular home visits. She lost over 100 pounds but never her smile when I came to visit. With counseling, Lola was able to give her a peaceful death at home.

As I reflect on the care and passing of these two special patients, it occurs to me that they were both on Medicaid. If our office policy had been not to accept Medicaid patients – as it   is for most physicians in the county – I would have been deprived of caring for Sharon and Evelyn.

I practice with four other family physicians in a rural town of 10,000 people. We have an open door policy to care for all segments of our community, and about 15% to 20% of our patients are on Medicaid.   Most of them, and most of our other patients, are considerate and sensitive human beings in need of health care. Yes, Medicaid reimbursement barely covers office overhead, and yes, we would each earn about $10,000 a year more if all our patients were fully insured, but we make a good living.   What my general practitioner uncle taught me is true: with low income patients, I will do the most good and derive the most satisfaction.

Unfortunately, even our openness to Medicaid patients has limits. Two neighboring communities of 35,000 each have lots of physicians, yet almost none of the primary care physicians in these two towns will accept new Medicaid patients.   As requests for care from Medicaid patients in these communities increased, we knew that we would soon have a much higher percentage of these patients and that the economics of our practice would suffer.   In order not to be overwhelmed, we chose not to accept out-of-town Medicaid patients.

Our ambivalence with Medicaid increased last year when we opened a satellite clinic in one of these larger towns. If we were the only primary care practice accepting Medicaid, a disproportionately high number of Medicaid patients would seek our care, and the practice would suffer financially. Accepting a certain percentage of Medicaid patients would have us still rejecting many.   We compromised by accepting new obstetrical patients on Medicaid and their families.

Our county is generally prosperous, and only 15% of the population is on Medicaid.   If everyone accepted these patients proportionate to the population, no one would be overwhelmed, and all our practices would still be successful.   This idea has been discussed and even tried halfheartedly over the years, but each new frustration from the Medicaid payment system seems to squash whatever altruism exists. Yesterday, a community activist called to propose that through the country medical society, we all try it again. Petition will be passed around asking all practices to accept up to 15% Medicaid patient. I think about how much richer our practices will be if we do.

David Swee was (and still is) a pillar of advocacy in family medicine education. As Chair of the STFM Education Committee David lead the development of a monogram on Teaching Family Medicine in Medical Schools (STFM, 1991). I contributed the chapter on career advising, a culmination of 12 years of service as the predoctoral advisor at the UC Davis.

Teaching Family Medicine in Medical School

Chapter 2, Career Advising

Published by:
The Society of Teachers of Family Medicine and
The American Academy of Family Physicians,
Kansas City, Missouri
Copyright 1991

Introduction

How medical students choose and how well they choose their future careers are of increasing debate and concern among medical educators. Some observers of this process estimate that as many as half of all medical students fail to make the best career choices by graduation (Pathway Evaluation Program, 1990).

Until the 1980s, as many as 30% - 40% of medical students expressed an early interest in family practice. This interest in family practice or any primary care field dropped significantly during the 1980s, causing many residency programs to go unfilled through the

Match. This decline in interest in family practice occurred at a time when the need for family physicians was increasingly recognized throughout the country, when there was an oversupply of physicians from the specialties which have had increasing student interest.

Medical student career advising is critically important both to helping students make their best career decisions and to promoting careers in family practice. Just as basic medical education and career development are the important dual processes of any medical school, a predoctoral program in a family medicine department should structure a career advising program as a dual component within the curriculum.

Family practice as a specialty choice has several distinctive characteristics which contrast with other specialty choices. First, the great majority of students who choose family practice come to medical school with this interest, and only a small number discover this interest during medical school (Babbott et al, 1988). Second, family practice is the only specialty in which there is a great loss of attrition of interest during medical school (Babbott et al, 1988; Markert, 1983). This loss of interest in family practice may be greater than 50% in some schools. Third and related to the first two, students will often receive considerable negative advice about a career in family practice by faculty in other specialties. These characteristics reinforce the recommendation that career advising should be an integral part of a family medicine predoctoral program.

Many descriptive reports and studies have looked at the important characteristics of schools with success in producing family physicians. These characteristics are: being a state-funded medical school, having a full department of family medicine, having a longitudinal program of family medicine courses and activities, and having a required clerkship in the third year (Harris et al, 1982; Rabinowitz, 1988). There seem to be key impact points at which student interest in family practice may be particularly vulnerable or can be reinforced. This chapter described the principles of career advising and a strategy for career advising programs which emphasizes continuity through all four years of medical school and highlights the timing of student activities. Table 1 illustrates the strategy for career advising with timing for key impact activities. This updates the work initially described in Scherger and Swisher (1986).

Table 1

A Career Advising Strategy
For Medical Students:
A Continuum With Key Impact Points

Year 1	Identify Student Interest	• Survey the potential interest in family practice among entering students
Year 2	Maintain Student Interest	• Identify student leadership for family practice interest groups, plan activities • Early preceptorships giving exposure to family practice role models
Year 3	Promote the Student's Best Career Decision	• Advising for specialty decision • Family practice clerkship
Year 4	Guide the Residency Selection Process	• Match Day – Assist unmatched students • Letters to assist students with applications

Principles of Career Advising

A career adviser has an ethical obligation to act only in the best interest of the student. Giving career advice requires more listening than speaking to get to know the student as well as possible. The adviser should be an active listener – open-minded, sensitive, and adaptable, and resistant to premature closure. The ultimate goal of any career adviser is to have students make the best possible career decisions. A student's career choice is the result of several composite factors; the student's origin, including family and hometown size; personality type; experiences prior to and during medical school; and personal considerations, including the influence of the student's spouse and family. Some of these operate automatically within the student and some may be influenced by a career adviser.

Student self-awareness regarding specialty choice can be enhanced through counseling. Most students can describe the physician characteristics that interest them most. These can be related to well-known characteristics of a particular specialty, although care should be taken to avoid stereotyping. The physician characteristics most associated with students choosing family practice include a desire to be a personal and primary care physician in a community, with an orientation to helping people with health problems which takes precedence over having an expertise in a certain area and a desire for variety in medical practice (Hafferty et al, 1988; Taylor, 1986).

Questionnaires have been developed to aid students in identifying their aptitude for various specialties (*New Physician*, 1984). The Myers-Briggs Type Indicator can also be used for this purpose (Harris et al, 1984).

Career advising by family medicine department faculty members will be interwoven with but not limited to educational experiences. For example, the department may offer an Introduction to Clinical Medicine course in the first year and have faculty and volunteer preceptors giving career advice. In the second year, the department may have no curriculum time but may continue its career advising activities through a family practice interest group. Since career advising is a team process using department faculty, staff and volunteers, continuing education within the department regarding the changes in medical practice affecting family practice is important.

A Strategy for Career Advising

An appropriate goal description for a predoctoral program would be to enable all students who should become family physicians to do so. How might this be accomplished? Which students and how many should become family physicians? How does the program retain those students who would be most satisfied as family physicians?

The answers to these questions will vary with each medical school, but there are generic strategies by which a program may *enable* students to select family practice.

Identify Student Interest

The first step of this strategy is to recognize those students with the potential for family practice careers in each class of medical students. This requires a method of identifying student interest in family practice. Most students who select family practice have this interest when they enter medical school (Babbott et al, 1988; Markert, 1983). A career advising program should begin with identification of the initial interest in family practice within a class of entering students. For example, if 60% of the students in an entering class are interested in primary care and 40% are specifically interested in family practice, there is great potential for nurturing family practice careers.

Identifying initial student interest in family practice allows the predoctoral faculty and staff to begin a process of communicating with and tracking these students during the ensuring four years. Ongoing communication with and tracking these students is critical in preventing attrition from family practice since students often receive negative input about family practice from academic faculty throughout medical school. Monitoring student interest allows predoctoral faculty and staff to identify the critical periods during which student interest is most vulnerable.

There are several techniques for identifying interest in family practice among entering medical students. At the beginning of the first year, a questionnaire which asks about career preference can be given. Some of the questions should be general enough to allow the student to indicate a preference for primary care rather than a specific specialty. There are efforts underway to collect this information on a national basis.

Family practice interest groups or pathway programs are used at many schools to identify career interest among entering students. During an orientation meeting, a brochure and presentation can be given to the entire class, describing the specialty of family practice and encouraging all students who are interested in becoming primary care physicians to join. For example, each year about 40% of the class at the University of California, Davis join the pathway program and most select family practice (Scherger et al, 1984).

At the University of Utah all entering students are given a Myers-Briggs Type Indicator. A seminar is held to discuss the relationship between personality types and career choices (Harris et al, 1984). Harris found that students currently choosing family practice differ from the personality type typical of the general practitioner (Harris et al, 1985).

A career workbook is given to all entering students at the University of Washington. This workbook guides students in identifying their initial career interests and in reevaluating their interests throughout medical school (Kirby, 1984).

Although the key impact point at which student interest in family practice is identified occurs early in the first year, this process should be ongoing throughout the four years, even up until the Match deadlines. Some students will develop a later interest in family practice, and the predoctoral program should be open to welcoming these students. Fliers about family practice activities should be sent to all students, and sign-up sheets can help identify both new and lost interest.

Maintain Student Interest

Maintaining student interest in family practice is a process requiring constant vigilance. The effort in the process is great and continuous because the environment in many academic centers is often derogatory toward family practice. A generalist specialty is the antithesis of many medical school faculty members whose careers are devoted to an expertise in a narrow field. Often medical school faculty have spent all of their professional careers in academia, and many simply do not believe that family practice is a viable specialty. These faculty believe it is impossible to be a competent generalist and do not hesitate to give this message to students at every opportunity.

Family practice faculty and residents must make an extra effort to present a positive image of family practice. Little value is gained by countering negative statements about family practice with negative statements about other specialties.

Student interest in family practice may be lost at any time during medical school. Activities to maintain student interest in family practice should begin in the first year and continue through the final year of medical school.

Several studies have been done to evaluate the effect of courses and pathway programs on career choice. These studies have shown that, with the exception of a required third-year clerkship, a single course has not affected career choice (Rabinowitz, 1988; Harris et al, 1977; Hale et al, 1779). Rather, longitudinal programs have resulted in greater numbers of students retaining interest in and choosing family practice as a career (Harris et al, 1982; Scherger et al, 1986). These longitudinal programs have
three common components which seem to be important in maintaining student interest in family practice.

1. Providing students with early clinical exposure.

Students entering medical school are eager to develop their clinical skills, and this enthusiasm is often dampened during basic science training. Family physicians can have a major influence on students if they are among the first teachers of basic clinical skills. Departments of family practice in Mississippi, Washington, California, Davis, and many other schools provide the instruction to first- or second-year students in introductory clinical skills. The primary care curriculum at New Mexico provides first-year students four months of community based clinical training.

2. Maintaining the student's perspective on medicine in the community.

Medical schools and academic centers can be confining environments. Students often describe becoming "locked into" a limited view of medicine after spending long periods in teaching hospitals. The contrast that currently exists between an academic perspective and a community perspective is illustrated by the common notion within academia that family practice isn't needed, while in many communities there is a manifest need for more family physicians, particularly within the growing market of health maintenance organizations.

3. Providing effective family practice role models.

Paiva et al (1982) underscored the critical importance of role models in affecting the career decisions of medical students. Coker et al (1960) suggested that for a discipline that has less prestige in medical school, the influence of role models and faculty advisers becomes especially important. Brearley et al (1982) reported that role models provided a major influence on students who selected family practice. Positive family practice role models, presented to students longitudinally during medical school, are the cornerstone of any career advising program in maintaining student interest in family practice.

A variety of courses or activities can be effective in giving students these three components for maintaining interest in family practice. Preclinical preceptorships, in full-time blocks or part time over a longer period, are described in *Predoctoral Education in Family Medicine.* The third year (first clinical year) of medical school is the most vulnerable period for a student's career interest in family practice and is the year when the student is most intensely involved with the academic environment. Family practice needs to be visible during this core clinical training. Many schools have required clinical clerkships in family practice that rotate students to community based practices. The clerkships at the University of Wisconsin and the Medical College of Georgia are exemplary models (Beasley, 1983; Hobbs, 1987).

If clerkship time in the community is not a part of the school's third-year curriculum, student interest can be maintained through a series of seminars or forum discussions on various family practice and community topics. This approach has been effective at California, Davis in maintaining career interest in family practice where there is no required family practice curriculum (Hale et al, 1979). The findings of Scherger et al (1987), which respond to many of the questions about family practice asked by medical students during this period, also will be helpful in maintaining interest.

Another effective way to maintain career interest is through student interest groups. These groups of students who share an interest in family practice may be organized at a single school or even statewide. These organizations may conduct regular conferences that provide current information on trends and career opportunities in family practice. The annual National Congress of Student Members, sponsored by the American Academy of Family Physicians, is also an excellent forum for students interested in family practice.

Promote the Student's Best Career Decision

Study results vary greatly with regard to when students indicate they made their career choices. The time of career choice also depends on specialty, with a choice of family practice reported as occurring much earlier than other specialties (Babbott et al, 1988; Markert 1983, Greer et al, 1989). However, since one half or more of medical students change career choices during the third year of medical school and since students must decide on a career early in the further year to take part in the Match process, the third year is a key time for career decision making.

A career adviser can help students discover which specialty best suits their personality styles and career goals. Any gap in a student's understanding of the specialties can be addressed by exposure to role models in various specialties. For the student interested in a community practice, a longitudinal experience on a clerkship with each considered specialty in the community would provide ideal in-depth exposure. Students' tight schedules usually limit the feasibility of this approach, but considerable insight can be provided by one- or two-day exposures to carefully selected role models.

Also, there are excellent reading materials which can give students insight into the various specialties. Taylor's *How to Choose a Medical Specialty* (1986) contains information obtained from a selected group of physicians within each specialty and highlights the important considerations for each. An article in the New Physician looked at "Seven Specialties Up Close" (*New Physician*, 1984).

Some students are not ready to make career decisions early in the fourth year. These students need to be supported and counseled by a career adviser until such time as they are ready. The fourth year can be used to obtain additional clinical exposure in the specialties being considered. Waiting until March Day gives the student an additional three to six months to consider a career choice but limits the available number of sites at which to train. Some students choose to wait an additional year so they can be more confident of making the best career choice. An extra year is a small price to pay for this decision.

Guide the Residency Selection Process

Career advising does not end with a choice of specialty. The choice of a residency program can be critically important in meeting the student's career goals and in achieving career satisfaction. Advisers should assist students in becoming the best residency applicants they can be. Advisers should also assist students in developing an appropriate range of residency programs which matches their career goals and academic standing (Hitchcock et al, 1989). Table 2 outlines the components of a career advising workshop for residency selection.

Table 2

Career Advising Workshop

A career advising workshop for residency selection should include the following:

- A general description of residencies by type – university based or community hospital based, public or private institutions – and the pros and cons of each.

- A general description of the components of a residency and how to evaluate for resources and quality – family practice center, inpatient settings, curriculum and faculty.

- Factors in choosing the location for residency with consideration given to family preferences and future practice interests.

- The appropriate number and range of programs to apply to – such as goals of sending for at least 12 applications, doing at least 10 interviews and ranking at least eight programs.

- Assistance with the application, including writing an effective personal statement. Faculty advisers can greatly benefit students by reviewing drafts of these statements.

- Assistance with choosing letters of recommendation and writing a letter of recommendation from the family medicine department which highlights the students' activities in family medicine during medical school.

- Assistance with preparing a curriculum vitae.

- Guidance regarding interviewing, follow-up communication and ranking.

For some students, the process of applying for residency begins early in medical school. First- and second-year students frequently request information regarding residencies, and many actually take time to visit programs to better understand the training environment offered by a specialty. The formal process of residency selection for family practice and most other specialties begins in May or June of the third year with requests for applications. Hence, the spring of the third year is an important time for specialty decision making and for advising students on the application process.

The dean's office of the medical school provides students with general information on residency selection, and some family medicine departments have provided specific formal guidance to students interested in family practice. The monograph *Strolling Through the Match*, published by the AAFP, is an excellent resource. A workshop which uses all of this material can assist students with the application process and validate their career interest.

The University of Tennessee, Memphis compiled the materials in *Strolling Through the Match*. A program at the University of Washington was the basis for an annual workshop given at the UMDNJ-Robert Wood Johnson Medical School since 1980. This workshop has been shown to improve students' chances in the Match process (Swee et al, 1986).

Match Day is a critical time for adviser involvement with those students who do not match. At this time of crisis, the unmatched student needs assistance in choosing among the options: accepting an available program, opting for an alternative such as a transitional year, or deferring residency training. Even students who do match, but with a program ranked low on their list, may need support and guidance.

Summary

Career development should be a major part of medical education. In many ways, medical school education has become the basic introduction to a career of lifelong learning in medicine. One can argue that what students learn about themselves as future physicians is as important as the medicine they learn during medical school. The fact that just 12%-13% of students choose family practice careers, despite a much greater initial career interest, suggests the need for career advising programs for students. A successful department may use the success it has preventing attrition away from family practice as a program evaluation. While not all students who express interest initially in family practice should choose this career, schools with well-developed career guidance programs retain about 75% of students with initial interest (Scherger et al, 1984; Bougler, 1980). In addition, some students who select family practice do not discover this interest until their clinical training. A visible career guidance program can greatly help these students as well.

Helping students with their career decisions is rewarded by having had a role in the career development of a group of physicians. Close contact with students throughout medical school is important. Students respond well to those who show interest in their futures. With a strategic approach, the predoctoral career advising program will enable those students who should go into family practice to do so and will help all students make their best career decisions.

References and Selected Readings are available in the text by STFM.

By 1991, the STFM Working Group on Family Centered Perinatal Care had grown considerably from its beginning in 1987. A team of us formed to write a two part article on teaching Family Centered Perinatal Care. I gathered Cheryl Levitt, Louise Acheson, Thomas Nesbitt, Cynda Johnson, Kathryn Reilly, Stephen Ratcliffe, Donald Marquardt, John Pfenninger and Wm. MacMillan Rodney for this effort. The Abstract is reprinted here:

Teaching Family-Centered Perinatal Care in Family Medicine, Part 1 & Part 2

Joseph E. Scherger, MD, MPH; Cheryl Levitt, MB, BCh; Louise S. Acheson, MD, MS; Thomas S. Nesbitt, MD, MPH; Cynda A. Johnson, MD; Kathryn E. Reilly, MD; Stephen Ratcliffe, MD, MSPH; Donald Marquardt, MD, PhD; John L. Pfenninger, MD; Wm. MacMillan Rodney, MD

Pregnancy, childbirth, postpartum, and infant care are a continuum in the family life cycle for which the family physician is especially qualified to provide primary, comprehensive care. The purpose of this paper is to document and share the controversies, wisdom, and knowledge about caring for women and their families before, during, and after pregnancy. Family physicians can be leaders in developing an appropriate perinatal care system for the community. The level of care the family physician chooses to provide is discretionary. However, the family physician should be invested in ensuring that all families receive the greatest benefit from pregnancy, birth, and the newborn experience. Interest in perinatal care in family medicine is increasing, as reflected by the growing numbers participating in the Society of Teachers of Family Medicine Working Group on Family-Centered Perinatal Care. The authors of this article, who are active in this working group, hope that this information is useful in designing a balanced curriculum and delivery system for perinatal care in family medicine training programs.

(Fam Med 1992; 24(4):288-98)
(Fam Med 1992; 24(5):368-74)

PART IV: MANAGED CARE AND FAMILY MEDICINE, 1992-98

During the 1980s health care costs more than tripled and an era of specialization played out to the marginalization of family medicine. By 1992, the payers were in full revolt and demanded managed costs, known euphemistically as managed care. Primary care physicians would serve as "gatekeepers" to manage the utilization of expensive services. Managed care was both good and bad for family medicine. Good because it increased the importance of the specialty, increasing student interest and family physician incomes. Bad because its goals and ethics conflicted with the physician as patient advocate. Some wondered if the Hippocratic tradition of medicine was at an end, replaced by corporate medicine.

Usually the optimist, I considered managed care as appropriate care and saw opportunities to modernize family medicine without losing its soul. Family physicians began to practice in different models and I thought all were good, dictated by the settings of their work. This essay was about these various models of practice:

Models of Family Practice

JABFP
1992;5(6):649-653

I recently drove to a rural area of Northern California to visit a group of family physicians. They are among the most popular of our clinical faculty with teaching and inspiring medical students. During dinner we talked about their practice. The four family physicians have separate offices in three towns along a 45-mile stretch of highway. They share call and are linked by the name of Intermountain Family Practice. One-half day each week they rotate offices to keep familiar with each practice. They meet every morning for rounds at the centrally located 20-bed hospital, where they are the only full-time medical staff. They see all the patients in the emergency department, deliver all the babies, including doing Cesarean sections, and perform many of the surgeries. A general surgeon based 1 hour away is available for elective cases and some emergencies. Our conversation was rich with stories of major trauma, harrowing transports in nasty weather, performing procedures under unusual circumstances (a chest tube in the office), and the frustration of getting outside specialists to accept referrals of low-income patients.

What was striking to me about this familiar story of traditional general or family practice was that all of these physicians were young, less than 10 years out of residency. What I was listening to was not the past but, rather, the present and the future of a model of family practice.

The Spectrum of Practice Models

Often I hear questions and comments today about the changing role of the family physician. Medical students ask, "What is the scope of family practice? What do family physicians do in the 1990s? What is the future practice model for family physicians?" Researchers study the "experts" looking to find what competencies will be needed for the future family physician and what competencies will be unnecessary.[1] Obstetrics, intensive care, and hospital surgeries have been considered unnecessary skills.

W. McMillan Rodney and William Close object, suggesting that a true generalist family physician is one who is able to set a fracture, deliver a baby, care for a sick child, run an office, and go to the hospital when necessary (personal communication, April 1991). Kaiser Health Plan is the dominant employer of graduates of the University of California-David program, and these family physicians rarely do any of these tasks. Their exclusive focus is office practice. My own practice is between these two ends of the spectrum. I am in a semirural area, remain active in obstetric care, assist at surgery and make as many house calls as I do hospital visits. Ninety percent of my time is spent in the office, however, and I frequently use consultants in caring for critically ill patients. Who are the real family physicians? Who reflects the future?

Twenty-five percent of the US population and most of our country's land mass are rural and are served by family physicians that are often alone in providing health care. These family physicians practice as they do as much by necessity as by choice. There is no reason why competent family physicians performing most of their own procedures could not practice in an urban area, and some do; but like urban cowboys, they are likely to be restless, frequently having to defend their privileges. The office-only family physicians are generally found in tightly run, large multispecialty groups, which by nature exist in urban and suburban areas. Intermediate family physicians, like myself, probably evolved from the traditional model to accommodate practicing with an increasingly sophisticated range of other specialists. Intermediate family physicians are found in all areas (rural, semirural, suburban, and urban) and often practice in single-specialty family practice groups or in multispecialty groups in which family practice has been a prominent specialty.

Discussions about the proper current or future model of family practice are generating unnecessary conflict within our specialty. Family practice has not transformed its practice model; it has expanded and become too broad to be defined by any singular model of practice. The spectrum of family practice has become so wide that practice models at either end are so different as to barely resemble each other in practice style.

Twenty years ago the picture of the practicing family physician seemed clearer than it is today. Even though rural family physicians would have performed more surgery than their urban colleagues, the style of practice was very similar. Virtually every family physician was in private practice and was active in the hospital. Most were in either solo or small-group practice. The early literature in family practice was able to describe a singular model of practice with minor variations depending upon physician training and community needs.

Currently, the practice options available to a residency graduate are numerous and divergent. Traditional private practice, solo or in small groups, continues in rural and urban areas, but differences in practice patterns are increasing. Table 1 displays the practice arrangements of 1991 family practice residency graduates compared with those who graduated in 1978.[2,3] While the single-specialty family practice group remains the most common choice, more graduates are joining multispecialty groups. There is also a decline in graduates choosing rural or small-town practice.

Table 1. Practice Arrangements of Graduating Family Practice Residents, 1978 and 1991

	1978 Graduates (n = 1340) Percent	1991 Graduates (n = 1559) Percent
Family Practice Group (two or more persons)	43.4	44.0
Multispecialty Group	7.4	12.2*
Solo Practice	12.7	7.8*
Emergency Department	3.6	5.1

	1978 Graduates (n = 1105) Percent	1991 Graduates (n = 1528) Percent
Rural or Small Town (<25,000)	50.4	42.1 *
Suburban or Small City (25,000-100,000)	39.5	44.5 *
Large Urban or Inner City	10.1	13.4**

*P < 0.01
**P < 0.02
Source: American Academy of Family Physicians.[2,3]

Table 2. Types of Patient Care in Family Physicians' Hospital Practices, 1990

	Rural (n = 932) Percent	Urban (n = 1636) Percent
Routine Obstetric Care	41.6	20.4 *
Multispecialty Group	14.9	2.2 *
Surgical Assisting	54.6	36.8 *
Major Surgery	11.2	3.1 *
Intensive Care Unit	71.3	54.8**

*P < 0.01
Source: American Academy of Family Physicians.[4]

Table 2 shows differences in selected types of patient care in hospitals by family physicians in urban and rural areas according to a survey by the American Academy of Family Physicians in 1990.[4] These differences are probably even greater today, because of continued changes in urban family practice, with more family physicians joining large multispecialty groups. Multispecialty group practice is the fastest growing practice arrangement, and many are competing for family physicians. Multispecialty practices with their own insurance plans increasingly rely on family physicians to provide primary care services. Some plans such as Kaiser generally limit the family physicians' role to the office, whereas others such as FHP (Orange County, California, and Salt Lake City) encourage a broad practice and surgical assisting. Some family physicians choose to work in urgent care centers or emergency departments, limiting their practice to acute, episodic care.

The American Board of Family Practice defines family practice as the medical specialty that provides continuing and comprehensive health care for the individual and the family. It is the specialty in breadth that integrates the biological, clinical, and behavioral sciences. The scope of family practice encompasses all ages, both sexes, each organ system, and every disease entity.[5] The family physician is defined as educated and trained to develop and bring to bear in practice unique attitudes and skills that qualify him or her to provide continuing, comprehensive health maintenance and medical care for the entire family regardless of sex, age, or type of problem, be it biological, behavioral, or social. This physician serves as the patient's or family's advocate in all health-related matters, including the appropriate use of consulting and community resources.[6]

These definitions describe the underlying philosophy common to all family physicians, regardless of practice model. While emergency department or urgent care practice does not qualify as family practice because of a lack of continuity and comprehensiveness of care, other divergent models are reflective of the specialty if the family physician takes responsibility for being the personal physician to a group of patients, providing and coordinating comprehensive health services. The challenges to the office-only family physician doing this may be just as great as for any family physician along the spectrum of practice models.

My purpose here is not only to describe the current diversity that exists in family practice today, but also to suggest that we more fully embrace our differences as a specialty. The Intermountain Family

Practice physicians, today's version of the able-to-do-it-all generalists, could feel forgotten by the rest of us. Office-only family physicians, particularly those not in private practices, might not feel respected by more traditional family physicians, who have generally been leaders in organized medicine. Disrespect of practice models within our specialty only divides us and limits the important contributions each model of family practice makes to our specialty.

This essay does not discuss other areas of variance among family physicians, such as special interest areas. Many family physicians focus heavily on such specific clinical areas as geriatrics or sports medicine. Others focus primarily on teaching, research, or administration. Fortunately for our specialty, most family physicians with special interests and expertise continue to practice broad family medicine and are resisting full subspecialization, as has occurred in internal medicine.

All family physicians, regardless of their practice models, have much to contribute to patient care and to the specialty. Family physicians who limit their practice to the office have an opportunity to develop a more sophisticated model of primary care. They have the time to develop state-of-the-art practices focusing on health promotion and disease prevention, those aspects of practice for which rural family physicians might simply not have enough time. Office-only family physicians might also have time to provide regular individual and family counseling and might more rapidly develop their skills in new office procedures, such as colposcopy and flexible sigmoidoscopy. Rural family physicians preserve the role of the true generalist in community care. Such family physicians are very busy providing the needed services to their community, do a wonderful job of teaching students and residents, and are grateful for the new developments brought to them from their regional referral centers. Intermediate family physicians like myself work to find a balance along the spectrum of practice models.

Residency Training

The Residency Review Committee for family practice has a singular list of essentials to which all residencies must comply. These essentials are broad and flexible enough to allow for training all models of family physician. The limiting factors are the resources of the residency programs. Should all residency programs be expected to train family physicians for the full spectrum of practice models? I suggest that for many programs, this approach is not possible. Are these programs inferior? Medical students coming from university medical centers are often surprised to learn that some family practice residency programs do an excellent job of training family physicians for remote rural areas. These programs are usually in community hospitals, where family practice is the only residency, and the residents are expected to provide a wide range of major surgical procedures. Graduates of these programs who choose to practice in an office-only setting will not use many of their skills. In contrast, as part of an effort to increase the number of family physicians, there is an effort to have health maintenance organizations (HMOs), such as Kaiser, develop residency programs. Should an HMO, which uses family physicians exclusively in an office, be expected to train residents for another model of family physician?

These issues and questions speak for a greater clarity of and appreciation for the various models of family practice and the nature and resources of training sites. It is hoped that most residency programs will be able to offer a sufficiently diverse training to allow the graduates the broadest range of practice options.

Medical Student Interest

The medical student interested in becoming a rural family physician is likely to be very different from the student interested in an office-only practice. Most students interested in family practice appropriately do not know which model they will practice, but they do have inclinations when the spectrum is discussed. Matching a student inclined toward a rural model with an office-only practice for preceptorship could turn the student away from family practice and vice versa. I suspect more medical students would choose family practice if they were aware of the rich diversity of practice models.

Their choice of role models, preceptorship sites, and application to residency programs should reflect their interests.

Organized Medicine

I have seen leaders of family practice organizations on the local and national level, who come from either a rural or intermediate practice, speak disparagingly of family physicians who limit their practice to the office of an HMO. The platform of candidates running for offices in organized medicine has been the preservation of traditional private practice and competition with office-only family physicians. In California, for the first time, a family physician who works for Kaiser Health Plan has been elected to the board of directors of the state academy chapter. With a large number of residency graduates choosing this practice option, to stay unified as a specialty, organized family practice should embrace these physicians.

Reimbursement

One of the ironies of present-day practice is the lack of fairness in how physicians are paid. Rural family physicians probably work hardest and place themselves in situations of much higher risk, but they could be paid the least among the practice models. Family physicians in private practice typically have incomes that reflect only what they earn, rather than what they are worth to the health care system. Family physicians in a large multispecialty group might work fewer hours and remain in the office, but they might well be paid much higher, reflecting their worth as case managers in an organized health system that financially rewards cost-conscious practice. These income imbalances could contribute to the animosity among family physicians in different practice models. Somehow we must work toward a system of physician reimbursement in which all family physicians, regardless of practice model, are paid according to their worth.

Continuing Education

Planning a conference to meet the needs of all family physicians is increasingly difficult. Rural family physicians might want to be updated on providing thrombolytic therapy for acute myocardial infarction, whereas office-only family physicians are interested in only primary care skills. Continuing education courses will be successful only if they address the diversity in their audience.

Conclusions

Family practice must have a clear and attractive image to motivate medical students to select the specialty and to encourage payers and insurers of health care to value family physicians for their worth. A goal for the United Sates would be a base of family physicians providing primary care in an organized health system with fair and equitable reimbursement for all physicians. The diversity of family practice models, demanded by different locations and community needs, clouds the picture unless all models of family practice are recognized and appreciated by teachers of family medicine and by leaders of our medical organizations. We have much work to do within our specialty toward this end before we can expect the outside world to understand and appreciate us.

References

1. Howokawa M, Zweig S. Future directions in family medicine: results of a Delphi study. Fam Med 1990; 22:429-33.
2. Report on survey of 1978 graduating family practice residents. Kansas City, MO: American Academy of Family Physicians, AAFP Reprint No. 155D.
3. Report on survey of 1991 graduating family practice residents. Kansas City, MO: American Academy of Family Physicians, AAFP Reprint No. 155Q.
4. Facts about family practice. Kansas City, MO: American Academy of Family Physicians, 1991; 118-9.
5. 1992 directory of diplomats. Definition and policies. Lexington, KY: American Board of Family Practice, 1992:iii.
6. Academy policy: 1991-92 compendium of AAFP positions on selected health issues. Kansas City, MO: American Academy of Family Physicians, 1992:23.

By 1992, the counter-culture phase of family medicine was over and the new specialty was maturing into a recognized mainstream discipline. A new type of leadership was needed in academic institutions and that formed the inspiration for this article:

The Second Revolution in Family Practice Has Begun

American Family Physician
1993;48(7):1238-1240

In his classic 1979 essay, "Family Medicine as Counterculture,"[1] Stephens described the first revolt in family practice, the specialty that preserved yet modernized the generalist physician in America. Stephens credits the success of the family practice movement in the 1970s with "reforms that were more pervasive and powerful than ourselves." According to Stephens, the broad social reforms of the 1960s and 1970s – agrarianism, utopianism, humanism, consumerism and feminism – "created the climate of public opinion that made it possible for family practice to success in an unprecedented way."

During the decade following the birth of family practice in 1969, the number of residents grew from a dozen to more than 300, and more and more medical students flocked to the specialty. The American Academy of Family Physicians established the goal that 25 percent of all medical students would enter family practice, but this goal was only half realized.

The 1980s were a different story. In what could be described as the decade of high-tech medicine, the growth of family practice stopped abruptly. The cost of health care in the United States skyrocketed, with minor public health benefits, and more Americans than at any time since the enactment of Medicare and Medicaid were deprived of access to basic health care. As medical students flocked to the subspecialties, the number of family practice residency programs plateaued and fill rates dropped. In a 1989 reflection on his earlier essay, Stephen lamented, "Our chief regret can only be that we were not able for our tasks. We have expended our energy on professional legitimation and enfranchisement rather than reform."[2]

Was health care reform and growth in family practice possible during the 1980s? Probably not, given the overriding social forces of less government and personal economic independence. The 1990s are a different story. Broad social forces are again at work and family practice is being caught up in them. The wind seems to be blowing in our direction again. A second revolution of growth in family practice has begun.

The current social forces that may finally bring about sweeping health care reform in the United States are social justice (equal access to basic health care), cost control and quality assurance through accepted standardization of care. With a new administration in Washington, Americans are open to legislation that will control the gross imbalances in American health care: excessive health care for some versus little or none for many; an oversupply of subspecialists versus a lack of primary care physicians, and excessive costs for even the most common of health problems. Family physicians are a key to correcting these imbalances.

What evidence is there that family practice will grow during this decade? As in the last 1960s, today a combination of forces – the public, government and academic medicine – is calling for more family physicians. Newspapers and magazines are carrying stores that call for more family physicians.[3-5] A life insurance company, in a letter to policyholders, advises "establishing a relationship with a family doctor" as a means of controlling health care costs.[6] Of course, the managed care model that is sweeping American health insurance requires such a relationship.

The Council on Graduate Medical Education, reporting to Congress as commissioned by the Department of Health and Human Services, has called for legislative action to produce more generalist physicians.[7] The cardiologist dean of a prestigious medical school writes: "It is becoming clear that the need to increase the number of primary care physicians in the United States is urgent. Patients increasingly require a personal physician who will be an advocate, guiding them through the complexities of a high-tech health care system. Also, people now recognize that primary care physicians can have a real impact on reducing health care expenditures by overseeing care that is responsible and appropriate."[8]

As family practice gets pulled into this time of reform, some critical questions arise. What will family physicians of the future do? With a managed care imperative in the insurance industry, will the family physician's role as patient caregiver be compromised by a need to restrict services to control costs? Will family physicians be trusted to provide high-quality and cost-efficient care or will medical decisions be micromanaged leading to a "Big-Brother-is-watching" form of practice? Will the scope of services rendered by family physicians be tightly controlled in the name of efficiency, neglecting the individuality of physician skills and the uniqueness of the doctor/patient relationship?

The answers to these questions and others depend on the extent to which family physicians place themselves in leadership positions during this time of reform. If family physicians become the victims of reform efforts, they will suffer the consequences of structural experimentation led by health care executives who cannot be expected to fully understand the nature of the family physician's commitment to individuals, families and the community. Already, discouraged physicians, including family physicians, are expressing a loss of control over their practices, a feeling of victimization during change.

I am, however, optimistic about our future. Even though large numbers of medical students did not choose family practice during the 1980s, some of the top students did, giving our specialty an unprecedented range of talent. Young family physicians have set up practices in rural America and are providing all the skills that their patients in isolated areas require. The shortage of rural physicians is placing family physicians in the spotlight. This role of family physicians needs to be nurtured. In urban areas, family physicians are assuming leadership of multispecialty groups and health maintenance organizations, and are leading new independent physician associations with the right balance of generalists and specialists. A growing number of family physicians are getting the M.B.A. degrees and are becoming executives in health care systems and in the insurance industry. In academic medication, primary care research has taken center stage with outcomes data that legitimize the role of the generalist physician.[9,10]

Will a growing number of medical students choose family practice and keep up with the growing number of residency programs? This is a critical question. However insulated by the protective walls of medical school, students also appear to be caught up in the forces for social change, and record numbers of medical students are expressing interest in family practice by joining the American Academy of Family Physicians. With reimbursement reform and the pressures of an intense demand for family physicians, economic parity of family practice with other specialties seems likely.

In 1985, Ransom[11] wrote prophetically about these times: "If family medicine can sustain its commitment and its unconventional approach for a bit longer, it may well assume leadership for all of medicine, both intellectually and in meeting patients' needs. This is not so because family practice seeks to correct a gross imbalance in the kinds of medical services available, or because family physicians are more humanistic than their technology-minded subspecialty counterparts. It is because family medicine will prove to be more effective at what people go to physicians for: help to get well, to feel well or to suffer as little as necessary."

Leadership is the key. Family physicians need not be victims of social change but can be leaders in social change by determining what managed care means and by training medical students and residents for the future. During this second revolution, family practice may achieve an enduring place in a new American health care system.

References

1. Stephens GG. Family medicine as counterculture. Family Medicine Teacher 1979;16(5)14-8.

2. Stephens GG. Family medicine as counterculture. Fam Med 1989;21(2):103-9.

3. Is there a family doctor in the house? Business Week 1992 Nov 2:124-5.

4. Tully S. America's painful doctor shortage. Fortune 1992 Nov 16:103.

5. Cimons M. U.S. needs more family doctors, study warns. Los Angeles Times 1992 Nov 9;Sect A:2(Col 6).

6. The cost of health care: ways to reduce the "ouch." USAA Life's Issues and Answers. 1992;2(2):1-2.

7. COGME's report to congress and HHS calls for more generalists (News). AAFP Director's Newsletter. 1992;Nov 19:1-4.

8. Shine KI. From the Dean. UCLA Medicine 1992; 13(1):2.

9. Bowman JA. The quality of care provided by family physicians.

J Fam Pract 1989;28:346-55.

10. Greenfield S, Nelson EC, Zubkoff M, Manning W, Rogers W, Kravitz RI, et al. Variations in resource utilization among medical specialties and systems of care. Results from the medical outcomes study. JAMA 1992;267:1624-30.

11. Ransom DC. Random notes: the unconventional future of family medicine. Fam Syst Med 1985;3:120-6.

In 1993 I became the first medical editor of a new journal, Family Practice Management. The mission was to help family physicians adapt to the changes brought about by managed care. I wrote 13 editorials between 1993 and 1997 and 7 are selected here:

Editorials – Family Practice Management:

Looking Back to the Future

Editorial
Family Practice Management (Premier Issue)
1993;1(1A):10-11

The year is 2018. An elderly family physician, residency trained in the 1970s, is giving a presentation at the annual meeting of the American Academy of Family Physicians (AAFP) to celebrate the 25th anniversary of the journal Family Practice Management. His topic is "Looking Back at Family Practice in the Late 20th Century." The speaker relates that the 1990s were a decade of transformation in American medicine, and a crucial one for the resurgence of family practice.

Those of you who were in practice during the 1990s remember it as the decade when American medicine changed fundamentally from a cottage industry of independent small businesses into the marketplace of health care systems that we're used to today. Before the mid-1990s, a patient receiving treatment for an illness before, during and after hospitalization might have 30 separate bills generated, most of which were usually paid by an insurance company after time-consuming individual processing. Per capita, the administrative cost of medical care in America almost equaled the entire cost of medical care in some other advanced countries!

This fragmented non-system, with its unchecked use of technology and specialists, caused such incredible inflation in medical care spending that the major purchasers of this care – the government and American business – demanded change. Over several years during the 1990s, various components of medical care joined together to coordinate care for defined population groups within defined budgets. Decades after its inception, managed care came into its own, and terms such as managed competition and integrated delivery systems were invented to describe this transformation.

The changes of the 1990s brought family practice back to a central role in American medicine. They helped produce an explosive increase in the number of family practice residencies and a corresponding upsurge in the number of family physicians trained. In fact, so many of the people in this audience were brought into family medicine by that upsurge that a large proportion of you can't even imagine what it was like to practice in a world where family practice was denigrated. Those of you who have been around long enough remember all too well the near extinction of the generalist physician during the post-World-War-II "age of specialization." To save the GP from extinction, family practice began as a specialty in the late 1960s and enjoyed a rapid growth in residency programs during the 1970s. This growth was stymied for more than a decade from 1978 until 1992 because medical students were lured into what were then the more lucrative and prestigious specialties.

As health care systems began to organize in the early 1990s, they found a physician work force terribly out of balance. Less than 30 percent of American physicians were trained to care for the whole person and manage common health problems! The sudden demand for more family physicians and lack of opportunities for limited specialists drove reimbursement for family physicians to a level of parity with that of the average American physician. At the same time, lucrative incomes for other specialties disappeared. Medical students, including many of you, recognized the tremendous demand for generalists. They flocked to become generalists, and the number of family practice residency programs swelled to over 500 nationwide.

By the end of the 20th century, more than 25 percent of American medical students were entering family practice, a doubling over a 10-year period. The number of family physicians swelled rapidly, and many subspecialists, no longer needed, retrained as family physicians.

Before the 1990s, most family physicians were either in solo practice or clustered in independent small groups. The various new kinds of health care organizations brought family physicians into systems with other specialists and hospitals. Even though many family physicians continued to work in small, community-based offices delivering personalized care, the management of those offices became more and more centralized as the sharing of facilities and services brought increasing economies of scale. Computers began appearing in exam rooms here and there as more and more patient records migrated into digital form. The process is not complete – I know some of you still use paper records today – but development of the medical information networks toward the end of the decade accelerated computerization immeasurably.

How did family physicians accomplish this transition? Physicians in independent practice often felt that merger meant takeover, and were threatened by the changes. Forming health care organizations required a cultural shift for many physicians, going from a physician-centered view of medical care – the idea that the doctor must be captain of the ship – to what has been referred to as the team-centered view – the idea that the physician is a team player and a multidisciplinary group thinker.

To its credit, the AAFP helped guide family physicians through this period of transition. Family Practice Management played a key role in educating family physicians about the many dimensions of change involved in the development of the new system. Many family physicians were leaders in the health care reforms of the 1990s, and articles they submitted to FPM helped their colleagues in traditional private practice make it through those years. Despite the sometimes almost intolerable pace of change, family practice was able to preserve itself as a specialty while not losing the reason for its existence: the idea of a personal physician caring for a community of individuals and families. Save those old issues of Family Practice Management. They chronicle a historic period for American medicine and family practice.

How American is Managed Competition?

Editorial
Family Practice Management
1994;1(6):14,16

Health care is a service industry. While it is common to point out its unique role in society, health care may in some respects be compared with other service industries, such as education, air travel and telephone service. Managed competition and a single-payer system are the most commonly cited structures for a reformed health care system. Other service industries in America provide examples of managed competition and single-payer institutions we may learn from. On the whole, what they have to teach is that managed competition seems likely to work better than a single-payer approach, but they offer some cautions about both.

Managed competition may be characterized as a marketplace in which multiple competing organizations offer services under a system of regulation designed to ensure a fair and honest market and a basic level of quality. While many politicians who favor the status quo or a single-payer system in health care are calling managed completion an untried model, there are already many examples of managed competition in America.

Consider air travel. While some countries have a single national airline, we have several competing private airlines (in effect, managed competition). The Federal Aviation Administration regulates the training and alertness of pilots and the quality of the planes (thank goodness), and both regional and national airlines compete for our business by balancing cost and quality. Does comparing health care with air travel trivialize it? I don't think so; after all, they are both life-and-death businesses.

As we contemplate a similar system for health care, it is instructive to consider how periods of regulation and deregulation have affected the airline industry. Deregulation under the Reagan administration resulted in many mergers and the loss of most small regional carriers. Now some small airlines are coming back, able to compete for price and service with the big national companies. Managed competition is never static; it will always change somewhat depending on which party is in power.

We once had a single-payer system for long distance telephone service – Ma Bell. In one of the most far-reaching business-related decisions of the 20th century, the American government, under challenge, chose to allow managed competition. Now AT&T, MCI, Sprint and others, compete for our business, balancing cost and quality. On a more regional level, there is managed competition for cellular telephone business. In San Diego, for instance, Cellular One, PacTel, USWest and San Diego Cellular all compete in offering quality at an affordable price. The cellular companies also strike deals with other businesses to capture market share. My new car phone is on USWest Motor Co. because Forde has a deal with them. My other portable cellular phone is with PacTel because the store at which it was bought (at the lowest price around) had a deal with them. Sound familiar? Managed competition is not without its challenges.

Rapid mail delivery is another example of the tension between a single-payer system and managed completion. Sending a letter or package by normal delivery uses what might be considered a single-payer system – the U.S. Postal Service. They are much maligned, but I think they are doing a reasonable job. However, if they were doing a great job of mail service, would Federal Express be so successful? For rapid mail service, we now have a managed competition market that has energized this entire industry. While the new companies compete over price and quality, the old companies, such as the postal service and United Parcel Service, are offering new services.

Education is a human service on par with health care in its social importance. In our public education system, we have a universal, tax-supported, single-payer industry. Private education alternatives exist for those who can afford them and flourish in areas where public education is weak. There is a growing movement to energize public education at the elementary and high school levels by creating managed competition. This has existed for a long time at the college level.

So as health care emerges from the status of a cottage industry to something bigger and more organized, there is much precedent from other service industries for managed competition and a single-payer system. Other countries vary in the degree to which human services are socialized in a government-run system or regulated in a private, competitive market. In order to guarantee universal access to a quality service with a basic level of benefits, some degree of government regulation is needed. Our current health insurance industry is largely unregulated and allows for distortions such as coverage only for the health organ systems of the body and an inability to get coverage when you need it most.

Whether health care in America becomes a government-run, socialized system or a private, competitive market is an open question. The managed competition model feels to many like an American approach to a service industry. It appears that under the Clinton administration, managed competition in health care will get a chance. I recognize its imperfections, but nothing's perfect. I hope it works.

Training Other Specialists in Primary Care

Family Practice Management
1995;2(2):11-13

The 100,000 or more surplus specialists and subspecialists in America are big news today. Managed care and the development of organized delivery systems are nudging the balance of primary care physicians and other specialists closer to the 50-50 ratio often recommended. Currently 70 percent of physicians in America are not trained to care for the whole person over time. Equipping physicians from other specialties to provide high-quality primary care is one obvious solution to the problem. One way that has been advocated is to train them to be family physicians.

In this issue of Family Practice Management, Richard A. Schwartz, MD, and Larry W. Johnson, MD, share their enthusiasm and the fruits of their early experience in what they call "recycling" specialists into family physicians – Schwartz from the unique perspective of a surgeon undergoing the recycling (see "Retaining Subspecialists: Making it Work," page 39). They describe a flexible curriculum that apparently meets the requirements for board certification in family practice. A similar program at the University of Tennessee developed by William Rodney, MD, has received considerable attention.

An alternative approach is exemplified by our program at Sharp HealthCare in San Diego. We have developed a primary care training program for OB/GYNs. The purpose of this program is not to turn OB/GYNs into family physicians but to give a carefully selected group of OB/GYNs the knowledge and skills they need to provide comprehensive primary care for women only. Our intent is to expand upon their training in order that they may continue to care for a group of women in a managed care environment.

The issue of training specialists in primary care is complex and inevitably colored by attitudes and emotions arising from many years of injustice against family physicians. The following arguments against training specialists in primary care are the ones most often heard:

1. They are doing it just for economic reasons and not out of a sincere desire to become personal physicians. Just wait until they learn how poorly primary care is paid!

2. Most other specialists would have difficulty living with the diagnostic uncertainty we family physicians have to deal with day in and day out.

3. Retraining physicians from other specialties would be a costly and impractical waste of resources; we would be better served by quickly increasing the number of new family physicians being trained, supplementing them with family nurse practitioners and physician assistants, who are much less expensive to train.

Each of these arguments contains a certain amount of truth, but none is persuasive in the end. Certainly some candidates for retraining approach it with the right attitude and can get used to diagnostic uncertainty. And is it truly more expensive to train a new family physician than to retrain a physician who already has practice experience? I wonder. Moreover, the fact remains that we are about to have a great surplus of specialized physicians who are not going to simply go away and drive taxis. Why not look at the bright side? The challenge of retraining a certain number of specialists, with the compassion exemplified by the article in this issue, constitutes a new opportunity for educators in family practice. Specialists have contributed enormously to the education of family physicians for decades, and now is the time for us to return the favor.

In 1893, William Osler expressed concern about the overspecialization of American physicians. He said we would be in trouble if we allowed physicians to begin their careers as specialists, rather than have a foundation of generalist training. Our current dilemma is a fulfillment of Osler's prophesy, and we must begin taking steps to correct it. These are the key issues regarding the training of specialists in primary care:

Selection of Candidates. As one residency director put it, "You can't make a silk purse out of a sow's ear, unless you have a silk sow." Somehow we need to evaluate the aptitude of specialists for primary care practice – and their attitude toward it. Are they willing to respond to all patient calls regardless of the problem? Can they practice cost-effective primary care? Do they relish the challenges of primary care? Are they committed to a new career? Surveys taken during medical school over the past 30 years suggest that most students who started out with a career interest in community-based family practice ended up specializing. Perhaps the interest in and aptitude for primary care can be reawakened in many candidates for retraining.

Curriculum Models. Medical school and residency are youth-oriented educational models that provide not only the necessary knowledge and skills for medicine, but also an important maturation process. Formal residency training may not be the most appropriate or efficient model for the mid-career transition from another specialty into primary care. Furthermore, some physicians will require much more training than others. Flexibility in curriculum is as important as clarity in the definition of the desired outcome. A physician from another specialty who wishes to become a fully trained family physician must certainly accomplish the equivalent of residency training. Others, such as internal medicine subspecialists or OB/GYNs, may simply wish to expand their knowledge and skills to allow for comprehensive care of their existing patients without changing their career identity. Wall and Saulz have described four possible pathways of training specialists in primary care.[1]

Assessing Clinical Competence. Other specialists wishing to practice primary care will be held to the same standards as traditionally trained primary care physicians. Since written board examinations have limited applicability to clinical practice, we need additional mechanisms for assessing clinical competence in order to evaluate new educational models. At Sharp, we use standardized patients as part of our formal evaluation, giving us a means of comparing the performance of our learners with medical students, family practice residents and family physicians.

Terminology. The language used for training specialists in primary care is awkward. Schwartz and Johnson refer to recycling physicians. Recycling may sound right for newspapers and aluminum cans, but it doesn't seem to fit professional people. Retraining is most often used, but applies only to a true career change and not to an expansion of skills such as might be appropriate for the OB/GYN or internist. A newly trained physician should be called a family physician only if he or she has successfully completed the equivalent of full residency training and is at least eligible for board certification. Primary care physician is a more general term referring to the first-contact physician who provides or coordinates care over time. Just as a pediatrician provides primary care for children and some internists provide primary care for adults, a more specialized internist or an OB/GYN, given the appropriate training, could provide primary care for a limited population.

With luck, the issue of whether and how to train other specialists in primary care will fairly soon be a nonissue. As our new health care models more clearly define the types of physician needed, medical students and post-graduate training programs should respond. The market will help fix the problem, although eliminating the perverse financial incentives to train hospital-based specialists will require legislative action. Meanwhile, we will go through an interesting period of creative medical education and credentialing as we help some of our colleagues meet the more clearly defined health care needs of our population.

Reference

1. Wall EM, Saultz JW. Retraining the subspecialist for a primary care career: four possible pathways. Acad Med. 1994;69(4):261-266

Are We Defined by Who We Are or by What We Do?

Editorial
Family Practice Management
1995;2(6):13

In the April issue, my good friend Wm MacMillan (Bill) Rodney, MD, challenged my earlier editorial, "A Procedures Bandwagon,"[1] and called for continued training and practice in a wide range of procedures in order to keep family practice "whole."[2]

While I generally support the training and practice of family physicians in procedures, I fear the notion of defining our identify by what procedures we do. Had Dr. Rodney been writing 25 years ago, he might have used appendectomies, cholecystectomies and hysterectomies as his examples of procedures that help define family practice. The first two of these procedures are more common for many patients than upper GI endoscopy. Are we already a severely "amputated" specialty in Dr. Rodney's sense? I don't think so.

We family physicians are defined by our relationship with our patients. This relationship may exist independent of most procedures. I agree that real family physicians are able to do things for their patients, but what we are called upon to do vary greatly by setting. I have chosen to continue to do obstetrics, vasectomies, family planning procedures and skin surgeries because I enjoy caring for young families and treating skin problems. If my practice setting didn't support this, I would probably not be there. I have chosen not to do flexible sigmoidoscopy (even though I was trained it it) because as yet I do not recommend this procedure for routine screening. I may change my mind on this as data accumulates. I order flexible sigmoidoscopies so infrequently that I would not be as skilled as my patients deserve. The same is true for me with colposcopy. I resist having women with mildly abnormal Pap smears undergo this procedure. Fortunately, I have family practice colleagues who perform both of these procedures, so my patients may receive this care in our office.

My concern, balanced with support for those in our specialty who promote procedures, is that we may become part of a major problem in health care today – the excessive use of technology. Just as the carpenter holding a hammer may begin to see more things as nails, we may give our colleagues inappropriate incentives to do more to our patients than they need, just to keep their skills. Examples include upper GI endoscopy for common reflux esophagitis and trigger point injections for fibromyalgia when a lifestyle change is what is needed.

One can be a whole family physician with just a small bag of examining equipment and the sacred trust known as the physician-patient relationship. What else we do may be important, but it will depend on our practice setting. Procedures are skills, not commandments.

References

1. Scherger JE. A procedures bandwagon. Fam Pract Mgmt. April 1994:17.
2. Rodney WM. Keeping family practice whole. Fam Pract Mgmt. April 1995:11-12.

The Window of Hell

Family Practice Management
1995;2(6):14-16

Change is stressful, even if it is for the better. Really big change can be hell. Health care in America has probably never undergone as rapid a change as it is going through now. I do not mean the medicine we practice, but rather the financing and structure of our practice. In order to control health care costs, the business of health care is being turned upside down – from fee-for-service to capitation. And because capitated contracts generally go to large delivery systems, the small independent businesses that have traditionally been the structure of health care are being transformed into larger and larger units.

The window of hell

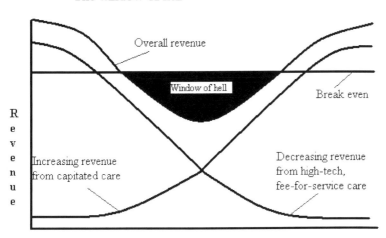

The transition from fee-for-service to capitation occurs faster than most delivery systems are able to change their structure. The organizations, designed for high-tech medicine and not yet ready to manage capitated dollars efficiently, see their fee-for-service revenues fall off faster than they can adapt, causing great pain and suffering. Success under capitation requires fewer hospital beds, fewer high-tech procedures, fewer specialists and more primary care physicians. Making all the changes necessary to arrive at this configuration is a daunting task for most newly formed delivery systems. If the organization succeeds in making the necessary adaptation, it gradually recovers from the pain. In the meantime, however, it goes through what a colleague has called "the window of hell" (see the illustration).

Sharp HealthCare, the large system in which I practice, is now passing through that window. In time, virtually all hospitals and multispecialty medical groups in this country will experience the window of hell.

Multispecialty groups usually have more subspecialists than they need for the population served. In the past, subspecialists generated their own demand; they were the "high rollers". Not true under capitation, when all services become costs rather than revenues to the group. Downsizing specialty departments is a difficult process, often described as "blood on the floor".

If hospital usage throughout the country declines as a result of capitation, we will need only 25 percent of the beds we now have. Hospitals are large employers, and downsizing or closing hospitals is a painful process. New integrated delivery systems that were built through the merger of hospitals and then multispecialty groups are ill-prepared for the rapid restructuring necessary for financial success under capitation.

Family practice groups may avoid the window of hell since their revenues have not depended on high-tech services. Exceptions to this may be family practice groups that have depended on profits from their own lab or X-ray services or the frequent use of procedures. On the other hand, even family practice groups that are poised for success under capitation may lack the capital they need to take full risk contracts. If they are forced to merge with hospitals or multispecialty groups to get the capital, they risk hitching ride through the window of hell themselves.

If your group is contemplating a merger with a hospital or multispecialty group, ask yourself how well prepared the system is for a capitated future and whether you should wait to merge until the system has passed through the window of hell. Family physicians with established practices bring patients, or "lives", to a delivery system, just what it needs to survive. If you sign on for a ride through the window of hell, make sure the initial financial arrangement is very good – including an appropriate capitation rate – since any increase in revenues is unlikely during the window of hell.

For our system, the window of hell opened noticeably when the percentage of capitated lives approached 40 percent. Money for bonuses, a tradition in the organization, suddenly wasn't there. Programs that didn't generate revenue began to be cut back. By the time capitation reached 60 percent, the system was facing serious financial problems and major cutbacks became necessary. Income for family physicians has remained stable, with most doing better under capitation than discounted fee-for-service. We will probably come out of the window of hell when capitation reached 80 percent, if we can have a growth in the total number of lives and can make the necessary changes. Delivery systems like ours are faced with the paradoxical challenge facing many industries today – improving service while downsizing.

There are ways to lessen the pain the window of hell. The wrong way would be to take advantage of fee-for-service revenues while they last, while at the same time working hard to be efficient under capitation. This schizophrenic way of delivering health care would be difficult to justify to the public or payers. The better way is to accept that costs must be reduced, that unnecessary care and wasteful overhead can no longer be tolerated – to prepare for capitation as rapidly as possible.

If you find yourself in the window of hell, my advice is to help your system through it. After all, you are part of the solution. Moving to another area in which capitation has not yet arrived does not make much sense. Who wants to live through hell twice?

Working for an Organization

Family Practice Management
1995;2(8):10-11

Physicians, in general, are an independent breed. A standard cliché is that you go to medical school partly to become your own boss. Private practice allows for such independent-spirited behavior. Physicians have traditionally been captains of their own ship.

All that seems to be changing, doesn't it? Rapidly, one way or another, physicians are becoming part of large organizations. Very few residency graduates are starting their own practices, and the number joining private practices is shrinking. Many are becoming salaried employees of large medical groups or health care organizations. This may say something about the lack of independent business spirit in the new generation of physicians, or it may say something about their lack of options in this regard. In any case, this new generation seems to be coping with the situation reasonably well. But what about the generation that has been in private practice for some time? Somehow, many of us are adjusting to a new reality – working for a large organization. I am, for one.

While I was "captain of a ship" for 14 years, I now work for a large organization. I was recruited to Sharp HealthCare in San Diego in 1992 to develop a new family practice residency program. Part of this process was to start a new faculty practice group within Sharp (now 15 family physicians in three sites). This was done through a combination of bringing in family physicians from private practice and recruiting new faculty from outside the area. While the overall results have been positive, the process has not always been smooth.

I want to share some observations and some insights I've gained in the process of adjusting. I will draw from a marvelous book by Peter Senge, The Fifth Discipline: The Art and Practice of the Learning Organization (Doubleday Currency, 1990), which says much about how organizations should work. I will also draw from the mistakes I've made in my transition to working for an organization. Why should I be the only one to learn from my mistakes?

My first mistake: I thought it would be easy. Since family practice is what health care organizations need most today, I thought the organization would make it quick and easy to establish a new family practice group. But my experience in small-group practice hadn't prepared me for the way any member of a large organization has to move at the speed of the whole organization and in paths the organization has laid out. Large organizations are complex, and their decision-making processes may be convoluted. Organizations have their own cultures and hierarchies, and each has different channels for information. And it isn't just that the decision making is a slow and complicated process: Just learning how it works (and how to make it work) requires considerable time and effort.

My second mistake: I assumed the organization would adjust to me. The culture of an organization is a complex set of behavior patterns, values and beliefs. Joining a large organization requires that you become part of this culture. Thinking you can change that culture is hopelessly naïve. Of course, the culture of any organization must evolve, and you may be an important part of this evolution. But ultimately you will be called upon to adjust to the organization rather than vice versa.

My third mistake: I assumed everyone would help me. Since family practice is so clearly needed and my role is to develop and expand family practice, I assumed I would have all the support and assistance the organization could offer. But change or development in one area usually means de-emphasis in another. Some in the organization will always be skeptical or threatened by change, and they may act in ways intended to prove them right at the expense of your success. Moreover, even with general conceptual support for what you do, everyone is very busy keeping his or her own house in order, and no one may have much time to assist you. It often feels that you will succeed (if you do) despite the organization rather than because of it.

In his book, Serge offers several "laws" of organizations. Five of them, in particular, strike me as applying directly to my experience and that of my colleagues trying to build something new within an existing organization.

Every problem was once a solution (that someone was invested in). Before you go after perceived problems aggressively, think about who may be threatened by your actions – for example, key specialists in an environment of surplus or overpaid specialists. Your goal may be increased reimbursement for family physicians, and this may have to come from monies now given to specialists. You will need a good relationship with key specialists in your organization to succeed.

The harder you push, the harder the system pushes back. Pushing your agenda or pushing for change is usually counterproductive. Learning the pace at which change takes place in an organization and the processes by which change proceeds is difficult and requires a great deal of patience.

Faster is slower. This follows directly from the above. If you try to accomplish something too fast and end up failing, you may not get another chance for quite a while. Slow and study progress toward a goal will achieve the desired result in the quickest way. Don't try to make things happen. Help them fall into place.

Cause and effect are not closely related in time and space. For the quick, analytical mind, this may be frustrating. Taking an historic perspective is important. The managed care changes of the '90s are a result of health care spending in the '70s and '80s, and not what someone is inventing today. This "law" also helps explain why the right thing sometimes seems to happen for the wrong reasons.

There is no blame. Criticizing someone in your organization merely provides evidence that you are a dysfunctional team or not a team at all. Assuming a victim mentality will compromise any chance of success you may have. Organizations are complex obstacle courses, even though almost everyone is simply trying to do the right thing. Your job is to work within the organization to accomplish whatever the organization wishes or needs.

Within an organization, any personal agenda takes a back seat to what the organization as a whole is doing or wants to do. However good they are, your ideas will seem bad if they are not in step with the organization's goals. If you push your ideas anyway, you will be seen as a problem, not a solver of problems.

Many family physicians are joining large organizations and for many different reasons. Joining a large organization may just make sense for your practice and your community. You may have leadership goals that can only be realized in a large organization. Regardless, understanding organizational behavior and culture is critical to your satisfaction and success. And if all else seems to be failing, just concentrate on taking good care of your patients. After all, that is what you went to medical school for. By pouring your energies into patient care, you'll be able to avoid frustration with the pace of change; by keeping one eye on organizational developments, you'll be able to seize opportunities to nudge things in the right direction.

Marcus Welby Returns

Family Practice Management
1997;4(6):11-12

A family physician medical director of a large managed care group recently told me, "Marcus Welby is dead." With a multidisciplinary team of health care workers in the office, extended hours for urgent care, a 24-hour nurse-on-call system and disease management programs, he said, the old-fashioned family doctor is no longer relevant. He predicted that family physicians will play a specific and limited role in the office and that people will have their relationships with institutions rather than specific physicians.

I don't think so.

True, health care is changing dramatically. The small, independent medical office with a do-it-all personal physician is being replaced by larger medical groups. Many people have a primary care physician designated on their HMO insurance card but have never met that person. Population-based delivery systems are designing new ways of "servicing the health care" of "covered lives". Many people, especially young, healthy adults, have expressed little interest in having a personal family physician.

Into the Machine

We are entering a very mechanistic phase of health care delivery. Efficiency – delivering quality service at the lowest cost – is the mantra of managed care organizations. Disease management programs and call centers are two of the latest examples of "advanced thinking" in managed care. One gets the impression that health care can be divided into bits and pieces that can be assigned to a variety of people and programs. The race is on to design the best system of care.

As I watch this whirlwind of change, I remember the aphorism that every problem was once somebody's solution. The mandatory gatekeeper was an early solution to controlling health care costs. It worked, but it created much unhappiness and put obstacles in the path of people who truly needed the care of referral specialists. The managed care industry eventually rediscovered how important choice is to many Americans.

Now we're watching a new solution play out. As family physicians are being assigned to office care in large groups, standardized schedules and measures of productivity are being developed. Primary health care is being chopped up into 15-minute units of service. Everything is neat and orderly, but physician morale and professional behavior are suffering, and the public is fearful.

If diseases and other health care needs actually existed outside of people, mechanistic systems like the ones now being built would work fine. But people and their health care needs are inseparable.

Sometime, and I hope soon, the managed care world is going to rediscover the nature of illness – how people experience being unwell. Even people with the same disease vary greatly in their illnesses and in how they seek health care. Hippocrates, Osler, Michael Balint, Gayle Stephens and, yes, even Marcus Welby understood the individual nature of illness and the degree of flexibility it requires of healers.

The wisdom of the ages has shown that two of the most

important parts of treating illness are time and the doctor-patient relationship. These two therapeutic tools are getting lost in the new delivery systems.

People make fun of Marcus Welby because the TV show suggested that he treated just one patient a week. Actually, I think this misses the point. I imagine Marcus Welby, and the team of residents and faculty who worked with him, treating many people a week. What the TV series showed was how Marcus Welby – by taking the necessary time and by exploring the family and social situation – was able to achieve one major therapeutic triumph every week. If only we could be so efficient and powerful! Maybe we could if we had the time, but to have the time requires control of and flexibility in our work environment – control and flexibility we just don't have today.

I fear that the mechanistic, standardized work role of family physicians will greatly reduce our therapeutic power. Short appointments are fine for dealing with simple problems, but for complex illness, the short visit leaves us spinning our wheels. The mechanistic solution turns out to be a problem in search of its own solution.

Into the Future

I have a prediction. The family physician's practice in the future will not be 24 or more visits per day on a standardized schedule of work units. Image this: The family physician sees 12 patients in a day. Each visit is an intense personal discussion and examination of the patient's health problems, often in the context of the family and social situation. However, with the collaboration of a nurse practitioner or physician assistant, a well-trained advice nurse, a well-trained telephone worker and email, the physician is able to meet the health care needs of 50 patients in one day. This family physician still takes responsibility for as many patients as the one now seeing 30 patients a day.

I spend much of my time now as a health care executive. Curiously, a busy 10-hour day for an executive is about eight appointments or meetings. After all, it takes time to sort out and process the problems of an organization. I also spend time as a mentor. A busy day advising students is about eight appointments.

After all, it takes time to sort out all the issues. Are our patients' illnesses any less complex? Do we not require just as much time to achieve therapeutic success? Certainly we physicians receive enough training to serve as executives or mentors in the care of our patients.

When I was in a private fee-for-service practice, where I could generate revenue only by seeing patients, I averaged 27 patient visits per day. Driving home, I often wished I'd had more time with the 12 or so patients that really needed me that day – time I couldn't give because I was busy attending to the needs of the rest.

While managed care today seems to be giving doctors less time with patients, I am optimistic that this will change. Spinning our wheels and not treating the complexity of illness is not only poor care; it's poor business in the long run. Physicians and patients are becoming progressively unhappier. But capitated care uncouples amount of revenue from number of visits, and team care unshackles the physician from routine complaints. Together, they have the potential to free physicians to concentrate on the patients who really need their help while not neglecting the rest. Marcus Welby returns!

The family physicians of the future will have many ways to care for their patients. They will have computers on their desks, at home and in their exam rooms. Much of their communication with patients will be electronic. (Think of the number of patients who would rather not leave the house, fight traffic, find a parking spot and survive the waiting room just to have a question answered or an obvious problem treated.) Each physician will have a talented staff helping to care for a population of patients. Each will have an intense personal relationship with those patients who want or need him or her. And, just maybe, each physician will achieve a major therapeutic triumph every week.

One editorial the AAFP would not let me publish in Family Practice Management fearing that it contained financial information that would suggest price fixing. However the California Academy of Family Physicians (CAFP) saw no conflict and the following was published in their journal and was reprinted in several other state academy journals:

What is a Family Physician Worth?

California Family Physician
1994;45(6):15-16

You are the family doctor. You respond to all of the health care needs of your patients – from head to toe, womb to tomb, day or night. You are trained and able to handle 85-95 percent of all of the reasons a person needs a physician. Middle of the night calls about chest pain, trouble breathing and fever in a young child are routine. In the new managed care environment, you have been "discovered" as the key to controlling health care costs. A person's desire to receive all of his or her health care from or through a family physician has become a requirement.

Reflecting on all of this responsibility and service one would assume that the family physician is valued with a significant chunk of the health care dollar. It is shocking to discover that the family physician traditionally receives as little as six cents to at most 10 cents of the health insurance dollar. This is typically half or less of the amount kept by the insurance company, half or less than the amount given to the specialists we prudently refer to, only a quarter of what goes to the hospital, and even less than what goes to the pharmaceutical industry for the drugs we prescribe. We are undoubtedly the most undervalued part of the health care system. In the new economic paradigm of budgeted health care, with capitated payments, we have an opportunity to change all of this.

How did this terrible imbalance occur? Actually, quite inadvertently. During the 1960s and 1970s, as family physicians kept their fees reasonable, other providers took advantage of the open checkbook fee-for-service medicine paid for by third-party payers.

This resulted in extraordinary health care costs in hospitals and by procedural specialists. During the 1980s, as attempts were made to control health care costs, all providers were discounted, including family physicians. The resource-based relative value scale (RBRVS) was government's attempt to fix the fee-for-service system, but all that resulted was some reduction in reimbursement for procedures and no increases for the family physician.

As we enter into capitated medicine, there is an opportunity to reconsider the value of all health care services. When capitation formulas are based on the traditional fee-for-service model, family physicians typically receive about eight to twelve dollars a month to care for an average adult (non-senior). With a typical monthly insurance premium of $120, this equates to six to ten percent of the premium dollar. With a typical active practice of 2,000 lives, and 50-60 percent or more taken by overhead costs, the family physician is locked into a fixed income that is at the low end of the physician's earning ladder. Should family physicians earn less than other specialists? Given our scope of practice and responsibilities, certainly not!

Determining the value of a family physician compared with other health services is somewhat arbitrary. Comparing physician services with hospital services, home health care, laboratory, X-ray and pharmaceuticals is like comparing apples, oranges and other varieties of fruit. Rational judgments can be made that take into account appropriate overhead costs.

Hsaio and his colleagues at Harvard attempted to develop a complex mathematical formula that determined the value of physician services. This resource-based relative value scale provides a more rational model for paying physicians than the historical fee schedules, which favored technology and procedures over spending time with patients.

The concept of RBRVS was that physicians enduring longer training and providing greater technical skill in more serious situations would receive higher reimbursement. The time with patients was also valued and, through the RBRVS formula, family physicians should have received 30-40 present higher earnings.

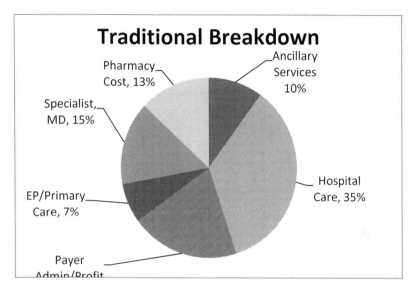

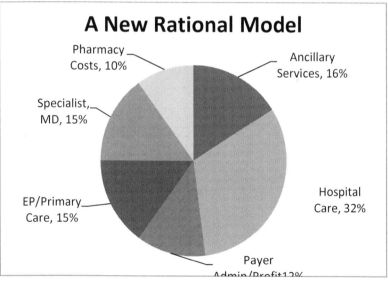

Figure 1

Figure 1 illustrates the traditional fee-for-service breakdown of the health care dollar and a more rational breakdown for the future. As you can see, the future model values the primary care physician, with half of the dollars going for physician services. This increase comes largely from a reduction in funds traditionally used for profit and administration. There is also some reduction in drug and hospital costs.

If a capitation formula is developed to give the family physician 15 percent of the premium dollar that would amount to $18 per member per month based on a $120 per month premium. The amounts would be higher for Medicare. A comparable amount would be divided among other specialists based on the frequency of use of these specialists.

If the modest shift in reimbursement proposed here were to occur, the financial situation for family physicians would change greatly. By earning 15 percent of the health care dollar, family physicians would have an average income at the median of all physician incomes (now at about $175,000/year). This is appropriate for the extent of our training and the nature of our responsibilities, particularly in a managed care environment.

This value is not going to be simply handed to family physicians on a platter. As a specialty, we must negotiate a proper level of reimbursement based on rational thinking.

There are two ways to increase reimbursement to family physicians in a capitated system. One is to give the family physician an appropriate capitated payment as illustrated in Figure 1. The other is for the family physicians to receive a lower capitation and the risk pool funds left over as a result of good case management. Either way, the family physician should be accountable and rewarded for providing quality, cost-efficient health care.

I propose two related slogans to carry this message. The first is "15 percent for 85 percent." This means the family physicians should receive 15 percent of the health care dollar for being able to manage 85 percent or more of the reasons a person goes to a physician.

Another would be "50 percent for 85 percent." This means that family physicians should receive 50 percent of the dollars going to physicians for providing 85 percent or more of the physician visits.

The enactment of these concepts does not require radical change and can be done without seriously hurting other components of the health care system. The low reimbursement of family physicians has been cited as a major reason why large numbers of medical students are not choosing family practice. Such a new valuation of the family physician is just and reflects our return to a central role in health care.

In 1995 I became president of the California Academy of Family Physicians and I wrote 6 columns over two years. One is reprinted here that focuses on restraint of the practice of family medicine in emerging health care organizations. We fought a battle in California with the support of AAFP around Caesarian section privileges for a well-trained family physician in rural practice. We lost that battle but it help mobilize the specialty around scope of practice issues:

Truth, Justice and the American Way

President's Message
California Family Physician
1996;47(1):7

Competition and choice are core American values. Our nation learned long ago that an energetic economy and high quality at a good price result if consumers are able to choose goods and services from private enterprises that have to compete fairly in an open market. Freedom to practice a trade is another core American value which allows anyone to exercise his skills in an open market.

The Sherman Act was passed by Congress more than 100 years ago establishing our anti-trust laws. It is illegal, even a felony, for a company or a group of individuals to act in collusion to drive out competition. Yes, this legislation applies to physicians and hospitals. For example, if a group of obstetricians in a community get together to prevent a qualified family physician from delivering babies, they are acting illegally. If the obstetricians did this as part of serving on a department of the community hospital, and the hospital supported this action, the hospital is also acting illegally.

Just such a case was ruled in favor of a family physician, Arlene Brown, this year in New Mexico. Dr. Brown was awarded triple damages, or $600,000, from a group of obstetricians and the hospital. Restraint of trade activities are not protected by peer review at the hospital, and the physicians generally do not have insurance protection for such illegal acts.

If appears that similar activities to limit FPs' scope of practice are unfortunately common today among physicians and community hospitals. As your Academy president this year, I hear about these instances, and they are occurring in rural and urban settings. The most common anticompetitive behavior encountered by CAFP is obstetric privileges. The California Chapter of the American College of Obstetricians and Gynecologists (ACOG) has been very supportive of family physicians doing obstetrics. While the collaboration has aided CAFP in its assistance to FPs with OB privilege problems, some hospital OB departments remain unyielding on the issues of FPs and obstetric care.

Defending family physicians with hospital privileging problems is complicated in part by the case of Hay v. Scripps Memorial settled in the late 1970s. James Hay is a family physician who sought D&C privileges at Scripps Memorial Hospital in La Jolla. When these privileges were denied with the hospital stating that only OB-GYNs could do D&Cs, the CAFP and the AAFP assisted Dr. Hay in his defense, claiming restraint of trade. Dr. Hay and the Academy lost this case because Dr. Hay had D&C privileges at another community hospital; hence he was not prevented from practicing his profession. It appears from this case that if there are multiple hospitals in a community, some of these hospitals may define themselves as "more specialized." If all the hospitals in a community acted together to prevent the privileges of a qualified physician, this would be illegal. By implication, if there is one hospital in a community, or just one hospital with certain services such as obstetrics, the medical staff and hospital should be open to all qualified physicians. Moreover, privileging should be based on training or experience and demonstrated competence, and not by specialty (AMA, JCAHO, AARP, and ACOG policy).

The California Academy of Family Physicians is committed to supporting all our members who are unfairly denied the opportunity to obtain privileges for which they are qualified. Quality of patient care should be the only concern in negotiating for privileges, and there is ample evidence that well-trained family physicians practice high quality care in all areas of family medicine including obstetrics.

In this time of oversupply of specialists, competition or privileges can be intense and specialists may be acting illegally against family physicians. We may need a legal case in California to heighten the awareness of physicians and hospitals regarding restraint of trade behaviors. Family physicians should not back down from practicing the skills for which they are trained. Truth, justice, and the American way (Superman!) are on our side.

Was managed care ultimately more helpful or harmful for family medicine? Many of the specialty's founders, most notably Gayle Stephens, felt that managed care and the gatekeeper role violated the ethics of good medical practice. As someone whose practice developed during the managed care period, I saw plenty of room to remain a high quality and ethical family physician. These two articles describe my position.

Does Managed Care Contaminate Practice?

In a properly managed system, patient advocacy and gatekeeping go hand in hand.

Family Practice Management
1994;1(1):94-100

To many, the transformation from independent, fee-for-service medicine to managed care contaminates the doctor-patient relationship. How can a physician be pure as a patient advocate when cost containment becomes an additional duty? Is managed care challenging the Hippocratic tradition of placing the needs of the patient above all other concerns? Are physicians losing their freedom to practice medicine autonomously in an office they control?

Some say managed care raises no more ethical conflicts than fee-for-service practiced, where the physician has an economic incentive to provide unnecessary services. And surely most physicians do their best to act purely in the patient's interest regardless of economic gain. But in managed care, acting in the patient's interest may result in loss of income, either for the physician or for the organization that employs the physician. Fear of loss may be a more pervasive economic incentive than greed.

Managed care does have its obvious advantages. Our traditional approach to health care has resulted in costs so excessive that they are crippling American industry, bankrupting local and state governments, adding to the federal deficit and severely limiting funds for other social services. The idea that our resources are limited is not a traditional American concept, but it is a fact of life. Managed care provides a means for rationally distributing limited health care resources. Managed care is here to stay, and on a societal scale it seems to have a lot to offer. The question is how we can make it work best for individual patients and physicians.

How managed care is applied in the exam room and how it affects the doctor-patient relationship have enormous implications for the ethics of medical practice and the survival of the Hippocratic tradition. When a person is ill and sees a physician, that person expects the physician to be focused solely on diagnosing and treating the problem. If a family has an ongoing relationship with a physician, the family expects the physician to care about their welfare above any other concerns. We cannot allow this trust to be violated in the economic shift to managed care.

In a 1991 article published in the Hastings Center Report, Marion Danis and Larry R. Churchill offer a perspective on the role of the physician in a society facing the reality of limited resources.[1] They argue for broadening the ethic of medical practice. Without abandoning the patient-centered Hippocratic tradition, they say, physicians should consider themselves citizens in a society that strives for social justice. Danis and Churchill argue that for too long physicians have been "dodging the dilemma" of balancing individual wants and needs with society's greater good. Physicians who are good citizens will want to provide high-quality care for their patients and will want to conserve health care resources to meet society's needs. In an interview last year in JAMA, Uwe Reinhardt noted this attitude among physicians and patients in some European countries where the limitations on resources for medical care are clearly recognized.[2] Of course, conserving health care resources may at times temper how much the physician can give an individual patient.

Consider a 60-year-old patient with new chest pain. The signs and symptoms suggest angina, but could also be caused by heartburn. If the physician is at direct financial risk based on his or her clinical judgment, the patient's care may be seriously compromised.

Workups for new-onset angina are usually expensive, and such costs should not come out of the physician's pocket. Rather, the physician should seek only the best care for the patient, while recognizing that resources are limited. This would mean aggressively seeking a cardiac workup for this patient but deferring it for a patient whose signs and symptoms suggest heartburn. The physician may be expected to follow clinical guidelines developed by a large entity (maybe the AAFP) and agreed upon by the physician's medical group. The physician is rewarded for providing quality care – not for limiting the quantity of care. If a heart transplant becomes the only treatment option left and is not available to the patient, the physician and patient share in this difficult situation.

Micromanagement or Macromanagement

Managed care is ethically feasible – and the Hippocratic tradition of medicine can be preserved – if cost-containment pressures can be made to act at a societal level rather than bearing directly on the doctor-patient relationship. In practical terms, this means that the managed care organization must avoid analyzing and trying to manage the actions of individual physicians caring for individual patients. This micromanagement is common in new managed care plans and is dangerous in its impact on physicians and patients.

Health economists and administrators think of primary care physicians as gatekeepers, and the concept may be useful when comparing a primary care doctor-patient relationship with open access to the health care supermarket of subspecialists. But to ask primary care physicians to think like gatekeepers in caring for patients creates ethical conflicts and contaminates caring for patients. After all, despite the increase in wellness visits, patients are a wounded humanity bringing their complex lives to physicians as illnesses.

If a managed care system wants good gatekeeping, it need only train or hire enough good primary care physicians and provide incentives for them to stay in the system: fair pay, a reasonable work load and opportunities to enjoy their practice and stay current. Primary care physicians are as well-trained as any physician to care for about 90 percent of the reasons a person seeks health care. This is possible because primary care physicians are experts in treating common health problems. The gatekeeper phenomenon is automatic with well-trained primary care physicians.

This is macromanagement rather than micromanagement: Create an environment that fosters high-quality, efficient care; set the necessary limits on the use of medical resources; then let physicians care for patients. Macromanagement even allows the physician to commiserate with the patient about the limits of available services.

Given the fact that terms like gatekeeper and case manager are useful to health care planners but have no place in the psyche of primary care physicians, the two perspectives need not be in conflict. Experienced and successful managed care systems appear to have resolved this dilemma. Physicians who practice in staff-model HMOs such as Kaiser Permanente or Group Health Cooperative of Puget Sound express an acceptable degree of freedom in serving their patients. They practice as "citizens" in a system of care: They do not have to claim responsibility for making the rules or setting the limits. They see their community of patients receiving consistent, quality health care.

Physicians: Leaders or Victims?

Managed competition is more than a proposal for health care reform: It is happening now. The Clinton administration appears to have embraced managed competition and must now figure out how to place the uninsured into such a system.

The full scope of managed competition, and its inevitability as the American model of health care, can be understood by dividing it into two parts: the mechanism of budgeting and reimbursement for health care on the one hand, and providers of care – physician groups, hospitals, etc. – on the other. The former is what is usually referred to when discussing reform proposals. Managed competition calls for multiple managed care plans operating in a given region, competing for contracts to provide health care to employer groups and other populations groups such as Medicare and Medicaid recipients. An organized delivery system under managed competition results from a level playing field of regulations produced by a local or central health care policy group. The Clinton health care reform proposal has captured the support of many groups in America because it offers the potential for universal coverage, standardized benefits, quality controls and efficiency coming from the market forces of competition.

However, it is the provider transformation going on throughout the country that makes managed competition inevitable. Our cottage industry of small, independent practices, hospitals and other health care enterprises is giving way to regional, integrated systems of care. These integrated systems are forming to compete as units of health care delivery with the goal of efficiency and quality comparable to or better than those of staff model HMOs. Soon, in most metropolitan areas, virtually all providers will be operating in one of several regional systems of care. Some systems are reaching out to rural areas, acquiring hospitals and physicians, to provide a broad geographic continuum of care. This new medical infrastructure, with its competing regional systems of care, makes managed completion the obvious model for health care in America.

One consequence of the development of this new infrastructure is that physicians are no longer autonomous captains of their practices, but rather are key participants in a much larger model of health care. Loss of control over the practice of medicine is the greatest source of physician discontent today. Physicians feel victimized as payers take greater control over clinical decisions. One physician writes that he now feels like the third party with patients[3] Getting approval for a medical service, usually from a person with less training than the physician, has become a daily irritant. Outright denials of service that the physician considered warranted seem like violations of clinical judgment – and they place the physician in a catch-22 situation with respect to liability. In the office, with our patients asking why and why not, the larger picture of social justice may be hard to focus.

Minimizing the micromanagement of medical practice will help, but what will help most is for some family physicians to take a leadership role in making sure the system works, not to protect their own interests or those of physicians in general, but to protect their patients and to protect physicians' ability to care for their patients.

Some physicians will be leaders in macromanagement, helping to set overall policies that balance quality and cost containment. All physicians in practice should take the lead to drive out the contaminants of micromanagement from medical practice. In turn, all physicians should act as citizens of the system, conserving health care resources for those who most need them.

If non-physician health care executives are left alone to design managed care systems based on economic data, with physicians as mere players, the mistakes will result in great physician dissatisfaction and a feeling of victimization. To the administrator, patients become a panel, while physician workload and productivity are determined in the aggregate. This administrative approach is workable only if there is reality testing regarding the actual practice of medicine, especially with difficult patients. Physician leaders, who can speak the same language as the administrator yet can also reflect the reality of caring for patients "in the trenches," are crucial to the success of managed care.

References

1. Danis M, Churchill LR. Autonomy and the common weal. Hast Cent Rep. 1991; 21(1):25-31.
2. Breo DL. Uwe Reinhardt, PhD – the economist as health evangelist. JAMA. 1992;268:1332-1336.
3. Is it still a privilege to be a doctor? [Letters] N Engl J Med. 1986;315:1097-1099.

Does the Personal Physician Continue in Managed Care?

The Journal of the American Board of Family Practice
1996;9(1):67-68

As health care in America transforms from a cottage industry of private physicians to large organized delivery systems, there is a fundamental question facing family physicians. Are we to continue as personal physicians to a group of families and individuals, or are we to become simply providers of primary care services? The dangerous aspect of this question today is that the transition from personal physician to provider of a limited range of services is occurring subtly and might not be apparent. Just as the frog about to be boiled does not jump out of the water if the heat is turned up slowly, so might the family physicians in a large medical group or delivery system experience erosion of the personal physician role without realizing the loss until it is gone. Unwittingly, family physicians might welcome some of the changes – having fewer fit-in appointments disrupt the schedule, giving up hospital work to hospital-based physicians, turning over after-hours calls to a nurse connection service. Family physicians might then realize that patients see them for only a part of their health care, and the patients have little identity with them as their personal physician.

The designers of new delivery systems, using a population-based perspective, conceive of multidisciplinary models of care that could replace the do-it-all personal physician. For example, case managers, usually nurses, are assigned to patients and families upon enrollment to ascertain health status and risk and direct the patients to a variety of services within the system, including a primary care physician. This early intervention and triage are felt to increase efficiency and prevent through early intervention the later use of expensive services. Why wait until the patient needs to see a physician to coordinate care?

Disease management is the latest concept capturing the imagination of large delivery systems. To ensure that patients with certain diseases, such as asthma and congestive heart failure, receive state-of-the-art care as soon as their conditions are diagnosed, they are referred to a multidisciplinary team of advanced practice nurses and other therapists led by a specialist medical director. This care is offered on an outpatient basis to prevent expensive emergency department visits and hospitalization and in a specialized way to allow "optimum management" of the disease. Oh yes, be sure to keep the primary care physician informed.

In this issue Weyrauch reports on the importance of seeing one's own physician or physician of choice.[1] Patient satisfaction is much greater when the personal physician, with knowledge of the patient and trust having already been established, is able to address the problems. Weyrauch did his research in a long-established and one of the largest health maintenance organizations in the country – Group Health Cooperative of Puget Sound. The patients are familiar with managed care and by and large have chosen this model. It is heartening to see that this group values seeing their personal physician as much as does the population at large. But is their care better? Patient satisfaction is important, but not enough. Research is needed comparing medical outcomes of patients receiving comprehensive care through a personal physician or a multidisciplinary system. We need to find out whether the personal physician has a healing power that cannot be replicated by a multidisciplinary team. Michael Balint,[2] Gayle Stephens,[3] and more recently Howard Brody[4] have given us the lessons and prose. Weyrauch's research is an important early step.

Many either-or questions have an ultimate answer of both. Multidisciplinary teams have real value as resources to enhance patient care. Family physicians acting alone have a dismal record in certain outcomes, such as rate of patients' receiving important preventive services. The family physician of the future will be required to orchestrate an even larger range of services, but will it be easier being part of integrated delivery systems? As patients receive more of their health care in different places from different people, the relationship with the family physician as personal physician could be attenuated. In the same way that young ducks or goats can imprint on a different species, our patients could attach to another place or person of care.

If lost in the complexity of new delivery systems, the personal physician might have to be rediscovered, because patients will, I hope, perceive the need. Health care will continue to be consumer driven. As a specialty, family practice must work heard to prevent this loss from happening. Osler said it is as important to know the person with the disease as which disease the person has. We will need to prove this maxim. We also need to be in the middle of health system design so a balance of personal physician and multidisciplinary services is achieved.

References

1. Weyrauch KF. Does continuity of care increase HMO patients' satisfaction with physician performance? J Am Board Fam Pract 1996;9:31-36.
2. Balint M. The doctor, his patient and the illness. New York: International Universities Press, 1957.
3. Stephens GG. The intellectual basis of family practice. Tucson: Winter Publishing, 1982.
4. Brody H. The healer's power. New Haven: Yale University Press, 1992.

During my twelve years in practice in Dixon and being the family medicine advisor for UC Davis, I had a medical student in my office most of the time. I put them to work, and consequently won the best clinical teacher award at UC Davis three times. My philosophy of medical students engaged in the health care team was shared by Bill Fowkes at Stanford and we wrote the following article. Some wrote pushback that we were fostering medical student abuse, but they clearly missed the point. Too much medical student education is observation.

It's Time to Put Medical Students Back to Work

By Joseph E. Scherger, MD, MPH; William C. Fowkes, MD

Family Medicine
1997;29(2):137-138

In the old days, medical students worked while they learned. They drew blood, took it to the lab, performed the complete blood count using a hemocytometer, and read the smear. They collected urine, sniffed it, spun it, analyzed it under the microscope, and plated the culture. They performed histories and physicals, which were confirmed by residents or faculty. Their note was often the definitive record. Part-time opportunities were available for medical students to work outside of medical schools as "externs," where varied tasks were assigned, including completing histories and physical examinations on patients scheduled by busy practitioners for following-day surgery, or even assisting in the operating room in a pinch. Medical students functioned as members of the health care team. Though not sanctioned and sometimes frowned on by traditional medical school faculty, the tasks performed by these students were valuable to the community hospital and were great learning experiences for the students involved.

Over the past 30 years, the role and responsibilities of medical students have changed. Medical student education, for the most part, has been separated from service. Funding for medical education expanded after 1965, and the medical student experience became gentrified. Even simulated patients have been used to give students a standardized experience. Medical students are not expected to perform any real patient care. Having students on the care team is often viewed as more of a burden than a help.

Whether medical education in the old days was better or not could be debated. Medical student abuse was more common in the days of heavy service and should be condemned. Service and education are both competing and complementary factors. Finding a balance between service and education is a continuing goal of medical education. However, the concept of education through service, which defines residency education, has been lost at the medical student level. We may not be able to afford this any longer.

The setting of medical education is changing dramatically in the 1990s. Hospitals are convenient places for medical student education; the patient is captive, and time and space are rarely an issue. But hospitals are no longer the place where common diseases are treated. More often, the diagnoses have already been made when the patient is admitted. Most health problems, even serious ones, are treated outside the hospital. Medical student education is shifting to ambulatory settings, where a schedule must be maintained to permit efficient patient flow. It is possible that the student may slow down the provision of care, decrease productivity, and increase costs. It has been suggested that, because of inefficiencies in the use of faculty teaching time, teaching in ambulatory settings may be as much as five times as costly as teaching in the hospital environment.[1]

Managed care organizations, which place efficiency of patient care as a top priority, are dominating the landscape. Can medical students be useful in ambulatory care, or are they a burden who slow down the process of care and require extra faculty time? The latter is the prevalent attitude today[2,3] and is causing great uncertainty about how medical student education can work in ambulatory settings under managed care. Who will fund medical student education, and what settings will tolerate having them are common questions today.

We believe that the process of medical student education in clinical settings needs to be reconsidered, with a return to a philosophy of education through service. Medical students can function as members of the health care team in ambulatory settings. Medical student education may then be palatable and even attractive in busy practices. If this is done appropriately, the quality of medical education will improve.

We have found that experienced preceptors in primary care settings not only enjoy having students but have found them useful. The literature suggests that medical students take extra time in the office,[3-5] but this has not been our experience nor the experience of other preceptors.[5] Also, the put-you-to-work approach has been well accepted by medical students; they like being useful as long as they are not over-loaded with patient responsibilities.

Even first- and second-year medical students can benefit an office. Community clinics have used preclinical students as medical assistants and patient advocates. The student brings the patient in from the waiting room, takes the vital signs, takes an expanded chief complaint history, and then stays with the patient while the physician is in the room. The student may escort the patient out and make sure all questions have been answered. If trained, the student may write the process note. An extra room is all that is needed, and the office staff and the physician appreciate the help. What a learning experience!

Third- and fourth-year students can be as useful to an office as a physician assistant. Additional training time is necessary up front to learn office procedures. The student then becomes an assistant provider with the physician. For example, with an intermediate office visit, the student may spend 30-40 minutes independently with the patient while the precepting supervisor continues seeing scheduled patients. What may have required 20 minutes of direct physician time with a patient could be reduced to 10 minutes of patient time and teaching (done together or separately). This saved time accumulates during an office day to allow more time for returning phone calls, completing paperwork, seeing extra patients, or finishing early. This benefit is not theoretical and is the experience of many preceptors. Community faculty who find that the presence of a student interferes with productivity or prolongs the working day probably need training in this mode of student management.

Medical students enjoy helping out and giving real patient care service. The preceptor should expect the student to read independently about patients seen and not have to give the student all the education around each encounter. Active learning has the student spending more time seeking information, while passive learning requires more time of the preceptor. This was a fundamental difference found by Vinson et al in showing that community preceptors had decreased productivity and more often used passive learning than academically based faculty.[5]

How we train medical students may need to be changed to make them functional members of the health care team in primary care settings. We would need to give students real clinical skills. (A radical concept?) Introductory courses in clinical medicine would include taking accurate vital signs and patient histories, along with basic office skills common to a medical assistant. More advanced courses would include problem-specific history taking, physical examination, prevention, and care of common health problems. We may need to reverse the order of medical education to start with basic knowledge and skills and reserve the most complicated patients for later. (Another radical concept?)

Putting medical students to work in patient care has legal and financial obstacles. The responsibility and payment for care is to the physician. We are not suggesting that the student is a substitute for the physician in this responsibility. The teaching physician must carefully supervise and be engaged with all patient care done by students. Patients must feel that they were cared for by the physician with the assistance of a student who gave them additional time. This is the art of clinical teaching in the ambulatory setting.

Funding for medical student education is critically important for medical school and department infrastructure, non-clinical teaching time, and teacher training. However, medical students should spend most of their time learning in clinical settings. If this time is a cost factor, then medical education may be more expensive than our resources allow, and most clinical settings will be reluctant to participate unless funded. If clinical education is able to pay for itself, medical student education can be much less expensive, and community practices and managed care organizations would be more willing to participate. We do not believe that this is just an economic issue and that medical students must become mercenaries. Medical education is enhanced through service, and an optimal balance of education and service is achieved even when medical students enhance office productivity. It's time to put medical students back to work!

References

1. Sostok MA, Luke RG, Rouan G. Confronting the costs of ambulatory care training. Acad Med 1994; 70:949-50.
2. Delbanco TL, Calkins DR. The costs and financing of ambulatory medicine education. J Gen Intern Med 1998;70(3 suppl):S34-43.
3. Vinson DC, Paden C. The effects of teaching medical students on private practitioners' workloads. Acad Med 1994;69:237-8.
4. Fields SA, Toffler WL, Bledsoe NM. Impact of the presence of a third-year medical student on gross charges and patient volumes in 22 rural community practices. Acad Med 1995;69(10 suppl):S87-9.
5. Vinson DC, Paden C, Devera-Sales A. Impact of medical student teaching on family physicians' use of time. J Fam Pract 1996; 42:243-9.

By the late 1990s leadership and standing up for your own department was not enough for family medicine. What some called "fortress family medicine" had become counter-productive in the new integrated delivery systems. Family medicine needed to integrate with other specialties and by doing that, family medicine increased its potential for leadership. I wrote about this new phase in the following:

Phase Three of Academic Family Medicine

Family Medicine
1997;29(6):439-440

The organization of health care continues to change dramatically in the United States throughout the 1990s. Independent private practice is being replaced by regional and national organized delivery systems. Academic health centers are realizing that they can no longer stand alone but must become part of something larger. New delivery systems are based on economic efficiency and require that components of health care, including the medical specialties, work together in a coordinated way. These trends have important implications for family physician and are changing the landscape for academic departments of family medicine.

Adjusting to the new health care environment, or a reluctance to do so, may be understood by taking a historical perspective. Academic departments of family medicine were formed in the 1970s during a time of social change and a rebirth of general practice as family practice. This initial phase of academic family medicine may be called the counterculture phase. During the 1970s, family medicine played a reform role in health care by focusing attention on the humanistic qualities of the physician and the nature of illness. Health care in the United States was subspecializing rapidly, and a reductionist biomedical approach to disease was dominant (and still is). Community medicine, medical ethics, prevention, and the biopsychosocial model were also part of this reform movement. The counterculture phase of academic family medicine was best described by Stephens.[1] During this period, newly formed departments of family medicine derived their value and presence by having different priorities than other departments, including humanistic education, social research, and community-based clinics.

During the 1980s, an evolutionary change became palpable among family medicine departments. The counterculture phase was wearing down, or wearing thin in the eyes of deans and other department chairs, and the question of parity was raised. Were family medicine departments equal to other clinical departments? Were our education, research, and clinical care up to academic standards? Maturing departments of family medicine began to focus on more traditional academic values, such as required clerkships, quantitative research, and clinical rigor.

Medical schools are often described as a collection of almost autonomous departmental pyramids, and family medicine departments began touting the strength of their pyramids with respect to curriculum time, quantity of research, and clinical volume. Geyman described well this phase of our development.[2] During this parity phase of academic family medicine, the counterculture role became attenuated, but elements of reform (now referred to as balance) remained important priorities.

Just as family medicine departments become proud of their parity status, the entire departmental structure of academic health centers has become dysfunctional. The transformation of fee-for-service to capitated financing for health care, with population-based budgets and financial risk for new health systems, requires coordinated multispecialty care. Departmental autonomy is now a problem rather than a strength for academic institutions.

The breadth of family medicine, which necessitates working with all other specialties in the care of patients, makes us ideally suited for a leadership role in new delivery systems, including those based in academia. The next phase of academic family medicine may be called the integration phase.

The heritage of the counterculture and parity phases of family medicine is important to our growth and identity but may be a liability for the 1990s. Many departments of family medicine are like islands in their schools. Soft, fragile islands in the 1970s became solid rocks in the 1980s, but islands nonetheless. Some family medicine departments even built empires, challenging the clinical turf of other departments. As academic health centers form into integrated delivery systems, such independent posturing of our departments may leave us behind or out of the newly formed academic systems.

Medical school deans and CEOs of academic health systems are asking all departments to integrate clinical activities. This is a time when giving up autonomy may result in increased strength and stature, rather than diminishment or dissolution. Integrated primary care coalitions of family medicine, general internal medicine, general pediatrics, and possibly general OB/GYN, may be synergistic in new coordinated clinical sites. Such synergy may also extend to educational time and research. Some have said that medical schools and academic health centers will become dinosaurs unless they understand the new managed care and become part of surviving integrated delivery systems.

Academic departments of family medicine, with a heritage of a balanced approach to prevention and illness and a newly realized academic presence, can pick up the mantle of leadership in those willing institutions. Secure with our identities, we can now adopt an attitude, philosophy, and behavior of integration with our other specialty colleagues. Taylor and a group of leading family medicine department chairs have described integration and institutional leadership as the ultimate success.[3]

Those academic health centers ready to join delivery systems are hungry for leadership that is not self-serving to its own specialty interests. I predict that the family medicine departments that will flourish in the next decade will be the ones that have shared the most with other departments in the collective success of new delivery systems in which medical schools and academic programs are able to exist.

References

1. Stephens G. Family medicine as counter-culture. Family Medicine Teacher 1979; 16(5):14-8. (Reprinted in Fam Med 1989; 21(2):103-9.

2. Geyman JP. Family medicine as an academic discipline: progress, challenges, and opportunities. J Fam Pract 1990;31:297-303.

3. Taylor RD. Colwill JM. Puffer JC, et al. Success strategies for departments of family medicine. J Am Board Fam Pract 1991;4:427-36.

Over my career I was very successful motivating medical students to reconnect with what led them to a career in medicine and become family physicians. The essence of my intensive sessions with students is captured here:

The 1-Hour Advising Session:
Helping Students Choose Family Practice

Reflections in Family Medicine
JABFP
1998;11(1):70-71

"Your job is to make sure that every medical student who should become a family physician does so." This job description was given to me by the late George Snively in 1981. George was chair of the Department of Family Practice at the University of California, Davis, and I was starting my teaching career. At least in part, this job description is appropriate for all predoctoral faculty in family practice.

Despite the recent resurgence of medical student interest in family practice, and despite the market forces that make family practice attractive, many students are still discouraged from going into the specialty. Student interest in family practice usually holds strong during the first 2 years, as activities in family practice interest groups are convenient and reinforcing. Also, basic science faculties generally do not discourage students from a family practice career. During the 3rd year, about one half of the students change their career interest, and attrition from family practice is common. We are all familiar with the discouragement medical students receive at the hands of some specialist faculty who still do not believe family practice is intellectually legitimate, and who seem oblivious to social needs and market realities.[1]

In the spring of the 3rd year, students are pressured to make a career choice so they can plan their 4th year and stay on track with residency selection. At this time many students who should go into family practice have the most doubts. Now is the time to undertake a "search and rescue operation" and to provide students with a 1-hour advising session.

If I can get students with family practice potential to come in for an appointment during this vulnerable period, the session usually goes something like this:

First I ask how they are doing and what their career interests are. A common answer is that they were considering family practice, but now they are on the fence in their choice between family practice and a couple of other specialties, for example, obstetrics-gynecology and pediatrics ("I like caring for the mothers and babies"). Sometimes a third specialty is being considered, such as psychiatry.

If students express a clear interest in a single specialty other than family practice, giving good reasons why they have "fallen in love" with this specialty above all others, I wish them well and end the interview by offering them any help I can. I try to make sure that they have at least a healthy respect for family practice.

If a student's interests are diverse and clearly directed toward becoming a personal physician, my motivation to help that student is intensified. After all, the decisions made during this period are crucial.

I ask the student why he or she went to medical school. A review of the student's career image before medical school is insightful and helps the student step back from the influence of recent experiences. Students can become jaded by recent experiences on clerkships and lose some of the ideals that brought them into medicine. They are often surprised when I, a fully trained physician, suggest that their early ideals are more objective and appropriate to career thinking than the feelings they are carrying from recent experiences.

When a student expresses multiple career interests, I suggest that family practice offers an opportunity to "have it all." That is when the doubts about family practice come forward. I listen to the student respectfully and provide a gentle response based on as much factual information as possible.[2] Arguing concepts, feelings, and opinions is rarely helpful. Rather, I say to the student, "Let me tell you about being a family physician."

I talk about the personal relationships, the intense experiences, how 2 days are never the same. I talk about the joys, the frustrations, but most of all the satisfaction of being a personal physician to people and families and in a community. I review with the student a typical day, week, or month. In some ways, this advising session is like a one-hour preceptorship.

After the student has been heard, after all doubts and feelings are put on the table, the student is ready to listen with keen interest. Often the student challenges whether the role of a personal physician is still possible. "What about managed care?" These fears are addressed compassionately. I explain that what is changeless about family practice, the role of being a personal physician to the family, is more enduring than any changes in practice structure and economics. If we somehow lose the family physician, it will have to be reinvented, because it is what families need first in health care. The student today represent the next generation.

If the student has listened intently and still expresses interest in caring for children and adults, I say, "You sound like a family physician." Often, there is a pregnant pause, a magical moment. I then suggest a real preceptorship as soon as the fourth year starts to test or reinforce what has been said. The preceptor is chosen carefully, matching the particular career interests of the student (e.g., women's health, adolescent care, sports medicine).

To engage a student in this manner is not salesmanship. It is an enabling process, intended to resurrect the career interest that has been covered up by narrow thinking and limited experiences. Of course, not all students from such encounters select family practice. The goal is to help all students make their best career decision, and students choosing other fields still appreciate the deep concern for their welfare.

Medical students deserve a positive, motivating view of the future. Most of the frustrations and problems of today will be gone or different when they finish their training. The best preceptors cut through the noise of current political and management issues and get to the essence of being a physician. Yes, this can be done in 1 hour.

References

1. Block SD, Clark-Chiarelli N, Peters AS, Singer JD. Academia's chilly climate for primary care. JAMA 1996;276:677-82.
2. Scherger JE, Beasley JW, Gaebe GI, Swee DE, Kahn NB, Rodney WM. Responses to questions about family practice as a career. Am Fam Physician.

PART V: THE INTERNET CHANGES ALMOST EVERYTHING, 1999-2005

Thomas Friedman in his book, The World is Flat, wrote that a new phase of human civilization started in 1995 with the introduction of the first web browsers. Computers and the development of the internet launched a new information age, and our world began to change. Of all service industries, medicine changed most slowly. Innovations that went through banking, travel, shopping and others transformed industries in a few years where the same changes, such as online services, took more than a decade in medicine.

I was fortunate to serve on the Institute of Medicine (IOM) Committee on the Quality of Healthcare in America in 1998. We wrote two groundbreaking reports, To Err is Human (2000) that launched the modern patient safety movement, and Crossing the Quality Chasm (2001) that pointed the way for a new health system for the 21st Century. From then on my leadership activities in family medicine would be dedicated to the transformation of how the specialty was practiced.

This short article in Academic Medicine came out of a precepting incident in 1999 that illustrated how teaching would be fundamentally different with the use of the internet.

The Internet – Don't Teach Without It

Academic Medicine
1999;74(11):1151

"Can a long-acting calcium channel blocker be used instead of an ACE inhibitor for microalbuminuria in a type 2 diabetic?" This question was posed by a third-year resident seeing an uninsured patient who could not afford an ACE inhibitor but had access to a calcium channel blocker through a "Meet the Need" program. I thought the answer was yes, but wasn't sure. The other preceptor on that afternoon thought he read something about that, but wasn't sure. None of the other residents knew. All the texts and other printed material in the office were outdated in answering the question. Less than five minutes on the internet provided three confirming sources that the answer was yes.

The days are over when we can practice medicine or teach "off the top of our head." Current quality standards dictate that we consistently provide the best care to our patients. David Eddy states, "The complexity of modern medicine exceeds the inherent limitations of the unaided human mind."[1] To provide optimal care, and to teach it in the ambulatory setting, access to electronic information is essential. The precepting rooms of all our residencies must have one or more computers for this purpose. The generation of physicians we are training will have these in their offices.

Reference

1. Millenson ML. Demanding medical excellence: Doctors and accountability in the information age. Chicago: University of Chicago Press. 1997. p.75.

In 1999 I was asked to be the editor of a new primary care journal started by the Massachusetts Medical Society. They had bought the rights to the name Hippocrates. This provided me a platform to express the transformations in primary care brought on by the internet. I started giving my e-mail to patients in 1997 and become one of the first physicians in America to use this platform of communication and care. To me, it was the new first tier in the doctor-patient relationship and transformed care based on episodic visits to a model of continuous access. The new journal lasted just 2 years due to a lack of advertising, another change brought on by the internet. Reprinted here are 7 of my articles in Hippocrates:

Email Enhanced Relationships:
Getting Back to Basics

Hippocrates
1999;13(10):7-8

My relationships with patients are being quietly transformed. Rather than episodic interaction during hurried office visits, I now have continuous communication. I feel like Marcus Welby again.

I began exchanging e-mail addresses with patients simply for convenience, theirs and mine. I knew how frustrating my office's telephone system had become, and I wanted patients to get right back to me with questions and information. I also wanted to share lab results without having to chase them down on the phone. After using e-mail for about a year, I realized that my relationships with patients had fundamentally changed. Communicating through e-mail had brought me closer to them, as in the early days of my practice.

When I started my practice 21 years ago, I had the luxury of taking a lot of time with patients. If they were sick with the flu or another self-limited problem, I called them the next day to ask if they were feeling better. Then, like the rest of us, I got very busy. Twenty-five to thirty patients a day consumed my time and energy. Driving home at night, I often wished that I'd had more time with the five or six patients who really needed to see me that day, but I was too busy servicing the rest of my patients' needs to make that happen.

Today, electronic communication provides a vehicle for transforming office practices. I envision a future where primary care physicians and their staffs are able to answer the daily needs of most patients electronically, freeing precious time for doctors to interact with those who require a more intimate level of care.

Many common acute problems can be handled electronically. The sinus pressure that occurs during a cold can be monitored through e-mail, and a patient can be reassured that nothing more serious is wrong. It's much easier to avoid antibiotics for URIs or an unnecessary referral when a patient hasn't gone to the trouble of coming in for a visit. E-mail is also ideal for following up on acute problems that take time to heal. If a patient with plantar fasciitis is given detailed instructions to resolve the problem after an office visit, a periodic e-mail exchange can help monitor progress and provide reinforcement. Acute positional vertigo generally takes six weeks to six months to resolve. E-mail can be used to gauge improvement after an office visit and can help detect worsening, which may be an early warning that something more serious is going on.

Electronic communication can provide continuous online management of chronic disease, replacing the need for episodic visits. Obese patients can email their weight and other data weekly, and can be coached online. Lipid disorder patients can receive periodic lab instructions and get feedback on their progress. L-thyroxine doses for patients with hypothyroidism can be adjusted easily through e-mail. Hypertension, diabetes, and asthma can all be monitored more closely, with less frequent visits, through electronic sharing of information. Patients with disabling chronic conditions, such as lupus, can communicate with their doctor and their consultant without the trouble of regular visits.

E-mail has also improved my relationships with consultants. I can send them messages introducing patients and providing important details about their conditions. This begins an electronic dialogue about their care. With the consultant's permission, I can copy these messages to patients, connecting them electronically with the consultant. This communication is especially helpful for postoperative care after early discharge.

Privacy and confidentiality are important issues with electronic communication. In the September issue of Hippocrates, our "Legal Brief" department reviewed the utility and pitfalls of e-mail communication with patients (see "You've Got Mail," September 1999). The cautionary guidelines of the American Medical Informatics Association (www.amia.org) outline the "informed consent" that should exist between physician and patient in the use of e-mail. These guidelines emphasize explaining the response time parameters for e-mail, being discreet, being careful, and, if in doubt, seeing the patient. I tell all my patients that e-mail with me is a warm line, not a hot line. They know I will see the message and respond in one to three days. Immediate access still requires the phone. I also tell patients I will treat our messages privately and confidentially, and that they will become part of the medical record. I tell patients that electronic communication is not guaranteed to be secure. However, password protected communication is probably as secure as phone lines and paper (which can readily be copied).

We all practice serious medicine on the phone at all hours of the day, with only partial documentation (or none at all), and under pressure to give immediate answers. If the phone were invented today, we would probably need to play an informed consent recording before talking to patients. If used wisely, electronic communication should improve quality and lower risk. It is essentially like the phone, but with a written record, and the freedom to respond more thoughtfully at a convenient time and place.

The critical enabling factors for an electronically enhanced practice are technology, financing, and control. Since information technology and usage are growing at an accelerated pace and Americans are comfortable with doing more things online, why shouldn't health care take advantage of the trend? I practice in Irvine, CA, and I haven't had any patients yet who couldn't give me an e-mail address, either their own or that of a trusted friend or relative — like in the early days of the phone. Colleen Connery at the University of Colorado in Denver told me that a survey of indigent patients at a community clinic showed 70% were able to provide e-mail addresses. Electronic communication will soon be as universal as television. A growing market of health care information technology will expand the sharing of information in ways we can only imagine.

An electronically enhanced practice is less expensive if it saves office visits and provides more service. This should capture the attention of health care payers and purchasers. The challenge now is to free the physician from a strictly visit-based reimbursement. Capitation, panel-size reimbursement, or salaries can allow for this. Even in a strictly fee-for-service cash practice, patients could be asked to pay a monthly fee, which would be automatically deducted from a credit card, in order to have continuous e-mail communication.

Finally, primary care physicians need to be given control over their schedules, with the flexibility to care for their patients in the most efficient way, meeting current standards for quality.

In the future I envision, physicians will have a more executive schedule for managing the 2,000 or more patients they must take responsibility for to earn their keep. Imagine a schedule with five or six time-intensive office visits daily, time reserved for e-mail, and for brief visits in which a physical exam is necessary. Wouldn't this be a better routine for everyone? Some of my patients have become passionate in their testimonials about having direct electronic access to their personal physician. It reminds them, and me, of the good old days of Marcus Welby.

Managed Care's Failure and Triumph

Hippocrates
1999;13(11):7

As the 1990s draw to a close, the consensus is clear. Managed care is a failure. The term has become the ultimate euphemism. The public and the medical profession are passionate in criticizing managed care. Congress and state houses are considering laws to protect patients from it.

What went wrong? A recent Gallup poll showed that 42% of Americans have "very little confidence" in HMOs, and 4% have "none", while only 17% have "a great deal" or "a lot". The public perception seems to be that managed care is a bureaucracy that puts profits above the health needs of its members.

Meanwhile, this summer a Henry J. Kaiser Family Foundation survey of physicians showed a similar antagonism toward managed care. In that study, between one and two thirds reported that, in their judgment, health plan denials of drugs or care resulted in adverse health consequences. Far outweighing any positive acknowledgement of the preventive services and practice guidelines promoted by these plans are doctors' frustrations with the administrative burdens, compressed patient visits, and reduced autonomy they suffer under managed care.

I have friends who are managed care medical directors. Early in the '90s, these were heady jobs filled with the excitement of transforming health care delivery. Now these physicians feel as though they don't have a friend in the world.

How quickly we forget. Why did managed care happen? Between 1970 and 1990, U.S. health care expenditures rocketed from $73 million to $700 billion annually, increasing at an average annual rate of about 12% up until 1990, roughly double the rate of inflation. American business, with double-digit annual increases in employee health costs, complained about being unable to compete in a global market. The federal government, picking up the tab for Medicare and Medicaid, experienced massive increases in the federal debt.

Along came managed care, with its aggressive cost containment, prepaid health care coverage, and shift of financial risk to providers. The cost efficiencies of managed care helped fuel the booming economy of the '90s, contributed to the federal budget surplus, and reined in the growth of health care expenditures, which have approached the rate of inflation in some managed-care markets this decade. Looking strictly at its impact on the economy, managed are deserves some positive recognition.

And what about quality? Perception has a way of clouding reality. Managed care, when done right, can improve the quality of health care. In HMOs, more patients receive necessary immunizations and screening services such as mammograms. Blood pressure, serum cholesterol, and blood sugar are better attended to in patients for whom these rally matter. In these ways, managed care is a triumph of American medicine. (Please keep reading and don't throw this journal into the fire!)

Now let's look at the problems. Unnecessary care and professional profiteering were rampant in the fee-for-service era. Managed care saved lots of money, but much of it went into corporate profits rather than into improving care and expanding needed services. While by some measures managed care has improved public health, the number of people without health care coverage has increased steadily in the past decade.

Managed care is an experiment in health delivery that fixed some problems and created others. The experiment is done, and the results are in. The '90s, I believe, should be viewed as the managed-care decade, a historical blip. However, what managed care started will be played out early in the coming century.

What we have learned about public and physician values during the managed-care decade will help shape the emerging health delivery systems. The physician-patient relationship, crucial to healing, requires a high degree of bilateral freedom to work. Patients should be able to choose their physicians, and physicians should be able to choose how much time to spend with a patient. Lab tests, drugs, and procedures, all expensive, should fit evidence-based guidelines whenever possible.

It is time to bury the term "managed care". The new American health care delivery systems that began to evolve under managed care will mature, reducing waste and providing unprecedented quality and service. Health care financing is likely to become population based with greater public assumption of risk and accountability. There will not be a return to cottage industry of independent private practice. Increasingly, evidence will guide the care that insurance covers, while the public pays directly for supplemental care. I believe these mature systems will restore our profession's stature and reward because they will allow us to deliver the services that patients demand and deserve.

The failures of managed care will recede from our consciousness. Like Harry Truman, largely reviled during his lifetime but honored posthumously, managed care will get its proper recognition by health care historians. The rest of us will be glad it's gone and benefit from what it started.

Teaching a Healthy Lifestyle

Hippocrates
2000;14(1):7-8

The rules are simple. They have been known for a long time. They are more important than ever.

A century ago, living a healthy lifestyle might not have given much assurance for a long and healthy life. If you acquired a serious bacterial infection or appendicitis, chances were you would die. We have conquered many of the causes of premature death that plagued mankind prior to the twentieth century. Now, as we enter the twenty-first century, good health and a long life are more than ever a choice.

Sure, genetics, infections, accidents, or cancers may end life early for some, but lifestyle factors now loom as the leading cause of premature death. Promoting a healthy lifestyle must now become a principal focus for primary care physicians.

Despite the extravagant claims of supplement manufacturers, good health does not come in a bottle. A "fountain of youth" craze seems to come over the population periodically, a hope for simple external solutions to what is an internal issue. The 1890s were the decade of patent medicines, with a proliferation of nostrums promising good health. Curiously, we saw a similar public fascination with unproved medications in the 1990s as pharmacies all over the country devoted expanding amounts of square footage to nutritional supplements that promised various health benefits. Truth and common sense usually prevail, and I suspect this current preoccupation will pass. Perhaps then we will have a more receptive audience for our teaching of the timeless rules of healthful living. These rules are straightforward – we heard most of them first from our parents – but coming from a personal physician they can be a powerful prescription. I offer these 10 simple rules as a reminder to ourselves and as a message to share with our patients.

Don't Smoke

I hate to lead off with a negative recommendation, but tobacco use is the number one cause of premature death in this country. We should not lose sight of that lest we let our guard down. With tobacco use rising again among high school and college students we must redouble our efforts to combat this social menace. We need to work hard to prevent and eliminate smoking one patient at a time – in the exam room, in our schools, and in our communities. Be active in smoking prevention and learn strategies for teaching patients how to kick the habit. See article which offers some useful fundamentals.

Be Active

The evidence supporting the health benefits of physical activity and the consequences of inactivity are so compelling that this rule rises to number two. Many adults have become more physically active in the last two decades, contributing to the decline in heart disease. However, a growing number of young people are not physically active, and obesity among children is on the rise. Work at home and on the job is less physically demanding today, and conscious choices must be made to walk and get other forms of exercise. Recent research shows that all physical activity counts and its benefits are cumulative. As we make time for exercise in our own busy lives, we should regularly inquire about out patients' activity levels and instruct them about being active.

Eat Right

Just what this means seems more confusing than ever, as "protein diet" books dominate the best-seller lists and carbohydrates are considered either a blessing or curse, depending on the diet. The real problem today is that an excessive amount of food is readily available, even to low-income Americans. Eating out can rival the cost of eating at home and is often easier. Jumbo-sized fast-food meals are commonplace. Unhealthy fat abounds in such foods as French fries, potato chips, and salad dressings. Eating right means not consuming more energy than you burn and making wise choices. The food pyramid is a big improvement over the four food groups and teaching its use promotes a low-fat, high-fiber diet, the healthiest combination. Effective nutritional interventions with patients must be sensitive to personal preferences, which may be culturally based. Start with the patient's own food diary and be flexible. Promote healthy eating.

Be Happy

I am not suggesting a false sense of bliss, but having a positive outlook does have health benefits. My first "patient" in this regard was my freshman college roommate. To him, life was a joyless, uphill struggle. He grew up on Long Island, the son of an industrial assembly line worker. I am proud to say that now with persistent counseling from myself and others he is a remarkably healthy and optimistic school superintendent. Depression is now regarded as a leading cause of disability worldwide. Mental health is critically important to overall health. In any way we can, we should model and promote positivity.

Relax

In the complexity of modern life, it is easy to be "all wound up." Do any of us have idle time? The body and mind need to relax, and probably more often than just during sleep. The integrative medicine article reports on the benefits of mediation, or deep relation. As with exercise, we need to make time for this fundamentally healthy activity. Promote relaxation with patients.

Have Purpose

George Engel suggested a biopsychosocial model for medicine in the 1970s. The growing evidence regarding spirituality and health suggests a connection. Purpose, or having a higher meaning to your life than mere existence, seems to be important for overall health. Explore this dimension with patients. For patients who don't have a social group or are not involved in their communities, for example, promote greater involvement.

Be Safe

Accidents loom large as a preventable cause of death, especially among the young. Instruct patients to wear seat belts or bicycle helmets, use infant car seats, and drive safely. Components of home safety such as smoke detectors, safe appliances and electrical wiring, gun locks, and fences around pools may be lifesaving. Safety lectures may be the last thing on a busy practitioner's mind, but accidents are the fifth leading cause of death in the U.S. Any effort physicians can make to prevent accidents is effort well spent.

Sleep Well

We should be spending between one third and one quarter of our lives in sound sleep. Poor sleep habits are common and the health consequences are becoming known. Most fibromyalgia patients improve with better sleep. Drowsiness kills on highways. We train our children to sleep, sometimes a challenging task, but as adults we often fall into poor sleep habits and lack a "parent" to set us straight again. We will have more emphasis on sleep hygiene as evidence comes in regarding the health benefits of good sleep.

Counsel Safe Sex

Many of the serious and incurable infections of our time, such as HIV and hepatitis B and C, are transmitted sexually. Being careful and using protection in sex is a health imperative for anyone not in a long-term, monogamous relationship. Teaching adolescents and adults a healthy lifestyle must include this precaution.

Use Moderation

My mother, like many, counseled "Everything in moderation." She was right. Moderation is important in several health-related behaviors. Light-to-moderate alcohol consumption has demonstrated health benefits. Alcohol should be consumed safely, which generally means at home. Moderate exercise makes the most sense for many, especially the elderly. Easting moderately means saying no to super-sized fries and desserts. Moderation is a wise principle to live by. Remind patients.

In this issue of Hippocrates, our cover article looks at the state of the nation's health and offers physicians tools for helping patients make important and sometimes difficult lifestyle changes. Prevention is one of the primary care physician's ways of saving lives. We may not see the results as clearly as in a surgical rescue, but we should take comfort in knowing that every time we have influenced a patient to live healthier, we may have added years to quality life. What greater reward can we have?

Have a healthy New Year.

Why do I Run?

Hippocrates
2000;14(6):8

Abstract: I can't preach a healthy lifestyle if I don't live it.

	1997	2000
Weight:	190 lb.	175 lb.
Total Cholesterol:	211 mg/dl	160 mg/dl
HDL Cholesterol:	37 mg/dl	51 mg/dl

Those are my vital statistics in the box. What made the difference? Twenty miles a week and a reduction in dietary fat.

As I am about to turn 50, my health becomes a high priority. The first weight and lipid panel, two years ago, frightened me. I had always been lean and healthy. Too many restaurant dinners and too little time for physical activity were taking their toll. One of my sons challenged me to get back in shape and run a marathon with him. He reminded me that I'd run three when he was a child. That was just the push I needed.

I learned from Galloway's Book on Running to train for a marathon by running just 20 to 25 miles a week. Such a regimen accommodates my busy life and my biologic need, as a runner over 40, for 48 hours of recovery between longer runs. After just four months of training, my weight was down and my lipids much better. Since the first marathon I ran with my son, on Father's Day in 1998, I have run three, including the Boston Marathon in April. I'm running another in June. Today I feel better than I did when I turned 40.

I resumed running for the health benefits, but to keep myself motivated, I need a concrete goal. A marathon to look forward to periodically serves that purpose.

The benefits of regular physical activity are well documented. Going from unfit to fit reduces all-cause mortality by as much as 44%. Besides reducing the risk of cardiovascular disease, regular physical activity reduces colon cancer risk, improves glucose control, increases insulin sensitivity, and lowers blood pressure. Recent studies in mice even suggest it may stimulate the growth of brain cells, thus reducing the risk of memory loss.

In the last five years research has proven that even moderate physical activity helps. We should counsel our inactive patients to include more physical activity in their daily routines – walking more, taking the stairs, doing things by hand. Structured exercise is the second step, and we should advise patients that making time for it may be just as vital to their health as eating and sleeping.

The mental health benefits of exercise are as important as the physical effects. The same son who encouraged me to resume running two years ago suffered a near-fatal auto accident on January 1, 2000. Running helped me deal with the stress of his tragedy and the hard work of helping him recover.

Being sedentary carries its own risks: It contributes substantially to the likelihood of coronary heart disease, Type 2 diabetes, and colon cancer – all potentially fatal. In 1992 the American Heart Association named physical inactivity as an independent risk factor for cardiovascular disease. Recent evidence shows that lack of cardiorespiratory fitness may be more of a health risk than obesity.

Promoting regular physical activity is a challenge worth taking on with all patients. We need to individualize our advice: patients will have their own ways of – and reasons for – being active. I do not entirely enjoy running marathons. They are painful, but the pain is quickly forgotten, I replaced by a sense of accomplishment. Sharing my marathon experiences with patients can help them find their own motivation for making exercise a part of their lives.

Breast cancer survivor Peggy Fleming calls exercise her "foundation of youth." The benefits have been known for centuries:

"Better to hunt in fields, for health unbought,
Than fee the doctor for a nauseous draught.
The wise, for cure, on exercise depend;
God never made his work for man to mend."
– John Dryden

A New Way of Practicing

Hippocrates
2000;14(8):8

Someday we will be measured not by the number of patients we see but by the quality of care we provide.

Someday we will be free to care for patients in the best way, determined only by their needs and not by financial incentives.

Someway patients will be able to communicate with us at any time, without the barriers posed by answering services and call centers.

Someday patients will gain ownership over their health and health care, with unlimited access to medical information and their records.

And when that day comes, we will be our patients' consultants, advisors, confidantes, and caregivers – that is, their true personal physicians, through renewed personal relationships.

This can happen now, starting today.

The medical office is a bottleneck of episodic care that does a poor job of healing. Overbooked appointment schedules, telephone barriers, crowded waiting rooms, impossibly brief visits with patients – these are the legacies of the late twentieth-century primary care office. In this book Health Care in the New Millennium, Ian Morrison likens us to hamsters running on a treadmill, and managed-care systems have asked us to run faster! With the power of the Internet, we are poised to break free of this inefficient system.

This doesn't mean we should do away with the office visit. Face-to-face encounters with patients are the most important things we offer. They are a precious use of time. But there is a new way of practice, slowly emerging and fully possible today. As Don Berwick, pediatrician and CEO of the Institute for Healthcare Improvement, says, "We need to free patients from the tyranny of the visit. The more you can move demand away from office visits, the more time you'll have to deal with patients who really need personal interaction."

Using the Internet, our patients can have continuous access to us, provide us with important health data, and set up visits. And we can meet their simple needs without seeing them in person. We can then use office visits more selectively, freed by the Internet to spend more time in person with the patients who truly need to be seen.

Mark Murray, MD, formerly a family physician at Kaiser

Permanente in Roseville, CA, and now an independent health care consultant, has championed open access for patient care because it enables us to do today's work today rather than putting patients off for two to three weeks on an appointment schedule. Dr. Murray points out that a physician caring for about 2,000 patients has about 40 patient interactions on any given day. Currently, 20 to 25 patients are seen each day in the office and the rest are handled by telephone.

Many of these interactions could be handled by e-mail. The physician and other office staff would spend one to two hours a day on the computer, interacting with 20 to 30 patients. Our offices could be much quieter, with 30- to 60-minute appointments given to the six to eight patients who really need to be seen. We would still use brief visits and telephone communication for a few patients each day as needed (see "Primary Care in 2010" in the March 2000 issue).

What is holding us up from this new way of practice? Reimbursement must be adapted to such a model. Prepaid contracts or capitation works better than fee-for-service because charging for e-mails may not be practical. We must be able to ensure privacy and confidentiality for e-mail communication. And our patients need guidelines for using e-mail appropriately (such as not using it for emergencies).

All of this is possible today. We need to seize control of our schedules and change how we work. We are a transition generation, trained in an office-based model and paid to see patients. Our job is to care for patients. With the Internet, this can be done. Negotiate flexibility in your schedule and in how you are paid. The next generation of physicians certainly will.

Virtual House Calls

Hippocrates
2000;14(11);8

Take two aspirin and send me an email.

Like so many apocrypha, the prescription "Take two aspirin and call me in the morning" just doesn't hold up. For example, exactly when in the morning is the patient supposed to call? The most inconvenient time for a patient to call me is between 7 and 8 a.m. The office is not yet open, and I am busy getting ready for the day, making rounds, or commuting to work.

After 8 a.m. isn't much better, but then it is the patient's turn to get frustrated: the flood of phone calls early in the day usually results in busy signals, prolonged holds, or exasperated staff members trying to fit in the patient's request.

I've found a way to avoid such chaos: email has become central to the development of my relationships with patients. Starting on page 39 of this issue, Laura Johnson Morasch, MPH, describes in detail how you can make the most of physician-patient email. Used well, the Internet builds communities, and email used well fosters new ways of communicating. The asynchronous nature of email has many benefits for patient-physician communication. Patients can express their concerns whenever they want, and even draft and revise messages before sending them. In addition, they can directly contribute to their own medical records. The physician or office staff can receive messages when convenient and, after doing any necessary research, respond. A back-and-forth dialogue is nicely captured for the record.

I can handle about two-thirds of my communication with patients via email. Each week I file twice as many email exchanges in the chart as I do visits and phone calls. Working on a salary and having capitated patients allows me to go all the way with this. But email can benefit even a fee-for-service practice.

For example, most lab and x-ray results can be communicated by email, which saves the time and cost of sending letters or making phone calls. Many common acute conditions can be addressed by email with patients whom the physician already knows, keeping colds, flu, and other minor problems out of the office.

Yet, for all its benefits, email communication is far from perfect. When the need for care is urgent, delays in seeing a message and responding can be a problem. Furthermore, not all patients can express their problems clearly in writing, which could trigger a physician response based on incomplete information. The physician must therefore always be on the alert for more complicated problems, and all patients are encouraged to keep in touch until the problem is resolved. Finally, not seeing or hearing the patient raises questions of authenticity and privacy. My rule: When in doubt, see the patient!

Compensation will become less of an issue in the future. There are different ways to charge for email communication with patients.

Healinx is a Web-based company (www.healinx.com) offering secure physician-patient email with an option for the doctor to charge a small amount for consultation. Healinx does all the billing and takes a small percentage as a fee. Blue Shield of California has announced a partnership with Healinx. First Health Group, a PPO in Illinois, is reimbursing physicians $25 for email communication with patients. Patients on capitation are ideal candidates because the time required and overhead costs are much less with email than with visits. Office visits remain important but can be reduced with email.

My patients love the convenience of email communication, and they regularly thank me for the accessibility and good service. Even though I get less email than I expect from patients, the more frequent communication that email offers brings me closer to those who do use it. Gaps in care are less frequent, which I believe reduces liability risk—thus negating any increase in risk that email might cause.

I strongly recommend that physicians maintain direct email communication with patients rather than delegating it entirely to the office staff. Frequent one-on-one contact by email brings back the closeness and accessibility implicit in the phrase "Call me in the morning."

Primary Care in 2010

Hippocrates
2000;14(3):27-32

It is a Monday morning in March 2010. FP Marcus Welby III, MD, and his wife Marcia, a general internist, begin their week. Marcia is jogging with friends, while Marcus feeds the kids – Marcus IV, aged 3, and 9 month old Marisa. He knows there are no urgent messages on the home computer from patients awaiting his attention because the red "alert" light isn't blinking, so he can enjoy this time with his children. At 7:45 am, when Marcia gets back from her run, Marcus heads to the office.

First, he checks the office computer for any weekend activity involving his patients, such as admissions, urgent care, or emergency visits. He also checks the ongoing evaluation and management tasks done by his staff and colleagues within the regional family care delivery system.

The data reveal an unremarkable list of minor injuries, infections, and requests for advice, each of which has been filed automatically in the appropriate patient's electronic record. Dr. Welby sees that one of his elderly patients, Mrs. Garcia, was admitted yesterday for an acute exacerbation of congestive heart failure. He enters the hospital database and reviews the admission note and nursing data, plus laboratory and X-ray results. He then video-links directly to Mrs. Garcia's bedside to talk with her, see how she is doing, and let her know he's involved in her care. He promises to stop by the hospital later than day or to see her at home if she's been discharged. Her advance directive and other relevant parts of her medical record are already downloaded into the hospital chart, so he doesn't need to worry that her attending will make decisions about her care in the absence of any vital information.

More Time with Patients

Dr. Welby then checks his schedule for the day. Six patient visits are booked – each 30 to 60 minutes long. Two of the patients are new, but between the regional health system's records and electronic questionnaire patients complete – with the help of the Welbys' practice staff – before their first visit, most of their history is already in his computer. He'll go over the high points with the patients when he meets them.

Two of today's patients are returning for annual visits. Each has a combination of chronic health problems: diabetes and hypertension for one, obesity and a lipid disorder for the other. Dr. Welby and his staff have managed these problems online over the course of the year. The patients enter weekly data on blood pressure, weight, glucose levels and the like; and the clinicians answer questions and adjust regimens through ongoing electronic dialogues. Dr. Welby will spend an unhurried, time-intensive visit of up to an hour with each of these patients, as he will with the two new ones. His extended visit includes the appropriate hands-on physical examination, but its focal point is the face-to-face discussion of the patient's overall health. Dr. Welby will explore the biopsychosocial, spiritual and family system dimensions of each patient's situation, getting to know them and firmly establishing a healing relationship that can then be reinforced during the year mainly through electronic communication.

Dr. Welby will perform a no-scalpel vasectomy on one of his patients today, a procedure he does weekly and teaches to residents. It is one of a variety of procedures he regularly performs. Colleagues in his practice, including his wife, Marcia, perform others, such as colposcopy and pelvic ultrasound.

His final scheduled visit is a counseling session for a family struggling with two rebellious teenagers. He delivered both children and has a close relationship with their parents. Together with a psychologist, Dr. Welby has been meeting with the family every two weeks for three months. The progress is good – the children's truancy has decreased, their grades have improved, and the family is enjoying more time together.

Besides these six scheduled visits, Dr. Welby will see four to six more patients in brief, face-to-face visits for acute problems not easily handled by email or video communication. With the office's open access scheduling system, these visits are arranged as the patients call in. Usually he sees same-day appointments at the end of the morning or in midafternoon.

A cornerstone of Dr. Welby's care for his 2,000 active patients is daily electronic communication. He spends up to an hour and a half each day in online patient care, interacting with 20 to 30 patients. They write him with inquiries and results, and he monitors or manages common acute problems, follows up on chronic ones, gives pep talks to patients working to improve their health, and reviews laboratory and other data. Virtually all patients by now have an email address or access to the account of a trusted friend or relative.

The practice broadcasts messages periodically to all patients with specific diagnoses. For instance, on this day, all patients with Type 2 diabetes will get a message about a new recommendation for monitoring liver function tests in patients taking a common drug. The system can automatically arrange the tests for those patients on the drug. Dr. Welby will also communicate electronically with two or three consultants that day, sharing patient data.

Staff and Colleagues

The Welbys' office staff is small but highly skilled. One front office worker, specially trained in communications and information management, interacts with patients, gathering data, scheduling appointments, and assisting patients with insurance information. The waiting room is gone, because patients no longer have to wait. It has been replaced by a library equipped with work stations where patients can update and review their medical records and view CD-ROMs and web sites the practice recommends for patient education. Some patients come by each day just to spend time there, even though most of the information is accessible from their home computers.

The office nurse also corresponds electronically with 20 to 30 patients that Monday, giving advice on common problems, arranging preventive services and lab work, and screening communications for Dr. Welby. The nurses are especially good at gathering data from patients, using a bank of questions drawn from guidelines and the Welbys' experience to help clarify such complaints as fatigue, abdominal pain, and headache.

A nurse practitioner shares the office with the two Drs. Welby, helping care for their patients and for about 600 others who specifically identify her as their primary source of care. Her schedule resembles Dr. Welby's except that she will hold two group sessions that day, one for patients with Type 2 diabetes and another for weight management. Ten to fifteen percent patients will attend these sessions, with several more linked by video. Because of the high quality of its patient management, the Welbys' office recently won two awards given by the local family care system: for lowest average Hb A1C and greatest BMI drop in the network.

Meanwhile, Dr. Marcia Welby enjoys an interim practice style that lets her spend time at home with her two young children while the baby is breastfeeding. She has office hours three afternoons each week, with four scheduled patient slots (like her husband's, these run 30 minutes to an hour) and two or three brief same-day appointments. Daily, from her home computer, she corresponds with 20 to 30 patients, so she can continue to monitor and manage them, as well as deal with common acute problems, without spending a lot of time in the office. Her practice specializes in the care of women and the elderly, and she is medical director of a senior care center. In that latter role, she manages care through daily electronic messages and uses a video link to "see" selected patients, as well as to participate in meetings and other administrative matters. She visits the senior center every two weeks and when patients are acutely ill.

Both Welbys are very active with the local hospice, and about twice weekly one of them makes a home visit. They share in the care of dying patients.

Getting There From Here

The vision of the future doesn't have to be implausible. We are at the dawn of a new century. How we deliver health care in America is ripe for radical change. Average life expectancy in the US increased from 47 years in 1900 to 76 years in 1999. Immunizations, antibiotics, and modern surgery – as well as improvements in diet and public health – have prevented scourges and extended life.

The 20th century also saw dramatic changes in how primary care was delivered, from house calls to the modern medical office with its episodic visits, hectic schedule, and multiple dissatisfactions for both doctor and patient.

Information technology has the power to change medical practice as much as the automobile and telephone did. As Bill Gates describes in Business @ the Speed of Thought, information technology will transform health care into an interconnected system that operates accurately and automatically.[2] At first glance, email may seem impersonal and a poor substitute for face-to-face contact. It's true, email can't replace necessary visits. But it can provide an alternative for handling routine problems, and it can enhance relationships by making communication between doctor and patient – albeit online – more frequent and more responsive to patient needs (see "Email Enhanced Relationships: Getting Back to Basics" in Hippocrates, November 1999).

Information technology will also allow primary care physicians to improve the quality of care. Electronic clinical decision support systems will automatically double-check all orders, including drug prescribing, and will routinely assist with diagnosis and treatment, alerting physicians to clinical guidelines from the moment the medical assistant enters the chief complaints into the electronic record. Michael Millenson, in his 1997 book, Demanding Medical Excellence: Doctors and Accountability in the Information Age, powerfully describes how computer technology must be routinely used to achieve medical excellence.[4] He quotes David Eddy, MD: "The complexity of modern medicine exceeds the inherent limitations of the unaided human mind."

In the future, primary care physicians could spend an extraordinary amount of time with their patients. Most human problems require substantial amounts of time for healing – both more time when we see them, and more care over the long interval it may take for a treatment to have its effect. We routinely spend half an hour to an hour on administrative and teaching appointments. Why should patient care get less? In a landmark book, Time to Heal, Kenneth Ludmerer, MD, calls the lack of time the greatest obstacle in today's healthcare system.[5] He cites compelling data that busy office schedules and short appointments reduce the quality of care and cause job dissatisfaction, burnout, and poor mental health among physicians. A new care model such as that described here can give the physician time to deal and can return satisfaction to primary care.

Three things need to happen to bring about this future vision. The first is information technology, which is available today and will likely become far more widely accessible in the coming decade. For those persons who will not have computers at home, kiosks will be available like public telephones, in addition to the computers available now in public places such libraries.

The second is reimbursement that supports such a model and does not depend on office visits. Fee-for-service, where the service is measured in visits, will become increasingly obsolete, replaced by better designed (and more realistically funded) capitation that pays for the overall care of the patient over the course of the year. The cost of innovations like email care and elaborate practice web sites could be defrayed with prepaid patient contracts for online access.

Finally, this model requires that physicians regain control of their work schedules. Physicians taking responsibility for 2,000 or more patients should have a more executive level of responsibility and be free to use the most convenient and effective means of serving patients' needs. Whether that means using nurse practitioners or email messages for routine care, physicians should be concentrating their efforts where their specific training and skills do the most good.

Marcus Welby III's fictional grandfather is well known to most baby boomers. Made famous by the hit 1970s TV show, he was the prototype of the primary care physician helping patients and their families with complicated problems. Marcus Junior practiced during the managed care era of the 1980s and 1990s. Frustrated with mandated busy office schedules that required him to see patients every 10 minutes, he stopped making house calls and even gave up hospital practice.

But if he can achieve this new care model, Marcus Welby III can return to something resembling his grandfather's style of practice, with its enhanced, personal patient relationships. Electronic communication, sharing of information and freedom from visit-based payment will allow him to focus on the important issues in his practice and make his routine care more efficient.

The future will not be handed to primary care physicians on a silver platter. Indeed, if primary care physicians stand by and let others implement information technology in health care, they run the risk of being relegated to the role of service workers on production-line schedules, while others in the emerging delivery systems provide electronic communication and information sharing. Primary care physicians must be proactive to make this future happen and preserve the time-honored tradition of providing comprehensive care through intense doctor-patient relationships.

The future rewards and satisfaction of primary care depend on it.

References

1. Davidoff F. Time. Ann Intern Med. 1997;127(6):483-5.
2. Gates, B. Business @ the speed of thought: Using a digital nervous system. New York: Warner Books;1999.
3. Linzer M. The physician worklife study: the results are in! Society of General Internal Medicine Forum. 1998;2(10)2 and 9.
4. Millenson ML. Demanding medical excellence: Doctors and accountability in the Information Age. Chicago: University of Chicago Press;1997.
5. Ludmerer KM. Time to heal: American medical education from the turn of the century to the era of managed care. New York: Oxford University Press, Inc.; 1999.

Medical schools are well known by their departmental silos. At the University of California, Irvine, where I served as Associate Dean for Primary Care and Chair of the Department of Family Medicine from 1996-2001, we had family medicine, general internal medicine and general pediatrics integrated into one primary care medical group, and we also did research and education together. The following article describes that symbiotic relationship:

The Primary Care Specialties Working Together: A Model of Success in an Academic Environment

Joseph E. Scherger, MD, MPH, Lloyd Rucker, MD, Elizabeth H. Morrison, MD, MSEd, Ralph W. Cygan, MD, and F. Allan Hubbell, MD, MSPH

Academic Medicine
2000:75:693-698

Abstract: In today's environment of decreasing resources and increasing competition among clinical delivery systems, survival and ultimate success require interdisciplinary cooperation and, if possible, integration. Academic leaders at the University of California, Irvine (UCI), have developed a collaborative model in which faculty in family medicine, general internal medicine, and general pediatrics cooperate extensively in education, research, and patient care. Generalist faculty jointly administer and teach both a four-year "doctoring" curriculum for medical students and an array of integrated curricula for primary care residents, including a communication skills course. Several primary faculties jointly developed a collaborative unit for health policy and research, now an active locus for multidisciplinary research. Other faculty worked together to develop a primary care medical group that serves as a model for interdisciplinary practice at UCI. Recently, the university recruited an associate dean for primary care who leads the new UCI Primary Care Coalition, reflecting and promoting this interspecialty cooperation. This coalition does not represent a step toward a generic primary care specialty; UCI's generalist disciplines have preserved their individual identities and structures. Yet interdisciplinary collaboration has allowed primary care faculty to share educational resources, a research infrastructure, and clinical systems, thus avoiding duplicative use of valuable resources while maximizing collective negotiating abilities and mutual success. (Acad. Med. 2000;75:693–69).

"Can the disciplines of family practice, general internal medicine, and general pediatrics work cooperatively rather than competitively in an academic setting?" Facing the prospect of primary care integration, a family practice department chair posted this question on a listserv of department chairs in family practice. The dominant sentiment was negative: "Been there, done that, doesn't work!" The cultures of these specialties and the departmental relationships in medical schools seem to work against cooperation.

Yet the competitive health care marketplace is moving toward functional multispecialty groups. A divisive group of physicians is ill suited to compete successfully with other clinical systems, and they are likely to miss opportunities for productive collaboration in education and research. In short, integration may be the most important strategy for the primary care disciplines today.

Interdisciplinary collaboration in academic generalism is not a new concept. For decades, educators have recommended integrating primary care teaching, research, and clinical practice.[1,2] On one end of the spectrum, some authors have advocated for primary care disciplines to merge into a single comprehensive specialty.[3,4] Others have proposed less complete forms of integration, such as multidisciplinary generalist curricula in certain courses or rotations,[5,6] a perspective reflected in the joint statement on collaborative generalist training issued by the American Boards of Internal Medicine and Family Practice in 1995.[7]

The literature on interspecialty integration documents formidable challenges.[8-10] These include traditional medical hierarchies, poor communication, lack of knowledge about other specialties, economic barriers, and lack of trust in the collaborative process itself. As Reynolds and colleagues[10] state, interdisciplinary collaboration requires unique efforts; it does not occur automatically within multidisciplinary groups, but necessitates working together to achieve both mutual and individual goals, maximizing the participation of all involved. Wartman et al.[11] learned this lesson in undertaking the national Interdisciplinary Generalist Curriculum (IGC) Project at ten U.S. medical schools. Collaboration on this project was time consuming and required meticulous communication and goal setting, even when broad-based institutional support was present.

Yet when interdisciplinary collaboration succeeds, the literature suggests it can yield tremendous benefits for all involved, including increased clinical efficiency,[12] better training for primary care learners,[13] and the enhanced research productivity that appears to be linked with strong professional networks.[14]

In this article we describe a medical school environment where the department family practice and the divisions of general internal medicine and general pediatrics cooperate extensively in education, research, and patient care. This cooperation did not happen overnight; rather, it evolved gradually over many years. No change was made to the academic structure; all three disciplines remain in separate departments. However, cooperation in the primary care education of medical students and residents, a unified health policy research unit, and a unified primary care medical group reflect the depth of cooperation and integration. Recently, the university recruited an associate dean for primary care (JES) to reinforce this integration and to represent primary care in the governing structure of the medical school. We now use the title the University of California Irvine Primary Care Coalition to reflect and promote this interspecialty cooperation.

The Primary Care Coalition is not intended to be a step in the direction of a generic primary care specialty.[3,4] Special identities and departmental structures have been preserved. However, we believe primary care is strengthened through both our diversity and our cooperation. Also, in working cooperatively, we are able to share educational resources, the research infrastructure, and clinical systems, thus avoiding duplicative use of valuable resources.

How and why did this cooperation among primary care disciplines come about at the University of California, Irvine (UCI)? It was not mandated from on high, nor was it forced by any departmental changes. It may reflect the particular attitudes and styles of the leaders in the three primary care specialties. Below, we describe the three major areas in which the specialties collaborate—education, research, and patient care—and how this collaboration was initiated, in the hope that our experiences will be helpful to colleagues in other institutions.

THREE AREAS OF COLLABORATION

Education

The cooperative effort in medical education grew from a knowledge of our strengths and a frank assessment of our weaknesses. As in the other two areas of cooperation, in education we were driven by the dual recognition that individually we had much to offer and collectively we had much to gain. This knowledge did not come as an epiphany; rather, it came gradually as a result of early efforts to work together.

The efforts of the senior associate dean for educational affairs to create a multidisciplinary, multiyear course on doctoring skills served as an initial stimulus for cooperation. This course spans all four years of the medical curriculum. The second-year component is the largest course in that year, including nearly 300 contact hours. It covers physical diagnosis and communication skills as well as such content areas as epidemiology, informatics, nutrition, human sexuality, medical economics, and ethics; it depends heavily on standardized patients for both instruction and evaluation. Obviously, no single department could run this curriculum independently. In the process of learning to work together to develop and teach this course, the primary care faculty discovered previously unrecognized advantages to bringing their collective skills to bear on curriculum development, course administration, evaluation, research, and clinical teaching.

The physical diagnosis component of the second-year course illustrates the benefits of this cooperative approach. Previously, this training had been led by internal medicine faculty and had been hospital based. With the advent of our cooperative approach, we began to bring patients with specific organ-system findings into our learning center as a programmed means of focused teaching. We invited family medicine and internal medicine faculty to train together as preceptors. Through faculty development and teaching together, the preceptors came to see themselves as a group of primary care physicians committed to teaching physical diagnosis. We developed curricula and core knowledge in subject areas that were independent of our own specialties. Students have given high ratings to the physical-diagnosis preceptors regardless of specialty, and they have done well on standardized tests of their skills. This same opportunity for shared expertise came through implementing faculty task forces to develop integrated, longitudinal curricula in medical economics, communication skills, evidence-based medicine, geriatrics, and palliative care.

Our experiences with medical students brought us to the realization that we might fruitfully work together to develop residency curricula. Certainly, the residency review committees' requirements for the individual primary care disciplines contain considerable overlap in such content areas as cross-cultural medicine, medical economics, medical informatics, evidence-based medicine, managed care education, and communication skills. In the past, each program's faculty felt responsible for developing their own curriculum for each of these areas, requiring considerable resources and expertise that was not always available in all programs.

We were convinced that we could achieve our independent goals and maximize our limited resources by working cooperatively together. We found that some of the residency programs already had considerable expertise in unique areas that complemented that of other programs. We divided up the tasks and shared the products. As we worked together we had to make certain compromises in program structures.

We needed to make sure that what one program developed, another could import. We also needed to ensure that the necessary audiovisual and computer resources were available to all programs. To a certain extent, we had to share budgets. But the experience of working together has made cooperation and interdependence preferable to going on our own.

Our communication skills course for primary care residents is an excellent example of the way in which collaboration can work. We adopted a training method in communication skills based upon the methods of the Bayer Institute for Health Care Communication. This approach requires trained faculty facilitators from family medicine, internal medicine, and pediatrics. When we present the course, we integrate residents from each of these disciplines and make the training available to all residency programs, including the surgical specialties. Residents and faculty are thereby encouraged to develop collegial working relationships and a larger pool of facilitators is made available.

Cooperation in educational affairs cannot be mandated. Faculty must see the advantage of working together. At UCI, we had to overcome our own particular departmental orientations and our traditional biases about what certain disciplines could or could not do. Broad curricula with interdisciplinary objectives provide an ideal environment for collegial growth and learning. Eventually, it becomes obvious that working together not only makes sense educationally, but also saves crucial amounts of time and resources. Cooperation also serves as a model of professionalism for our students as they prepare to work in practice environments that emphasize teamwork.

Research

Research collaboration among the primary care disciplines began at UCI in 1991 with a proposal to establish a health policy research center. At that time, relatively few faculty members in general internal medicine, general pediatrics, and family medicine conducted research. This was not surprising, since UCI fostered these disciplines to meet the need for better primary care teaching and patient care, not to address research issues. Therefore, those faculty members who were involved in research faced several obstacles to competing in the larger research arena. Two problems were particularly evident: first, the lack of an effective research infrastructure within these disciplines, and, second, limited opportunities for collaboration with investigators from other fields. The latter issue was of particular concern, because the focus of most of the research-oriented faculty was health policy research, an area in which multidisciplinary collaboration is particularly important.

To overcome these barriers, several faculty members from the primary care disciplines, along with additional investigators from the social sciences and health economics, developed a proposal for a multidisciplinary research unit that would focus on health policy issues. The unit would provide an infrastructure for collaborative research, including space and administrative staff with expertise in contract and grant development and administration. The proposal included a request for only a limited amount of funding, with the expectation that most resources would come from extramural sources. Because several of the proposal's authors had large federally funded grants at the time, this did not seem to be a false hope.

In 1993, after extensive evaluation by the appropriate deans, the Committee on Research, the vice chancellor for research, and an extramural advisory committee, the Irvine Research Unit in Health Policy and Research (HPR) became officially established at UCI. Initially, the unit included a director (FAH), eight faculty members, and a small administrative staff. The faculty members were from the College of Medicine, the School of Social Ecology, the School of Social Sciences, and the Graduate School of Management.

As HPR gained a reputation for its work in health policy research, additional faculty members joined the unit. In 1999, HPR had 21 members—the majority of whom were from the primary care disciplines of the College of Medicine. Their areas of expertise included anthropology, biostatistics, community health, epidemiology, family medicine, general internal medicine, geriatrics, marketing, medical economics, medical education, medical ethics, sociology, pediatrics, and public health. Interaction among the members has resulted in numerous innovative multidisciplinary research projects that have received funding from federal, state, and local agencies.

The HPR unit has also provided an educational environment for undergraduate and graduate students to learn how to conduct health policy research. Once exposed to the research environment, many of the students have chosen to participate in other projects in the unit. Most of the students are enrolled in the School of Social Ecology, the School of Social Sciences, or the Graduate School of Management. However, some of our medical students and residents have also found the time to participate in HPR research programs.

The HPR unit fosters research on a variety of health policy issues. Initially, most of the research addressed problems that affect medically disadvantaged populations, including the poor, minorities, children, and the elderly. For example, the research program in pediatric injury prevention and control has addressed the epidemiology and prevention of childhood injuries, with particular emphasis on Latino children. The research findings have led to changes in laws regarding the use of seat belts and riding in the beds of pickup trucks. Another example is the program in cancer prevention and control. Faculty members have worked together on a variety of studies aimed at identifying and addressing the cancer-control needs of Latinos, Asian Americans, Native Americans, and American Samoans in Southern California and evaluating culturally sensitive programs to improve cancer prevention in these special populations. As HPR has evolved it has developed research programs in other important health policy arenas, such as health care delivery systems, the cost of medical care, and medical education.

The challenges associated with running a multidisciplinary research unit such as HPR are complex. Funding depends largely on extramural support and consequently the number of administrative staff varies according to funding levels. In addition, collaboration among faculty members from different disciplines doesn't always go smoothly. Furthermore, space requirements sometimes exceed the unit's capacity to provide an adequate working environment for everyone.

Despite these challenges, HPR has been a success by most measures. It has provided a research infrastructure and has facilitated collaboration among health policy researchers. Moreover, it has led to increases in both the number of primary care physicians involved in research and the number of funded projects. These successes could not have been accomplished without collaboration among the primary care disciplines of the College of Medicine.

Patient Care

The process of organizing and managing a faculty medical practice offers an ideal opportunity for fostering cooperation and improving integration among academic primary care faculty, as leaders in other health systems have found.[15] The highly competitive Southern California health care market provided UCI's departments of family medicine, internal medicine, and pediatrics with the impetus to develop an innovative interdisciplinary practice organization, the UCI Primary Care Medical Group (PCMG). This organization has allowed UCI (1) to compete more effectively with local medical groups; (2) to expand its pool of clinician–educators; and (3) to elevate the stature of the primary care disciplines within the larger UCI Health System and College of Medicine.

Before the mid-1980s, UCI's primary care faculty practices were organized along traditional departmental lines. The small faculties of family medicine, general internal medicine, and general pediatrics devoted less than 20% of their individual and collective efforts to patient care. Because clinical faculty practiced at what had formerly been the county hospital, the majority of their patients was either underinsured or uninsured and was cared for in the medical center's multispecialty and community teaching clinics.

In order to attract commercially insured patients to UCI, all clinical departments were encouraged to expand their faculty practice commitment and to recruit more clinically oriented faculty. To support the growth of its primary care patient base, the university entered into its first fully capitated managed care contract in 1984 with the enrollment of some 800 university employees. One of us (RWC) was chosen as the medical director of the faculty practice's managed care component, and he quickly became aware of the shortcomings of our departmentally structured primary care practice. These included an inadequate number of faculty clinicians, a lack of adequate incentives, a low valuation of patient care relative to education and research, an insufficient practice infrastructure, and the physicians' lack of practice-management expertise. Patients were not satisfied with many aspects of the existing practice structure and functioning. They expressed dissatisfaction with physician availability, urgent care access, phone and messaging systems, confusing billing systems, and cumbersome utilization-review procedures. Many faculty, particularly those with strong clinical orientations, were unhappy with the practice environment, and several key faculty had resigned out of frustration.

In 1985, we initiated a series of informal meetings of internists and family physicians in an attempt to improve relationships among primary care colleagues who had previously had little interaction and to identify areas of mutual concern. A joint utilization committee began to meet. This committee included key clinical leaders of both departments and it served as the main forum for fostering cooperative problem solving. In 1986, a leading family physician was selected as the assistant medical director, further strengthening the developing trust among the two disciplines.

Although this informal working relationship did improve some aspects of the practice environment and infrastructure for primary care faculty, many problems persisted. Lack of an integrated practice organization hampered our ability to address key issues: capitation, faculty recruitment, practice staffing, and physician availability and scheduling. Our resulting inability to negotiate with the hospital and the dean's office placed the primary care disciplines at a significant disadvantage in competing with specialty colleagues for resources. Instead, we found ourselves competing, usually ineffectively, against one another for the investments we felt were necessary to develop our departmentally based primary care practices.

In searching for a more effective primary care delivery system for UCI, we began to look to the larger community, where managed care had fostered the development of several large primary and multispecialty group practices. With the support of the chairs of both family medicine and internal medicine, we created an extra departmental practice organization to take responsibility for managing the faculty medical practice of the two primary care departments. With support of the dean and the hospital director, we hired a practice-management consultant, and a subcommittee of general internists and family physicians worked for four months to create a practice model and business plan. Ultimately, the plan was endorsed by the key leadership of the university and the PCMG began operation in 1992.

Key elements of the new practice organization included:

1. The designation and empowerment of a PCMG president to be responsible for overseeing all aspects of primary care faculty practice.

2. The establishment of PCMG as a separate business unit reporting to the dean of the College of Medicine.

3. The creation of a PCMG governing board consisting of key leaders from the primary care departments, the medical center, and the health system.

4. Joint faculty recruitment by the PCMG and the academic departments, with salary support provided by the individual entities proportional to their clinical and academic responsibilities.

5. The development of an equitable incentive-based compensation system applied uniformly across all participating primary care departments.

6. The creation of a practice management subcommittee consisting of practice medical directors and key medical center personnel as a forum to improve practice infrastructure.

7. The implementation of a regular set of practice-site meetings and membership forums to ensure open communication, solidify group identity, and direct team building.

8. Commitment by each member of the PCMG to a minimum of 10% time to their departmental teaching responsibilities.

Our experience with the integrated primary care group practice has been very favorable. Our number of capitated patients has grown to nearly 35,000 enrollees, of whom 13,000 are commercially insured; the remainder is part of the capitated Medicaid program. In addition, we have attracted many other patients with Medicare and private insurance. Patient satisfaction has improved dramatically, and our practice infrastructure has greatly improved. The group has been able to recruit and retain exceptionally trained clinician educators and currently has over 50 full- and part-time clinicians, including three nurse practitioners. The general pediatrics faculty joined the group in 1996, further strengthening the ability of the PCMG to negotiate with the medical center and health system. Two new ambulatory care sites have been added, while older sites have benefited from major remodeling and facelifts. The PCMG has also been able to secure improved support for faculty involved in supervising residents and students at all of our university teaching clinics.

In spite of these successes, the UCI PCMG is confronted by a number of ongoing challenges. These include:

1. Dependence upon the medical center and health system to cover the regular budgetary shortfalls that result from low capitation allocation and a high proportion of indigent

patients.

2. Attraction of the sickest and most costly capitated patients to our specialists; many of these patients are then transferred into our primary care group. This results in the group's treating a disproportionate share of high-acuity capitated patients, which in turn exposes the group to losses on capitated contracts.

3. Faculty providers' relatively high use of technology and high-cost drugs in patient care, resulting in utilization rates that exceed capitated budgetary allowances.

4. Low faculty productivity compared with community based counterparts. Because the group receives health system budgetary support, the productivity of its clinical faculty is under close scrutiny, and changes in the compensation plan are being considered to help address this concern.

5. Educational needs competing with clinical time. The college and departments are continually soliciting the PCMG faculty to expand their involvement in student and resident educational activities. Although rewarding for the clinical faculty, these activities do not generate professional fees and may adversely affect patient access and satisfaction. The PCMG struggles constantly to ensure an appropriate balance of academic and patient care activities.

In spite of these problems, we believe the UCI model of integrated faculty practice has been extraordinarily successful. Despite changes in leadership in the dean's office and new department chairs, this integrated practice model continues to receive support throughout the institution. In fact, the cooperation and integration of UCI's primary care physicians has become a model for interdisciplinary practice development in both medical and surgical areas at UCI.

Conclusion

At the University of California, Irvine, cooperative efforts among primary care departments in education, research, and patient care began separately but simultaneously. We believe there are two reasons for their linked successes. First, all three disciplines were in strong but not dominating departments. If one department had been dominant, then that department would have had little reason to cooperate and integrate with the others. Second, all three primary care disciplines benefited by cooperating in all three spheres; in other words, we all had something to gain. Since each department had its own strengths and corresponding interests, and since each department was willing to share what it had, we were all able to see that cooperation would ultimately strengthen each discipline. The integrated activities of the office of medical education, the health policy research unit, and the primary care medical group all grew out of that cooperative spirit.

Every medical school has its own history and balance of power among departments. In today's environment of decreasing academic resources and managed competition among organized clinical delivery systems, survival and ultimate success require interdisciplinary cooperation and, if possible, integration. We hope that our positive experience serves as an incentive for other medical schools to move toward greater cooperation among the primary care disciplines.

References

1. Geyman JP. Training primary care physicians for the 21st century: alternative scenarios for competitive vs. generic approaches. JAMA. 1986;255:2631–5.
2. Bulger RJ. Generalism and the need for health professional educational reform. Acad Med. 1995;70(1 suppl):S31–S34.
3. Benson JA. Isn't it time for one family of generalists? The case for an American Board of Physicians. J Am Board Fam Pract. 1990;Apr–Jun, 3 suppl:29S–37S.
4. Colwill JM. Education of the primary physician: a time for reconsideration? JAMA. 1986;255:2643–4.
5. Freeman J, Cash C, Yonke A, Roe B, Foley R. A longitudinal primary care program in an urban public medical school: three years of experience. Acad Med.1995;70(1 suppl):S64–S68.

6. Schatz IJ, Realini JP, Charney E. Family practice, internal medicine, and pediatrics as partners in the education of generalists. Acad Med. 1996;71:35–9.

7. Kimball HR, Young PR. Educational resource sharing and collaborative training in family practice and internal medicine: a statement from the American Boards of Internal Medicine and Family Practice. JAMA. 1995;273:320–2.

8. Inui TS. Stand and deliver—together. J Gen Intern Med. 1994;9:S1–S2.

9. Petersdorf RG. If I were dean. J Am Board Fam Pract. 1990;Apr–Jun, 3 suppl:39S–48S.

10. Reynolds PP, Giardino A, Onady GM, Siegler EL. Collaboration in the preparation of the generalist physician. J Gen Intern Med. 1994;9(4 suppl 1):S55–S63.

11. Wartman SA, Davis AK, Wilson MEH, Kahn NB, Kahn RH. Emerging lessons of the Interdisciplinary Generalist Curriculum (IGC) Project. Acad Med. 1998;73:935–42.

12. Weitekamp MR, Ziegenfuss JT. Academic health centers and HMOs: a systems perspective on collaboration in training generalists [sic] physicians and advancing mutual interests. Acad Med. 1995;70(1 suppl): S47–S53.

13. Kimball HR, Young PR. A statement of the generalist physician from the American Boards of Family Practice and Internal Medicine. JAMA. 1994;271:315–6.

14. Hitchcock MA, Bland CJ, Hekelman FP, Blumenthal MG. Professional networks: the influence of colleagues on the academic success of faculty. Acad Med. 1995;70:1108–16.

15. Urbina C, Voss C, Seeger K, et al. Interdisciplinary ambulatory education and service in primary care at the University of New Mexico. Acad Med. 1999;74:659–62.

While the internet changed the dominant method of communication to an online platform, the essence of the doctor-patient relationship and the Hippocratic tradition of care were not only preserved but enhanced. These three articles describe my perspective on better care through the use of the internet.

What Patients Want

The Journal of Family Practice
2001;50(2):13.

In the movie "What Women Want," Mel Gibson's character Nick is transformed by being able to hear women's thoughts. What if we could hear our patients' thoughts? As they sit in the waiting room, talk with the staff, look around the office, listen to us, and depart, our patients are undoubtedly sizing us up: Is this the physician I want to entrust with my health? How might we change if we really knew what patients want?

MANAGED CARE AND PATIENT VALUES

Managed care has done much to teach us what patients do not want. The principles of managed care are fine—appropriate care delivered with consistent standards. The trappings of managed care tend to violate core patient values, such as the ability to choose physicians and being able to trust their physicians' decisions. Patients have rebelled, as insurance plans have directed them to certain primary care providers and require that the physician's decisions be approved by a higher authority.

The 2 articles in this issue from The Health Institute in Boston validate the core elements of the physician-patient relationship and show that these elements have eroded in the past few years.[1,2] No matter how much administrators try to define and dissect medicine into units of service (relative value units), patient care is fundamentally based on human interaction. Diseases do not come for treatment, people do. Although industrialized health care systems think management, people want healing. Healing requires healing relationships.

GIVING PATIENTS WHAT THEY WANT

So what are we to do with these data showing that the relationship elements of care—trust, interpersonal treatment, knowledge of the patient, and communication—are what patients want and that these elements have been eroded in recent years? Health care is a service industry consuming more a trillion US dollars every year. Ultimately, those who succeed will do so by giving patients what they want. Family physicians should be satisfied by these validating studies and realize that the core relationship elements of care are critical for their success. Gatekeeping brought us back to the frontline of care in the early 1990s, but that is not what patients want. Being true personal physicians is what sustains us in the long run. Today's health systems must relearn this. When we entered medicine years ago, we were taught some timeless adages that are validated by this research and need to be continually reaffirmed:

• Patients want the 3 "As"—accessibility, affability, and ability, in that order.

• Patients do not care how much you know until they know how much you care.

• It is much more important to know what sort of patient has a disease than what sort of disease a patient has.[3]

• The secret of caring for the patient is caring for the patient.[4]

How do we operationalize these principles in the 21st century? Will the new information and communication technologies be used to make care more personal or impersonal? We can use electronic communication to enhance our relationships with patients by making us directly available and continuously accessible to them. As for managed care and the problems causing the negative findings in these studies, everyone involved with health care payment and administration must realize that continuous relationships based on trust are critical for effective care. Now is the time to develop new structural features in our practices to give patients what they want.

References

1. Murphy J, Chang H, Montgomery JE, Rogers WH, Safran DG. The quality of physician-patient relationship. J Fam Pract 2001;50:123–29.
2. Safran DG, Montgomery JE, Chang H, Murphy J, Rogers WH. Predictors of voluntary disenrollment from a primary physician's practice. J Fam Pract 2001;50:130–36.
3. Osler W. Aequanimitas. Philadelphia, Pa: Blakiston; 1904.
4. Peabody FW. The care of the patient. JAMA 1927;88:877–82.

E-Mail "Visits" Can Save You Time

Medical Economics
2004;81(18):37-38,41

Some physicians have started using e-mail to communicate with their patients, but most of them are doing it as an add-on to their busy visit schedules. To take advantage of e-mail's efficiency, it should be integrated into the schedule, replacing the many unnecessary visits that all offices log. By using e-mail this way, physicians can save time and take better care of more patients. Here's how:

Currently, most health care communications occur in face-to-face visits or over the telephone. Offices have multiple phone lines flashing at the same time, with patients being put on hold just to enter the system or get a simple question answered. Physicians are frantically trying to see patients and respond to phone messages at the same time.

Yet a great deal of clinical communication does not require doctor and patient to be present at the same time. To answer a question about how to take a medication, for instance, the physician doesn't have to be in the same room or on the phone with the patient. E-mail provides an asynchronous form of communication in which physician and patient can correspond when it's mutually convenient. Patients don't have to wait on hold, and doctors and staffers don't have to play phone tag with patients.

Online communication has its limits, to be sure. Messages can be misunderstood or used inappropriately. But telephone communication has drawbacks, too, and it's become the principal means by which most after-hours care is provided.

Many physicians are also concerned that e-mail with patients might violate HIPAA regulations. But secure online messaging systems that comply with HIPAA privacy rules are now available from several vendors. These systems can be used only to protect your e-mail or they can be imbedded in an interactive practice Web site.

And from a liability viewpoint, online communication is better than telephone calls because it's self-documenting. E-mails can be printed out easily and inserted in the patient record, or copied to electronic medical records. Patients must understand, however, that they should never use e-mail in an emergency.

Old Schedule		New Schedule	
AM		**AM**	
8:00	Complete physical (plus a brief acute	8:00	Log into practice Web site to respond
15	patient with a rash, double booked)	15	to messages triaged from on-call
30		30	physician and front desk. Respond to
45	Follow-up hypertension, diabetes	45	15 patient messages, including
			follow-up hypertension, diabetes,
			asthma, weight loss, and travel
			medicine issues.
9:00	Follow-up pneumonia	9:00	
15	Follow-up abnormal chemistries from	15	
	annual exam		
30	Counseling for weight loss,	30	New patient evaluation, electronic
	dyslipidemia		history form completed.
45	Elderly patient with memory loss	45	
10:00	New patient, family planning	10:00	
15		15	Follow-up hypertension, diabetes
30	Established patient, travel medicine	30	
45	Follow-up hospitalization for	45	Acute patient, rash
	congestive heart failure		
11:00	Two patients fit in with cough,	11:00	Meeting with married couple to
	congestion		discuss genetic health issues
15	Follow-up depression	15	
30	Follow-up asthma	30	
45	Catch up on charting and phone calls	45	Check e-mail and respond to four
			patient messages
PM		**PM**	
12:00		12:00	
15	Hospital committee meeting	15	Hospital committee meeting
30		30	
45		45	
1:00		1:00	
15		15	
30	Repeat of morning schedule until 5	30	Repeat of morning schedule except
	pm, finish charting and phone calls at		that new patient evaluation is first and
	6 pm.		45-minute session practice Web site
			ends the workday at 5 pm.
	Patients seen.......................26		**Patients**
			seen........................10
	Phone calls.......................12		**Phone calls.........................4**
	Total patients cared for........38		**Patient e-mails....................36**
			Total patients cared
			for.........50

How to Modify Your Office Schedule

Online communication has the potential to transform the nature of today's office environment, making it much less stressful and harried for both doctors and patients.

Rather than seeing 24 to 30 patients a day, and dealing with nearly as many phone calls, a physician could care for the same number of patients online in 60 to 90 minutes. The rest of the day might be spent seeing 8 to 12 patients who have complex needs in unhurried visits that last 30 to 60 minutes each. If a patient problem required two hours of face time that could be accommodated without stealing time from the care of other patients.

Used to seeing all your patients, you may fear a loss of intimacy if you e-mail most of them. In my experience, however, more-frequent electronic communication enhances the patient-physician relationship, and visits are more rewarding when less rushed.

A major advantage of a schedule that integrates e-mail into the workday is that office visits are reserved for those who really need them. Longer appointments for these folks are much more professional than brief, hurried visits, in which patients with complex problems are rarely given the services they need.

Listed above you'll find examples of an old and a new office schedule. Even though fewer patients are seen under the new schedule, more receive care. The front and back office staffs are also able to deal with more patients each day in a less hectic manner, thanks to the asynchronous communication offered by e-mail.

How to Address Financial Issues

Although some insurance companies have begun paying for e-mail on a limited basis, it's unlikely that this will become widespread or that it could totally replace the income lost by having fewer visits. A monthly user fee could help make it possible for practices to offer e-mail service on top of office visits.

Capitation and other prepaid reimbursement systems offer more flexibility in matching finances to the way care is delivered. Under capitation, doctors don't depend on visits for revenue, and the most efficient methods of care are desirable. Heavily capitated practices have an incentive to provide more care over the phone. The same is true for e-mail, and physicians in these practices should try using e-mail more often with their capitated patients.

Since visits are an expensive way to deliver medical services, this new model of office practice should be far more efficient than the current one. When I began giving e-mail access to all my patients seven years ago, my cost per patient went down considerably. There were not only fewer visits, but also fewer tests. It turns out that it's easier to reassure patients that they don't need a test or a prescription by e-mail than it is when sitting face-to-face with them.

While current reimbursement methods are not propitious for practices that do a lot of e-mail consultations, this new model promises to provide better care at lower cost. It offers even more to patients and doctors when combined with electronic medical records and the latest clinical decision support tools. Together, these new knowledge management and communication methods can vastly improve how we delivery care.

Concierge Care for Everyone

Editorial
San Diego Physician
2005;92(7):3

The conservative, market-oriented chairman of the Federal Reserve Bank, Alan Greenspan, stated on his retirement that his greatest fear for America was the cost of the Medicare program. With 78 million baby boomers becoming over 65, twice the number as today, the unfunded Medicare mandate for this generation is estimated at $67 trillion! What is a trillion dollars? To put that into perspective, one million seconds ago was last week. One billion seconds ago was the early 1970s when Nixon left the White House. One trillion seconds ago was 30,000 BCE! The current federal deficit is approaching $10 trillion. A doubling of the Medicare population, and business as usual, will certainly bankrupt America for our children.

Medicare is already in crisis. Current estimates show that Medicare will run out of money in 2019, just 11 years from now. Reimbursement cuts are being proposed, a mindless method of reducing costs that will certainly be counterproductive. Most hospitals are already losing money on patients that only have Medicare. Physicians are in the same situation and are fleeing from taking Medicare patients. Further reimbursement cuts will make this access even worse as emergency rooms, not equipped to manage the chronic diseases of seniors, face further overcrowding.

Healthcare researchers estimate that medical waste makes up 30-35 percent of healthcare costs. Price Waterhouse Coopers recently estimated this at 50 percent! Medical waste is expenditures that provide no benefit to the patient. Even using the lower 30 percent figure, for the $500 billion Medicare program, the waste is $150 billion! Add the $300 billion Medicaid program, and we have about $250 billion of taxpayer-funded medical waste in this country. Saving the Medicare program should begin with reducing medical waste. How much money will we keep borrowing to pay for unnecessary and overpriced tests, procedures, and medications?

Medical care is a dance among people, the medical profession, and the overall healthcare system. This dance has become overly expensive as we have medicalized normal parts of living, such as aging and death, and have made common health problems overly expensive. When a third party pays the bills, what happens in the patient-physician relationship becomes unrestrained. Restraint must come before we bankrupt America and leave a problem for our children that is beyond solution.

In 1981 when Ronald Reagan took office, he appointed the 34-year-old David Stockman as federal budget director. Stockman's job was to apply "tough love" to the federal budget and reduce spending by 30 percent. The government should only pay for socially necessary programs. No frills, no fat, and no payment to compensate for poor human behavior. Stockman did just that, although what finally passed Congress were lesser savings. Unfortunately, Medicare was considered untouchable during the Reagan years, and the escalation in costs rivaled the rate of today and the federal deficit tripled.

Will Durant in his 11-volume Story of Civilization states that one factor in the decline of ancient Egypt was that healthcare became "overspecialized." The Greek and Roman civilizations declined in part due to slothful human behavior and a sense of entitlement to its maintenance. America is already the most overweight developed country in the world, and Medicare is planning for three million bariatric surgeries a year! I know about the cost effectiveness data supporting bariatric surgery, but come on, would entitlement to this procedure using taxpayer dollars pass a voter referendum?

It is time to apply "tough love" to Medicare. If we provided only healthcare that was evidence-based, cost effective and necessary for health, we would save hundreds of billions of dollars. We could provide that for everyone, the foundation of a healthcare system, and let people pay for or buy supplemental insurance for everything else they want.

None of the candidates for president is expressing anything close to this bold vision for fixing Medicare. They only want to tweak our current failing system. Cut reimbursement but still provide for almost everything under the sun. How stupid. This is a recipe for continued social decline. The richest country in the world with the best medical schools and higher education can do better. We can provide necessary healthcare for all Americans, not just the seniors and disabled, be affordable, and have the best healthcare in the world. Right now we need to focus primarily on reducing the waste in the system and a lot of tough love.

Concierge medical practice is a recent, growing trend among physicians, especially in primary care. Its success grows out of a combination of frustrations and opportunities. The frustrations are felt by both physicians and patients. Physicians are frustrated by too many insurance hassles and reimbursement for care that is underpaid and undervalued. In today's health insurance climate, primary care physicians have to see more patients just to meet a growing overhead and maintain an income that has not risen in years. Sometimes quality of care is compromised by seeing too many patients.

The frustration among patients is the inability to easily access their primary physicians for care when they want it. Patients are put on hold for extended periods, do not speak to who they want (usually the physician), and find getting even routine healthcare services a great hassle. Many health insurance plans restrict the choice of physician. Even when a good physician is found, there is often an extended waiting period for what is often a hurried visit.

Out of these mutual frustrations comes the opportunity to offer highly personalized services at a premium cost. Having a primary care physician always available, easy to reach, and able to give all the time desired for care is a luxury that many will pay for directly, bypassing health insurance. This concierge level of service allows the physician to have a low practice overhead, since there is no billing, to limit the number of patients cared for, and to have the freedom to spend as much time with patients as they need and want. The going rate for concierge care, reflected in the national medical group, MDVIP, Inc., based in Boca Raton, Fla., is $1,500 – $1,800 per year.[1] Rather than 2,000 or more patients, the primary care physician limits the practice to about 600 – 800 patients. The physician enjoys an unhurried and more personalized practice, while patients have a physician readily accessible. The physician's income may actually increase using this model.

While the long-term market opportunity of concierge practice is unknown, the number of physicians "dropping out" of traditional medical groups and starting these practices is impressive, including in San Diego County. What can we learn from this trend?

Concierge practice is filling a need caused by our dysfunctional healthcare system. The process of delivering high quality health does not need to be user unfriendly for the patient and frustrating for the physician. It does not need to be impersonal, with multiple barriers between the patient and physician. This current situation of mutual frustrations has grown out of 40 years of interference in the patient-physician relationship, especially in third-party payment for care. Many medical groups have also created much of their own service problems. Telephone-driven appointment schedules contribute heavily to the frustration of patients getting care when they want it.

There are alternatives methods available today to make healthcare much more personal and user friendly and not necessarily at a premium cost. The hallmark of concierge care is patients having direct access to their personal physicians. While the cellular telephone has been the original method of this in concierge practice, online communication for all problems except emergencies is a good alternative and avoids the interruption of synchronous communication. The medical practice of Alan Dappen was described in a recent issue of San Diego Physician, a new communication model of care affordable to almost anyone.[2]

The best use of new health information technology will bring highly personal and well-informed healthcare to patients at all times. An electronic health record will be accessible to patients in their home, as a personal homepage that documents their healthcare, arranges for their preventive needs, and offers an abundance of medical information to help manage their chronic illnesses. The modern electronic health record will be intelligent in automatically giving the patient customized health information. Most importantly, this electronic record will be a means of communicating directly with the physician and all the staff members of the healthcare team. This new health information age will bring highly professional services right into the patient's home and will make the traditional processes of care obsolete. All medical groups, including community clinics for the underserved, will participate as the new standard of care.

Concierge care is a call for the return of professionalism in medicine. It is growing because of widespread problems in healthcare delivery today. We will not solve all these problems and try to resuscitate an outdated model of practice. We will move on to newer and modern methods of intelligent and highly personalized care. Concierge care at a premium cost will give way to universally customized and digitalized care with greater efficiency, leading to lower costs for many services. Other service industries like banking and travel have already done this. Today's concierge practices are like the early automobiles that were only available to the wealthy. We have the opportunity through new tools and methods to bring concierge care to everyone. The next ten years will be very exciting and challenging in health care, and San Diego is postured to be a leader in developing new care models.

References

1. www.mdvip.com
2. Dappen, A. "A New Communications Model of Medical Practice." San Diego Physician. March 2005: 12–13. www.doctokr.com.

At the 2005 Annual Spring Conference of STFM in New Orleans, I had the honor of giving the Blanchard Lecture. I used this opportunity state an imperative for the redesign of how family medicine was practiced. The article from this presentation helped set the stage for new models of care.

The End of the Beginning: The Redesign Imperative in Family Medicine

This commentary is a condensed version of Dr. Scherger's 2005 Blanchard Lecture, presented at the Society of Teachers of Family Medicine 2005 Annual Spring Conference in New Orleans.

Family Medicine
2005;94(5):6-7

Family medicine is facing its greatest danger since its inception 38 years ago. While the value of family medicine and primary care is well documented, the current model of practice is outdated, the hassles of insurance and paperwork are choking career enthusiasm, and reimbursement is low. There is an urgent need for radical change in family medicine if it is to survive in the US health system. In the first decade of the new millennium, we have exposed the quality chasm in American medicine — the difference between the care people could receive and the care that is delivered.[1] Cost inflation has resumed as managed care has faded. Consumer-driven health care has arrived with both good and bad consequences—good in that there is a call for more patient centeredness in decision making and bad in that people are bearing more of the costs of their care to the point that basic care is unaffordable for many. The decade of health information technology has been declared, and evidence of the transformation of delivery systems with modern tools and methods is underway. In the face of all this change, will it also be a time of transformation in family medicine?

A big question looms over primary care as health systems develop disease management programs and interactive Web sites where patients can arrange the services they need. Is family medicine simply a range of services, or will it be based on personalized relationship-centered care? If relationship-centered care from a personal family physician has value and is to continue, family medicine will need to come up with new models of care that are effective in the patient-centered and information-rich health systems of the future.

The Value of Family Medicine

The value of family medicine has been well documented. Stange and a team of investigators performed direct observations of family physicians in practice and documented many added values such as the care given for other family members and other problems during a single office visit.[2] Greenfield and Rosenblatt performed studies demonstrating high-quality care by family physicians in rural environments,[3,4] and Starfield's work on the importance and quality of primary care is well known.[5] Phillips, Green, and others at the Robert Graham Center have provided data to support family medicine's value to America's health, while Epstein, Miller, Crabtree, and others have shown in qualitative studies the importance of relationship-centered care.[6] All of this work shows the value of our specialty, but we should not focus only on our value when there are serious problems to address.

The Problem with Family Medicine

So what is the problem? The problem is not who we are or what we do but how we do it. The problem is that our current process of care is ineffective and obsolete. Why? Because the brief-visit model is an acute care model—whereas today, in addition to acute care, we also provide preventive care and chronic illness management, and we strive to do this using the biopsychosocial model and with a family systems orientation. The brief-visit acute-care model no longer fits these tasks.

Outcome studies show that current office practice with brief visits is a poor way to manage common chronic diseases. McGlynn et al found that with brief visits, patients only receive the currently recommended care for chronic conditions about half the time.[7] Similarly, community surveys of hypertension management show that while about two thirds of patients know that they have hypertension, only about half are receiving treatment, and only a quarter have their hypertension controlled.[8] Why? Because 15-minute visits every 3 months don't work for controlling hypertension. Trying harder with the same ineffective model will not work. Indeed, one definition of insanity is doing things the same way over and over and expecting a different result each time.[9] We must redesign our care model to achieve better outcomes.

Thus, the basic engineering problem of primary care is the bottleneck of the brief office visit. A typical daily office schedule for a family physician shows a long list of patients to be seen, each with preventive health care needs, a variety of health problems and comorbidities, and biopsychosocial and family dimensions. The family physician faced with this list of patients has a wealth of resources to offer, but that physician tries to address each patient's complex needs in only 15 minutes. Physicians are the only professionals in society who attempt to do complex work in brief visits. Attorneys don't, architects don't, and engineers don't. Students see us work like this and run the other way.

The result is that Morrison and Smith have described primary care as "hamster care."[10] Primary care physicians are like hamsters running on a treadmill while productivity- oriented medical directors tell us to run faster—so fast, in fact, that many think the number of visits has increased in response to productivity demands. Not so. The actual number of visits per week in primary care has steadily fallen in recent years.[11] What has changed is the nature of the work, including more paperwork, which has compressed the time available to spend with individuals patients.[12]

The Problem With Residency Training

Some of our inability to deal with these problems starts during residency training. Stop a busy third-year resident racing through a clinic of 10–12 patients and ask about the biopsychosocial model. Response: "You've got to be kidding!" Ask "What is the family genogram?" Response: "Give me a break!" Ask the resident just to tell you the patient's story. Response: "Look, I have three patients waiting." We are still training hamsters to provide care! We are dis-educating our residents! We forget that entire civilizations and societies collapse from within if new energy is not brought to them,[13] and we may be engendering the "society" of family medicine in our residency programs.

We should immediately eliminate the visit number requirements for our residents. Instead, we should look at the population of patients they care for, their caring interactions, and their quality outcome measures. Most importantly, we should give our residents the time to become effective healers.

Why Don't We Change?

So, what keeps us from changing? There are two processes holding us back—complacency and powerlessness. The complacent among us feel that the problems are external to family medicine. They feel we are in a cycle and that nothing needs to be done because over time, family medicine will come back in style. The powerless, on the other hand, feel they have little control over their work environment, especially in relation to patient schedules, productivity, and finances. The truth, however, is that family medicine as it has been practiced up to now will not come back in style, and time alone will not change things for the better. Further, we are not powerless to make things change — we need to change things ourselves.

How We Can Change

The future of family medicine depends entirely on the quality of care we deliver. In fact, family medicine will be an anachronism if we do not meet today's quality of care standards, and we cannot do that unless we change how we work. We can take a lesson on how to change from Womack and Jones, who studied the Japanese model of change used by Toyota.[14]   They found that the Japanese use two words for change processes: kaizen, which means continuous incremental improvement, and kaikaku, which means radical improvement.

Both kaizen and kaikaku are necessary for success over time. Kaizen, built into the workflow, creates continuous improvement cycles. Periodically, however, it is necessary to step back and implement kaikaku (radical change) to come up with new models, for without kaikaku you may become obsolete even with incremental kaizen change. Many of the individual elements of the Future of

Family Medicine report—open access scheduling, group visits, and even the electronic health record—are kaizen (incremental change) in which the basic care model is not changed. It is time for kaikaku in family medicine.

The New Model

The new model of family medicine as described in the Future of Family Medicine report has many elements.[15] I want to focus on the first one and discuss it alongside the first rule of change in the Institute of Medicine (IOM) report, Crossing the Quality Chasm.[1] The first rule in the IOM report is that "Care is based on continuous healing relationships." The key word is "continuous," which is in sharp contrast to the current use of episodic visits.

The first element of the new model of family medicine is a "personal medical home." In patient-centered care, the personal medical home is not the physician's office or clinic. The personal medical home is the patient's home. We need to reach into the patient's home and provide continuous access to services to help patients manage their health and illnesses.

With new health information technologies, all patients will have a "home page" that contains their health information and that provides them with access to medical knowledge and services. The various health information technologies, including electronic health records, knowledge management for clinical decision support, and secure communication for Web messaging and remote care, can be combined into one product that is intelligent and communicative and that can create a revolution in how we provide care.[16] Family medicine should embrace these new technologies as a means for delivering higher-quality and more efficient services. It is inappropriate to shun these technologies because of concerns that all our patients do not have access to them, for even patients who do not currently have a computer at home, Internet access can be obtained at public libraries and other sites.

In addition to adopting technologies, we must adopt a planned and systematic approach to chronic care. Ed Wagner and his team in Seattle have developed a model for chronic illness care that reflects the best of community-oriented primary care.[17] It involves productive interactions between informed, activated patients and a prepared, proactive practice team. Note that "productive interactions" is the operative term and not visits; not all interactions have to be office visits. Further, the planned care is provided by a team, and team care, done well, may achieve outcomes far superior to that of a single physician.[18] Family medicine should embrace these new methods of care and be leaders in their development.

Real World Examples

How do we implement these new methods? Here are three real examples of how this might occur. First is the case of Alan Dappen in Virginia, who dropped out of a highly respected family medicine group to form his "doctokr" practice, which uses a new communication model of care.[19] All patient communication begins with a telephone call or e-mail, and patients are seen only when necessary. He has about 1,000 active patients and handles about 20 patient messages each day. He sees four–five patients each day in unhurried visits and makes one–two house calls each week. He charges patients for his time, regardless of how it is delivered. His practice has a Web site and patient newsletter. Dr. Dappen's experience mirrors mine, in which I've found that 40%–60% of patients' needs can be handled by e-mail.

The second example is Greenfield Health in Portland, Oregon.[20] Led by Charles Kilo, a general internist who originally directed the Idealized Design of Clinical Office Practice project for the Institute for Healthcare Improvement, Greenfield Health's practice uses secure Web messaging, telephone, and selective use of office visits. The five physicians spend half the day seeing patients in visits that are 30 minutes or longer. They spend the other half day messaging with patients via the e-mail or by telephone. In a day of patient interactions, by volume, 20% are through in-person visits, 40% are via Web-based email, and 40% are by telephone. The practice has a regular electronic patient newsletter, and the office is used for patient education classes. There is an affordable annual fee to be a member of the practice, based on a patient's age, with a discount for other family members.

The third example is on a larger scale. Kaiser is rolling out Health Connect, a new platform in which patients may communicate with their providers, receive customized health information, arrange for services, and review their health record — all on-line without the need for an in-person visit. Harvard Care Group has developed "Patient Site," which offers similar services.[21]

By using these new tools and methods, a new model of family medicine emerges. Family physicians take responsibility for a population of patients. We manage our patients' needs and demands efficiently and effectively. We prioritize our patients' health problems and use a team approach to their care. We take the time to be effective, and we change our concept and application of productivity. This new model of family medicine can have more caring interactions with patients each day and fewer visits. We work in real time through open access, doing today's work today. Patients get all the time they need and receive excellent care.

Finances

Any discussion of new models of family medicine should include a comment on finances. Today's fee-for-service reimbursement and productivity measurement based on visits and relative value units hold back innovation. There are emerging methods of reimbursement that fit the new model, and Task Force 6 of the Future of Family Medicine project has published a report that predicts better reimbursement for family physicians that use the new model.[22]

Reimbursement methods for the types of care I've described fall into three groups: fee for service, prepaid or contracted care, and a combination of the two. Fee-for-service reimbursement includes payment for all services, including Web messaging, and there are services available that do this automatically. Prepaid contracts include unlimited communication with the physician for a monthly or annual fee, which can be less expensive than many of the things that our patients already pay for, such as health clubs and storage facilities. Combination models have prepaid fees for Web messaging and telephone communication and fee-for-service charges for office visits. Finances follow innovation; the new models of care described here are better, faster, and cheaper—the dream of any redesign engineer.

What Next?

The radical change I am suggesting is hard work. It requires strong leadership, and a focus on continuous learning of and teaching about new methods of care. It will require building the capacity for change, using data to drive the improvement. We will need to start with pilot projects and, after achieving incremental improvements of office systems (such as implementing e-mail with patients, open access, and an electronic health record), then move toward the redesign of all systems.

Family medicine is embarking on a project to develop model practices through a national demonstration project. The American Academy of Family Physicians is launching a new company, a practice resource center, to execute the demonstration project in up to 20 practices, including some teaching practices. Hopefully, these new practices will be like the original 15 family medicine residency programs and serve as catalysts to a new future.

We are witnessing the birth of modern medicine. Within 10 years, it is likely that nearly all patients will have a personal home page that contains their medical information and that provides access to services they need. Our current handwritten paper charts and episodic visits will seem like they are from a primitive past. Where will family medicine be when this comes to pass? Will we be in the back rooms of medical office buildings churning out patients? Or will we be front and center in the new methods of relationship-centered care? Will we have the vision and courage to transform our specialty for this new modern age? I am optimistic. I think we can do it. I think we will do it. We must do it. Let's do it.

References

1. Institute of Medicine. Crossing the quality chasm: a new health system for the 21st century. Washington, DC: National Academy Press, 2001.
2. Stange KC, Jaen CR, Flocke SA, Miller WL, Crabtree BF, Zyzanski SJ. The value of a family physician. J Fam Pract 1998;45: 363-8.
3. Greenfield S, Rogers W, Mangotich M, Carney MF, Tarlov AR. Outcomes of patients with hypertension and non-insulin-

dependent diabetes mellitus treated by different systems and specialties. JAMA 1995;274:1436-44.

4. Rosenblatt RA. Family medicine in four dimensions: developing an ecobiopsychosocial perspective. Fam Med 1997;29(1):50-3.

5. Starfield B. Primary care: balancing health needs, services, and technology. New York: Oxford University Press, 1998.

6. Miller WL, Crabtree BF, Duffy MB, Epstein RM, Stange KC. Research guidelines for assessing the impact of healing relationships in clinical medicine. Altern Ther Health Med 2003;9(3 suppl):A80-A95.

7. McGlynn EA, Asch SM, Adams J, et al. The quality of health care delivered to adults in the United States. N Engl J Med 2003;348:2635-45.

8. Meissner I, Whisnant JP, Sheps SG, et al. Detection and control of high blood pressure in the community: do we need a wake-up call? Hypertension 1999;34:466-71.

9. Berwick DM. Escape fire: designs for the future of health care. San Francisco: Jossey-Bass, 2004.

10. Morrison I, Smith R. Hamster health care. BMJ 2000;321:1541-2.

11. Mechanic D, McAlpine DD, Rosenthal M. Are patients' office visits with physicians getting shorter? N Engl J Med 2001;344:198-204.

12. Ludmerer KM. Time to heal: American medical education from the turn of the century to the era of managed care. New York: Oxford University Press, 1999.

13. Diamond J. Collapse: how societies choose to fail or succeed. New York: Viking Press, 2004.

14. Womack JP, Jones DT. Lean thinking: banish waste and create wealth in your corporation. New York: Simon & Schuster, 1996.

15. Future of Family Medicine Project Leadership Committee. The future of family medicine: a collaborative project of the family medicine community. Ann Fam Med 2004;2(suppl 1):S3-S32.

16. Kilo CM, Leavitt M. Transforming care using information technology. Chicago: Health Information Management and Systems Society (HIMSS), 2005.

17. www.improvingchroniccare.org.

18. Lawrence D. From chaos to care: the promise of team-based medicine. Cambridge, Mass: Perseus Publishing, 2002.
19. www.doctokr.com
20. www.greenfieldhealth.com
21. https://patientsite.caregroup.org
22. Spann SJ, Task Force 6, and Executive Editorial Team. Report on financing the new model of family medicine. Ann Fam Med 2004;2(suppl 3):S1-S21.

JOSEPH E. SCHERGER, MD, MPH

PART VI: NEW MODELS OF CARE, 2006-2013

Slowly but surely the information age and the internet began to change how health care would be delivered in the 21ˢᵗ century. Three transformative applications began to take root: A change from episodic to continuous access to communication and care, strategic proactive care through the use of information technology, and patient self-management through internet applications with patients having their health records. Better access to information enabled evidence-based medicine at the point of care of the patient. I served as editor of the San Diego Physician, the publication of the county medical society, from 2005-2009 and had another platform to express these transformative changes. A selected group of these monthly editorials is reprinted here:

Evidence-Based Medicine and Clinical Practice

Editorial
San Diego Physician
2006;93(4):3

Human beings have four ways of knowing.[1] One is reason, based on remembered experience, education, and reflection. Another is intuition, grounded in experience and based on wherever that "little voice" comes from. Another is faith, based on our beliefs. And finally, there is scientific evidence, based on careful study using dispassionate methods to achieve objective knowledge. Human beings, including physicians, but especially patients, vary greatly in which of the four ways dominate their knowledge. Whether we want to or not, we all use some blend of these four ways in knowing the world around us, including what we know in medicine. Whether any of this knowledge is true is beyond the scope of this editorial.

Evidence-based medicine (EBM) is defined as "the conscientious, explicit, and judicious of the current best evidence in making decisions about the care of individual patients".[2] What a lofty goal! Science-based medicine is what we all learned in medical school. Superstition dominated medicine until the 17th century when the age of Francis Bacon, Galileo, and Newton launched the scientific revolution. You would think by now that all of an advanced society like the United States would be firmly in the grips of a science-only approach to medicine. Yet, unscientific knowledge is flourishing today. My wife and I enjoy shopping at our local health-food market because we like the food, but I am amazed at the advice I hear thrown about by the "trained" staff about which latest supplement is sure to cure one's ills. The pharmacy is no better. Big on display is a popular remedy for the "flu" called Airborne. Very little, if any, science is behind the combination of ingredients. But to give it validation, it was "developed by a school teacher!"

It is true that we do not have scientific evidence for most of the clinical questions we face every day. We cannot practice medicine in 2006 based only on science. However, our clinical judgment is only selectively based on what science we do have. Even the best university professors I work with will often trump science with their beliefs or experience. It is human nature!

Evidence-based medicine will always find resistance in medical practice because it is about human beings caring for other human beings. Objective facts are respected by human beings to varying degrees. We are, by nature, subjective, and our beliefs and experience make adherence to facts that are contrary to those very difficult to accept. Most physicians have learned to accept the primacy of science in medical knowledge, but the public-at-large is a very different story. And to make matters worse, we keep changing what is true in medicine.

The spectrum of scientific medical knowledge can be divided into two groups: the absolute and the relative. Absolute medical knowledge is easier for everyone to accept. It is like the earth is round and rotates around the sun, even though our senses tell us otherwise. Absolute medical knowledge is common in infectious disease, such as with strep throat or the AIDS virus, for example. There are nonbelievers, but they are few and usually on the lunatic fringe. But most scientific medical knowledge is relative and subject to change. Are eggs good for you or not? Does fiber help prevent colon cancer? What about hormones after menopause? I am convinced that much of the knowledge generated by the Women's Health Initiative's (WHI) randomized, controlled trials will turn out to be false. Of course, that is based largely on my reason, intuition, and beliefs!

Some physician investigators have devoted their academic careers to pursuing evidence-based medicine. I admire them. But, I must admit, I also feel a little sorry for them. They will perpetually buck up against human nature and its dependence on the other three ways of knowing. When EBM hooks on to a new, absolute truth, that is great ... a true breakthrough. Unfortunately, relative truths are far more common and subject to change.

What baffles me most today is the comeback that belief in medicine has made in the last five to ten years. It seems to mirror the comeback of many religions. One of the most fascinating areas of sociology deals with the stresses of war and poverty, and how belief systems play a role in culture and human nature. I believe we inadvertently foster belief in medicine through the media's constantly reporting the changes in our relative scientific knowledge. Belief is ok if it does not harm. Sometimes it reflects a return to superstition, which seems not to want to go away no matter how intelligent we are supposed to be.

The second part of the definition of EBM is this: "The practice of evidence-based medicine requires the integration of individual clinical expertise with the best available external, clinical evidence from systematic research and our patients' unique values and circumstances".[2] That is a more practical ideal. As intelligent and scientific physicians, we keep an eye on absolute and relative knowledge, and combine it with our reason and honed intuition. Then we face our patients and realize that they may have very different ways of knowing. The art of medicine is applying the right judgments and using the right words to help our patients benefit from the best of what is known. Given human nature, this is a never-ending quest and will never be replaced by computers loaded with all possible scientific knowledge. I wouldn't mind having one of those around though.

References

1. Robinson DN. The Great Ideas in Philosophy, 2nd Edition. The Teaching Company. Chantilly, VA. 2004. www.TEACH12.com.
2. Centre for Evidence-Based Medicine. Glossary of EBM Terms. www.cebm.utoronto.ca.

Future Office Practice
Painting a Portrait

Editorial
San Diego Physician
2006;93(7);3,5

The new model of office practice cares for a population of patients with robust information systems and continuous healing relationships…Office practice has been fixed in a routine of visits as the unit of care for so long that major change is needed and likely given the impact of information technology.

Office practice is about to change in a big way. Medical office practice today is much like banking before ATMs and online access to accounts. Remember when we had to stand in line to deposit checks into our account, and get some cash? Remember when we checked the balance in our accounts once a month by pencil and calculator (a modern invention)? Patients face these types of inconveniences regularly as they try to find out how they are doing with their preventive services and chronic health problems.

All service industries except medicine have advanced into an age of ready access to information and services. Medicine is about to catch up. Health Information Technology (HIT) is maturing and becoming more affordable, and the tipping point is being reached in its widespread application in office practice. Will the future be similar office visit schedules as today, just with computers? I think not. HIT will be a disruptive technology which is likely to change how most common health services are delivered. Here is a portrait of what I think the office practice model will be like after 5-10 years of rapid process change.

The new model of office practice cares for a population of patients with robust information systems and continuous healing relationships. The care team takes pride in achieving high levels of patient satisfaction and excellent clinical outcomes whenever possible. Patients are actively involved in their care. Face to face visits occur selectively, time intensively and include family and group visits. A continuous platform of care, secure and web based, is the dominant means of coordinating patient care needs and communication among patients and caregivers. The practice is a personal medical home for patients, accessibly both physically and remotely through the patient's home page on an electronic health record. Primary care physicians attend to the broad, comprehensive needs of patients while specialist physicians focus on the organ system or disease process the patient might have, such as the cardiologist with heart failure, the rheumatologist with lupus patients, the neurologist with seizure disorder patients and the urologist with patients with prostatic hypertrophy.

As population based providers of care, new model physicians play a unique role in the communities they serve. The primary care teams across a health care delivery system have knowledge about the health and heath needs of a community which were never before realized. Specialist physicians can see the progression of disease processes in the community. Pooled patient information allows for a regional health information network which is able to respond to community needs in prevention and chronic illness care. Planned care to populations of patients will be rich with information and options for providing care.

There are new skills and practice elements required by this new model of office practice. These include:

Management of a Population of Patients

The new model of office practice allows physicians to manage both the population of patients as a whole and the individual patient. New model physicians are proactive in reaching out to patients to achieve high levels of preventive services and chronic illness management. They have the tools to provide this care in a continuous way. They are incentivized through pay for performance reimbursement based on achieving high levels of successful care to populations of patients.

Patient Centered Care

The traditional paternalistic model of the patient-physician relationship is replaced with patient centered care in which patients are taking an active role in their health and health care. With patient centered care, physicians serve their patients with continuous respect for the patient's autonomy and self-control. Personal physicians are advisors and caregivers on the patient's terms whenever possible. There are times when a physician must step in and assertively provide patient care, such as in medical emergencies and with major illnesses, but this is always done with the utmost respect for the patient's needs and desires. The practice has a patient centered, relationship oriented culture that emphasizes the importance of meeting patients' needs, reaffirming that the fundamental basis for health care is people taking care of people.

Personal Medical Home

The office practice serves as a personal medical home for each patient, ensuring access to comprehensive, integrated care through an ongoing relationship. New online communication methods allow for a continuous connection between the patient, family and the office practice team. The services provided by the practice are readily accessible to the patient. The office system of care available in person and online becomes a home for health care to the population being served. Patients feel connected and have a sense of ownership of all the resources available for their care. The physician is a steward for the patient and family in this medical home.

Best Knowledge at the Point of Care

Physicians should use the best scientific knowledge in the care of patients. Physicians are committed to evidence-based medicine and have the skills to evaluate the quality of medical information. Since the complexity of modern medicine exceeds the inherent limitation of an unaided human mind, knowledge management and clinical decision support tools are used routinely at the point of care. Patients consistently receive the best available clinical care. Currently, access to the best knowledge at the point of care is the goal through currently available electronic systems. Soon, best knowledge will be imbedded into the electronic record and will help guide patient care. Increasingly, some routine care will be automated for the patient to receive best practice upon request.

Continuous Access to Multimodal Communication

Quality of care is achieved through a continuous healing relationship. This requires that patients and providers have access to secure communication at all times. The care team in the office handles patient messages in a timely manner, and important health information is proactively given to patients. Nurses, other office staff and physicians respond to patient messages and proactively communicate with patients through a secure online portal, by telephone and by arranged patient visits.

A New Platform of Care

The convergence of these skills provides a new platform of care which makes the previous model of office practice obsolete. The new platform of care offers an electronic health record available from any computer including by the patient in their home (their personal health record). This record has imbedded evidence-based knowledge management to guide clinical decisions. Secure online communication is imbedded in the electronic record, allowing for access to all patient information with online or telephone communication. A version of this new platform of care is being rolled out by Kaiser Permanente through their Health Connect system of care. They will be the equivalent of the first bank in an area to provide online banking services, and other practices will have to catch up to this new service model.

Fewer and More Time Intensive Office Visits

With physicians having productive interactions with patients online and by telephone, fewer office visits are needed in caring for a population of patients. Office visits in the new model are scheduled selectively and time intensively based on patient needs (6). Brief visit office schedules are replaced by flexible and time intensive schedules. Physicians will spend from 30 minutes to more than an hour in the care of complex patients. The number of office visits is reduced, but the overall number of productive interactions with patients increases from the traditional brief visit model of care.

Group Visits

Physicians use group visits to consolidate care with patients having similar conditions, such as obesity and diabetes, and to create a dynamic where patients help each other. When organized well using the entire care team, with appropriate coding and billing for services, group visits may become an important part of a modern office practice. Technology applications allow for a virtual presence of some patients, or possibly an entire virtual group visit.

Teamwork and Interpersonal Skills

The new model of office practice requires a high level of teamwork and interpersonal skills for the physician. Traditional practice was a physician "craft" with office staff as ancillary. Successful wellness care and chronic illness management requires that the entire office staff be engaged in the care of patients. The physician not only communicates well with patients, but also with the entire staff in a collaborative care manner. Everyone knows their responsibilities and the responsibilities of others, and the team "huddles" at the start of every patient care session.

Financial Practice Management

The new model of office practice must be financially successful. Physicians realize the financial aspects of all the care activities they provide. The new platform of care requires financial contracts and policies which support it. Prepaid services such as for online care should be considered as part of the contracts with patients and insurers. While there are new delivery methods in the new model such as online communication with patients and group visits, there is much efficiency created which should allow for the new model to enhance revenues. In the words of design engineers, it should be "better, faster and cheaper". Models of the new office practice will reflect smart financing of care, highly efficient, affordable and successful.

Many leaps of faith have been taken in presenting this new portrait of office practice. This presentation so positive to be almost Pollyanna. However, the only constant is change, and we tend not to see the magnitude of long term changes. Office practice has been fixed in a routine of visits as the unit of care for so long that major change is needed and likely given the impact of information technology. Just look how much banking, travel and other service industries have changed. There will be lots of problems, battles to fight, and threats to our role as physicians. What is presented here is a portrait of a better future we can have if we work for it.

Listen, Observe, Think, Speak and Act (Not Keyboarding): Optimal Activities for the Modern Physician

Editorial
San Diego Physician
2006;93(8)3

When I looked at the four residents keyboarding away silently, with their backs to me and each other, I had an epiphany. This will go away!

I walked into the residents' work room for my afternoon of being the attending physician. Four residents were busily working away on computers. They were all in their cubicles catching up on patient data, reviewing lab work, adding notes, checking orders, seeing what might have happened recently with their patients. While their diligence and hard work impressed me, there seemed to be something wrong with this picture. Is this the way the modern physician works?

Computers are a great advance for medical practice. Now, for the first time, all of the patient's information is in one place and readily available. Critical functions like checking lab work, writing new orders, requesting consultations, comparing the past with the present, are all done rapidly with points and clicks. At UCSD, we use the new Epic record system and no one would go back to paper. We all have a sense that we are now in modern 21st century medical practice, and that the paper ways were indeed primitive. Having access to the entire patient's data throughout the system makes clinical decision making much more informed.

When the patients are brought into the visibility of their consultation reports, lab results, x-ray reports, flow sheets of their vital signs, they are duly impressed. As we prescribe medications accurately, with automatic checking for spelling, dosing and drug interactions, then have the prescription autofaxed to their preferred pharmacy, it seems magical. All patients leave with a printed summary of their visit, with confirmation of their diagnoses, orders and all their instructions.

After the patient leaves, the real keyboarding begins. Where do we find time to accurately document the visit in the "progress note"? With other patients waiting, we put off this "charting" to a later time. With access to the patients' records from any computer, including at home, we defer completing the charts to the evening, or the next day, or whenever. Every clinic session comes with its burden of documentation which must get done while we remember it. The In Box of patient messages and reports grows just like our e-mail, and keeping up requires "keyboarding time" filling up much of our waking hours. Did we go to medical school and residency to spend our life pounding away on computers?

When I looked at the four residents keyboarding away silently and with their backs to me and each other, I had an epiphany. This will go away! This is the primitive early computer era. Working with computers should not require keyboarding. We are not at our best as physicians typing into machines. We are at our best when listening, observing, thinking, speaking and acting.

The art and science of medicine are using the best medical knowledge gained from many sources over time to render excellent clinical judgments for patients using well developed communication and relationship skills. The time honored methods of clinical excellence are careful listening and observation, thinking assisted by knowledge of both the diseases at hand and the patient, and acting on this as a healer. We physicians are at our best standing up or sitting with patients and using these clinical skills. We must be fully present with our patients to do this well.

The complexity of modern medicine exceeds the inherent limitations of our human minds. We simply cannot store all necessary medical knowledge and retrieve it for patient care accurately at all times. We may have vast knowledge about our established patients, but we cannot remember accurately all their important clinical information. Paper records are woefully inadequate for information retrieval. This is where computers come in. Computers are essential for modern medicine. Not only do they make the patient's clinical information readily accessible, but they may combine this with the best of medical knowledge to guide clinical decision making. Computers are the new "third element" in the exam room and at the bedside.

But will we always have to keyboard our way into the computer's vast resources? Certainly not! I can keyboard as well as most in my generation (which isn't saying much). I often reflect that my most important class in high school was typing. Forty words a minute has been a useful skill throughout my professional life. Of course the younger generations put me to shame. Keyboarding is now taught in the third grade and the residents move much faster than I can. They even answer questions and talk about other things without stopping their hands on the keys! To them, keyboarding is second nature. However, when keyboarding, they are really not listening, observing, thinking much or acting except through the machine. There is a better way and I hope it comes soon.

There will be a future when we will be able to talk with our machines. Like Hal in 2001 A Space Odyssey, our computers will seem alive to us. We will talk to them, ask them questions, and have them look things up instantly. They will assist us greatly, almost completely, in the medical knowledge part and with patient information. We will be uninterrupted in our listening, observing, thinking, speaking and actions with patients. Like Dr. Bones in Star Trek, we will have the power to heal aided by superhuman tools while we stay completely human with our patients.

Voice recognition technology is now about 98% accurate. It learns with the voice of its user. I can't wait until it becomes standard in clinical medicine with our machines. The use of the internet and clinical uses of computers took off just a decade ago. We are still very early in this revolution. I hope to be alive and still working we our use of computers is beyond the keyboarding era. They will be great companions but I want to use my hands for healing.

Email is Old:
Live Video is the Future

Editorial
San Diego Physician
2006;93(11):3

My thinking that email with patients is on the cutting edge of health care innovation was dampened recently when my 28 year old son told me, "Dad, email is old".

Physicians providing email communication with patients is growing slowly. Recent reports state that "only" 25% of physicians in 2006 are offering email services. This is remarkable because the percentage five years ago was closer to 5%. In the realm of diffusion of innovations, around 27-28% penetration if often a "tipping point" where an innovation cannot be stopped and will sweep society. I believe this will happen with email and physicians, most likely through secure web portals.

I began giving my email to patients in 1997, mostly as a convenience and to avoid the terrible telephone system where I worked. After about a year I realized that I had discovered an important innovation for patient care, a new platform of communication which enhanced the physician-patient relationship. I joined with other early physician users of email and began speaking and writing about it, studying the early data on its use. Five years ago I received a lot of push-back from physicians. Email would be an uncontrolled extra burden that would not be good for patient care. Now, most physicians see it as an inevitable part of the internet age.

My thinking that email with patients is on the cutting edge of health care innovation was dampened recently when my 28 year old son told me, "Dad, email is old". He went on to explain that email was the past, not the future. Live video is the future.

My son is living proof of this. His serious girlfriend recently moved to Indiana University to pursue a PhD in English. He is a graduate student in film studies at San Diego State. Every day they communicate with each other live and "in person" using their Apple computers with a built-in video camera. Three times a week they have dinner dates. My son sits at his computer, nicely dressed from the waist up, with a nice dinner in front of him. His girlfriend does the same from Bloomington, Indiana. At my son's apartment she is larger than life on his monitor, sharing dinner and close conversation. The images are as clear as a CNN interview from multiple locations.

Imagine the health care applications! Video visits and providing remote care, having the advantage of all the senses except touch. A common criticism of email is that it is typed text, with no voice, no visual, and no emotion. Information is obtained by email, but the limitations are enormous. Video becomes the next best thing to being there, and makes email seem obsolete indeed! Imagine caring for patient in their homes by video or even in remote areas such as oversees. I can easily see the Mayo Clinic or the Cleveland Clinic expanding their reach around the world. Why not us in San Diego! Pacific Rim, here we are, ready to care for you!

When you are living through history it is easy not to appreciate the magnitude of some historic events. As I write this, the big business story of the week is Google buying YouTube for 1.65 billion dollars. Why did they do that? The simple answer they gave was, the future of the internet is video. Notice on Google home page the icon for video now shows up next to images. You may think I have gone off the deep end, but I think the Google purchase of YouTube was a major historical step for the internet age, and will also have enormous implications for health care.

Just imagine what video means for our medical records! Not just static information anymore. Want to document the progression of someone's Parkinson disease? Watch the videos of the patient's gait or arm movements at rest and while eating. With Alzheimer's patients, take a look at the behavior which happens at sundown. Look at the child's behavior, is it really ADHD or a need to get out more and play. Life, documented, becomes a series of video clips. A camera records our office visits. The applications are endless and mind boggling. Those moving pictures in the Harry Potter stories become real after all.

So, fellow physicians get those electronic health records with a secure communication portal and start emailing with patients. That will be just the beginning of the future of online and remote communication. Evisits, which of course must be financed as part of care, have an incredibly exciting future. Email may be old to the new generation of adults, but it is finally coming to health care.

Someday soon, we will have continuous access to our patient's life situation, at home and at work. This may sound like an Orwellian big brother, but not if it is patient driven. How limited we are today by only seeing our patients in the office. Caring for patients the 21st century way is just beginning. One hundred years ago it was horse and buggy. Someday, our great-grandchildren will look at 2006 office practice the same way. Email is only a primitive beginning. Email is old.

Google for Diagnosis

Editorial
San Diego Physician
2007;94(3):6-7

"The complexity of modern medicine exceeds the inherent limitations of the unaided human mind." David Eddy, MD

There was once a time when medical students and residents were expected to memorize the information required to practice good medicine. Physicians would attend continuing education courses to keep this memorization up to date. Patients would expect their physicians to be completely knowledgeable about their medical problems. Those days are gone, yet the expectations still linger on.

In November 2006, the British Medical Journal (BMJ) published a study, "Google for a diagnosis …"[2]. Two authors from Australia took 26 of the challenging case records published in the 2005 issues of the New England Journal of Medicine. Google searches revealed the correct diagnosis in 15 (58 percent) of the cases. The online responses to this article were legion, sometimes emotional, and revealing how timely the topic of Internet search for diagnosis is.[3]

The Internet has changed how we do about everything. Dictionary.com is must faster than grabbing the book off the shelf and looking for the right page. In my medical office, copies of reference books will not be replaced. Online reference materials are better, faster, and cheaper.

For a decade, the Internet has become the place to go for information. Until recently, we had our list of favorite websites, and we might spend time "surfing" the Web for information. We would have our online list of reference materials, like a new virtual library. As Battelle has described in his popular book, The Search, all that has changed to using Google or one of its rivals like Yahoo. These search engines make 10 billion decisions in a second and eliminate the hit or miss of limited reference sources. Search may even be rep lacing popular Web references like UpToDate and First Consult.

The question of using Google as an aid in diagnosis brings speed and practicality up against evidence-based medicine. Google and similar search engines were never designed for evidence-based medical diagnosis. They simply put us in touch with the world's information, based on frequency of use and general accuracy.

For many years, there has been a quest for computerized diagnosis decision support systems (DDSS). One such product is Isabel (www.isabelhealthcare.com). Isabel claims to be able to help physicians reach a correct diagnosis in 96 percent of cases. I looked over Isabel and was impressed, but it was not near as fast as Google. If I want to make a difficult diagnosis accurately, I would use Isabel. If I wanted information, I would use Google.

Some responders to the BMJ article touted PubMed as the website of choice for medical science as an aid in diagnosis. One physician used PubMed for the same 26 cases and found important diagnostic information on 23 (88 percent). I suspect this took most of a day to do. PubMed is a great site for the National Library of Medicine and brings up a list of articles, but may not readily help decision making at the point of care.

Google is not resting on its success. Google Scholar gives you access to the world's scientific information. Google Health, like Yahoo Health, is a vast medical library of information. The entire world's knowledge is now democratized, everyone has equal access, so patients will use these searches for self-diagnosis and treatment.

So, where does this leave diagnostic decision making in 2007? I would say this. Think off the top of your head at your peril. In seconds your patients can know whether your thinking and advice are on target or off base. Medicine today is about knowledge management and clinical decision support. Tools for doing this better are amazing but still in their early days. We all need digital brains to help us on a routine basis.

Balance speed and practicality with evidence and good medical knowledge. Google will not be with you in court if you use them to make a wrong diagnosis or pick a wrong treatment. Our job is to put information together in the care of patients for accurate diagnoses and the correct treatments. This is what both medical education and medical practice are about today.

Do not practice medicine without a computer on and connected to the Internet. Better yet, have this in every exam room, with a screen that can be view by the patient. Gone are the days when patients might not have faith in you if you needed to look things up. Now, patients may wonder about you if you do not look things up! We all need clinical decision support. No longer do you need a library of websites to wonder through. Search is fast and simple. Google may the place to start, but not necessarily the place to end your search.

Will We Ever Simplify American Health Care?

Editorial
San Diego Physician
2007;94(4):6-7

"Americans can always be counted on to do the right thing ... after they have exhausted all other possibilities." — Winston Churchill

We know the statistics well. Forty-seven million Americans go without health insurance, equivalent to the population of about 20 states. Even more are underinsured and face financial ruin if they get a major illness or injury. For those who have insurance, the plans are a patchwork of confusion and uncertainty. Paul Krugman of The New York Times refers to the health insurance industry as a "racket" (2/16/07), with plans negotiating their deals and avoiding payment. Consumers (a.k.a., people) are absorbing more of the costs of the care (a.k.a., "skin in the game") but have little understanding of what healthcare costs are or should be.

Our bold governor is making national news with his plan for covering all Californians. Massachusetts is doing the same. Every politician gunning for the presidency in 2008 is formulating their plan for universal coverage. When I look into the plans, all I see is confusion. The mosaic of SChip, HDHPs, HSAs, HMOs, PPOs, Medicare, Medicaid, employer plans, and individual plans is a bewildering array of options — all hard to understand. Is this the American solution? It may reflect the current American landscape for healthcare financing, but I do not see it as a solution to be proud of.

Providing and financing healthcare to a diverse population of more than 300 million people is about as complex as anything you can think of. But, do complex problems require complex solutions? We know from complex systems science that dealing successfully with the "zone of complexity" requires following "simple rules" to guide behavior [see Appendix B, "Redesigning Health Care With Insights from the Science of Complex Adaptive Systems," by Paul Plsek, from Crossing the Quality Chasm: A New Health System for the 21st Century (2001)]. An American solution to healthcare should be more simplicity — not more complexity — in its design and application.

I have a plan: All Americans receive the healthcare they need. This would be done in a simple, straightforward way with a choice of excellent providers. Americans could also receive the healthcare they want, above those needs, if they want to pay for it directly or through insurance. Two categories of healthcare, two payment mechanisms — how simple. I do not think of the healthcare that would meet people's needs as a single payer, but rather as a single solution. This foundation of healthcare meeting all Americans' needs is publicly supported by the more than two hundred million Americans who pay taxes — hardly a single payer!

So, you ask, how do we separate the healthcare that people need from the healthcare that people want? Keep it simple. Preventive medicine would be all the things the U.S. Preventive Services Task

Force says that we should receive based on the best available evidence. Universal coverage of needed immunizations (polio yes, zostavax no). Everyone would be eligible for the recommended screening tests for the early detection of disease (mammograms yes, body scans no). Counseling for smoking cessation and healthy behaviors would be abundant. Care of acute and chronic illness would be driven by current best evidence, and, where evidence is lacking, the best expert opinions not biased by industry. Transparent, publicly trusted authorities would provide a foundation of needed healthcare for all Americans, with providers delivering these services at fair reimbursement. Keep it simple, and administrative costs would be low. We could do this for a fraction of the $1.9 trillion we currently spend on healthcare.

But many Americans would not want to stop there! We crave choice, freedom, and getting what we want. No restrictions on the healthcare we want, as long as we are willing to pay for it, either directly or through insurance. You want only brand name drugs, some plans will guarantee that for you. If you want the freedom to choose therapies or surgery beyond the foundation of scientific need, there will be supplemental plans or providers competing on price and quality ready to serve your needs. Bariatric and plastic surgery continue to flourish.

Here are more examples of need versus want. We all watch television and see that every time a professional athlete gets an injury of almost any kind, an MRI is done. Many Americans expect that the good care of any musculoskeletal injury requires an MRI. Imaging costs have been the fastest rising sector of healthcare spending in the last few years. We have excellent clinical guidelines as to when imaging is appropriate and necessary (e.g., the Ottawa ankle rules). These would be followed in the publicly funded need category, and people could still get their wanted MRIs in the want category.

Sleep studies are big now, and it seems almost anyone who snores or sleeps next to such a person wants one done. The obesity epidemic has been coupled with a snoring epidemic. We need good objective clinical guidelines for when sleep studies are needed. Everybody else who wants a sleep study is in the want category.

New drugs are coming out at a rapid rate, and all are expensive. Four-dollar pills are now the norm for new therapies for hypertension, dyslipidemia, and diabetes. More than 40 percent of adults over 40 have one or more of these problems. We know what good control is, and this can be achieved inexpensively or expensively, depending on lifestyle and choice of therapies. The "need" category would have rational clinical guidelines for appropriate and cost-effective use of medications. The want category would be whatever new brand the patient or physician wants to use.

Sound simple? It is! Of course, the devil is in the details, and the application of this need versus want could be very political. I can think of excellent people to serve on the "healthcare based on needs" panel, like the current U.S. Preventive Services Task Force. The important thing is that for those Americans who select or can afford just the need coverage, the best healthcare in the world will still be delivered by the best providers in the world if the system is designed right with fair reimbursement.

How do we pay for this? Currently, a conservative estimate is that 30 percent of healthcare expenditures in the United States are waste, benefiting no one. Thirty percent of $1.9 trillion is $570 billion — more than enough to pay for this transition. American employers would be relieved of paying for the cost of expensive healthcare for their employees while they try to compete in a global market. Employers could choose supplemental health plans in conjunction with their employees as an added benefit.

What I am proposing could be anywhere between terrible and great, depending on our leadership and how the need category is applied. Americans should be so proud of this system that they will demand good leadership. The need category should be at a level of care of many current plans such as Kaiser. The need category and the want category would both be seen as positive and highly American. Is this socialized medicine? Only if you want to call it that. Do we have a socialized highway system with private toll roads? Do we have a socialized police force with private security for those who want additional protection? Do we have socialized television with additional private choices through cable? It is just semantics. Americans know and understand two levels of service. Those flying coach do not sneer at people flying first class.

Is this just a dream? Maybe. As we know in the world of new technology, if you can think of it, it is possible. I say to today's leaders who want to reform healthcare: Simplify, get rid of all the waste, and give all Americans the healthcare we need.

Time Management Today

Editorial
San Diego Physician
2007;94(6):6-7

Remember reading articles about how we would all have increased leisure time as new technologies simplified our work? Well, new technologies have made lots of things easier, but most of us are working harder than ever. Overwork has become endemic in our society. An alarming number of people, even physicians, are forgoing vacations in order to meet the demands of their work.

Life is short, and not enjoying life while working is tragic. Good time management is a key to having your life and work organized for personal satisfaction. All of us wish to have a sense that we have control over our lives and work schedules.

The Internet and online communication have changed how we work, but not necessarily our work schedules. Many of us are working on our computers late at night doing the emails we did not get to during the day. Time spent online by today's professionals, including physicians, is moving past the one-hour mark to up to two hours a day. As online patient care becomes more common, this time will increase further. No wonder that physicians resist communicating with patients online if it is done in addition to a busy office schedule of patient visits.

This leads to my first time management recommendation: Work-related online communication and Web-based activities must be scheduled into the workday, and not be added to an already busy appointment schedule. Time spent online has crept into our lives over the past 10 years since Web browsers and email became commonplace. It is now time for all employers to recognize that work done online is a core part of the work and should be scheduled like everything else. Whoever manages your schedule should put in the necessary time for online work, and that means you if your schedule is under your control. Of course, it helps if you have a payment model that supports working online. We physicians should not give away patient care done online like we have for telephone work.

How many hours are there in a week? I ask this of patients frequently and rarely get an answer. We all know by reflex there are

24 hours in a day and seven days in a week. But few of us have thought about the 168 hours in a week, even though we tend to plan our lives by the week. Most of us on Sunday take a look at our calendars and see what we are doing this week. Since most days are not identical, it makes sense to organize our time by the week.

How shall we plan these 168 hours? I like to start with five hours devoted to exercise. That first priority might surprise you, but spending five hours a week in exercise makes you fit and more likely to live longer and healthier. Five hours sounds like a lot, but when you think there are still 163 hours left, there is no excuse not to exercise that amount of time. Your life depends on it.

Plan five hours of exercise into your week as a top priority.

Since most of us average seven hours of sleep a night, 49 of the 168 hours goes to restful sleep. This is important for health and recharging our energy sources. Give two hours a day to eating, an important activity that should not be rushed, and so 14 hours a week for eating. Five plus 49 plus 14 is 68 hours. That leaves 100 hours a week for everything else.

One of my favorite books from the 1970s was Richard Bolles' The Three Boxes of Life and How to Get Out of Them (Ten Speed Press, 1978). He called the three boxes work, learn, and play. His main point was that people overly compartmentalize their lives into working, learning, and playing. Often when doing one, they wish they were doing another. It is part of the "thank God it's Friday" mentality. We live with less satisfaction when we feel ourselves in such boxes. Rather, Bolles recommends an attitude like the saying, "If you love your job, you never have to work a day in your life." He argues that if you find pleasure in your work, your learning, and your play, you will always be happy and not even think about being in a "box."

As a working physician (I read Bolles as a student), I would label the three activities as work, learning, and personal/family time. If we have chosen wisely, they should all be pleasurable. That gets me back to those 100 hours left in the week. Don't schedule them as boxes! My second time management today recommendation is: Your life should be a well-balanced and well-prioritized blend of work, learning, and personal/family time.

If you asked me how many hours a week I work, my honest

answer would be, "I have no idea." I don't think about it. I know it varies some from week to week. What I care about, and monitor internally and externally with the help of my wife and children, is whether or not I am in balance. Am I spending too much time at work or learning at the expense of my personal and family time? If so, make an adjustment. My wife does like me to work hard because we have lots of bills to pay. I enjoy my work so that is ok. The key is to refine a balance of those three activities for whatever phase of life you are in. If you are out of balance, make adjustments. My wife helped me limit my evening computer time so we had more time together before going to bed, a very nice adjustment indeed.

This leads me to my third recommendation for time management today: Live a life of choice, doing the things you want to do with the right amount of time and energy. There are more forces than ever trying to control our lives. Most physicians today work in medical groups with fixed schedules and productivity demands. Realize that we chose to be wherever we work. If you are not happy, change. Take risks if necessary. Living a life of your choosing is critical to your life satisfaction, and critical to those who love and depend on you.

No article on time management would be complete without some words on prioritizing. We all have lots of things we can do each day and each week. Make lists of the things that must get done and give them an "A" priority. "Do what you have to do" is what my inner voice says, which keeps me doing A priorities. "B" things are tasks you should get done if you can, but are not critical. Something on the B list one week may be on the A list next week. "C" things are tasks that you may get to if you have extra time. I have lots of C things that may wait until my retirement! Actually, holiday weeks not spent on vacation are often good times to get some C work done, like clearing out old files. I'm often amazed at how some people have trouble with such prioritizing, putting off an A task while doing something that is of C priority. This leads to misery and even failure. Prioritizing work, learning, and personal/family time is a critical life skill and must be developed in order to live a satisfying life of choice.

So, in summary, exercise, sleep, and eat well to be healthy. Work, learning, and personal/family time are the three blendings of a happy and well-managed life. Don't wish you were a member of the "leisure class." Those people rarely look happy anyway.

Consumer Directed Health Care Abroad

San Diego Physician
2007;94(9):6-7

A new medical magazine arrived in the mail. Big deal. Then I took a look at it. Issue 1 of The International Medical Travel Journal. I was flabbergasted by what I found inside. I knew that places like India were attracting "medical tourists" from the United States for less expensive surgeries and other treatments. I was not prepared for what I found inside, and I would like to share with you a sampling of articles and current offerings.

Singapore aims to attract one million medical tourists by 2012 through the efforts of Singapore Medicine [www.singaporemedicine.com], an initiative of the Economic Development Board of Singapore, Singapore Tourism Board, and International Enterprise Singapore. In 2005, the number of visitors who came to Singapore expressly for healthcare reached 370,000. A growing number of medical and surgical specialists offer a complete range of consultative and treatment procedures. Medical travel agents are standing by to help you.

Vietnam opened its first medical-travel resort, Medicoast [www.medicoast.com], in February 2007 in the popular seaside town of Vung Tau. The resort offers pediatrics, obstetrics, eye surgery, orthopedics, nutrition advice, general surgery, and cosmetic dentistry.

Tourism officials in Thailand are optimistic the number of medical tourists will reach two million by 2011. The Thai medical-travel industry has several advantages: "First is the quality of doctors, second is price, and third is that patients do not have to wait to see a good doctor."

The South Korean government and private hospitals are collaborating to attract overseas patients. The priority target for international patients is Korea's advanced techniques in LASIK operations, Oriental-medicine treatment, plastic surgery, backbone surgery, artificial fertilization and implant treatments.

India and Taiwan are relaxing visa restrictions to help promote medical travel, and the options are extensive and rapidly growing.

Turning from Asia to Latin America, a recent San Diego Union Tribune reprinted a Miami Herald article about Americans traveling to Panama, Mexico, Costa Rica, Columbia, Argentina, and Chile. The article states that United Nations figures show that travel and tourism is now the world's largest industry at $4.4 trillion, more than defense, manufacturing, oil, and agriculture. Medical tourism is the hottest new sector in the travel industry.

This is not just about Americans traveling abroad for less expensive medical care. Annually, about 50,000 British patients travel out of the United Kingdom to escape long waiting lists and out of fear of contracting hospital infections. The most popular destinations are India, Hungary, and Turkey. In Germany, a new website is offering "e-auctions" for medical treatment: www.arzt-preisvergleich.de. The site asks patients to post how much they have been quoted for a treatment from one physician, allowing other physicians to offer to beat the price. When physicians compete, you win!

A new Irish Internet start-up [www.revahealthnetwork.com] describes itself as a matchmaking site for those interested in having medical treatment in other countries.

If you want to avoid the Third World, try Switzerland. The five-star diagnostic center, The Diagnostic & Prevention Center (DaP) in St. Moritz [www.dap-center.ch], claims to be the first European medical resort of its kind. DaP offers a range of packages to suit each client's needs. Clients are expected to come from all areas of Europe, particularly Italy, Germany, and the United Kingdom. Like with Swiss banks, strict confidentiality of results will be maintained.

The list goes on: Bahrain, Dubai's Healthcare City, Israel, South Africa, and even (this will make you smile) Iran. Not to be totally outdone, the United Kingdom's largest private hospital, London Bridge Hospital [www.londonbridgehospital.com], is getting into this.

Of course this type of activity has been going on in the United States for many years. Cleveland Clinic [www.clevelandclinic.org] and Mayo Clinic [www.mayoclinic.com] have large international caseloads. New York hospitals advertise all over the world. I have witnessed the efforts of the University of California medical centers. But the problem in the United States is our prices for medical care. Despite the higher costs for almost everything in Europe, healthcare costs run about half that of the United States. In the Third World, pockets of excellence can operate at a small fraction of U.S. prices.

What about accreditation and liability? These issues are being covered. Our own Joint Commission [www.joincommission.org] now accredits international hospitals and facilities. Interestingly, India added Australian hospital accreditation as an option. The quality international centers make transparent their liability coverage, and patients can purchase their own policies to guarantee the results.

The days of rich Arabs coming to the United States and paying top dollar are coming to an end. The world is rapidly becoming flat for quality medical care. The private healthcare market in the United States facilitates Americans going abroad for care. With the rise of consumer-directed healthcare, and patients paying more of the costs, medical travel is likely to steadily increase unless we can be competitive at home. Health insurance plans in the United States are even beginning to cover medical travel since the costs are lower.

San Diego, as a major Pacific Rim destination, has a real opportunity to become a hub for medical tourism. Not only are we "America's Finest City," we are arguably the "World's Finest City." As our patients think about traveling abroad for care, we should seize the opportunity and become a destination for medical travel. Think of those HMO and PPO rates we accept. Many people in the world will pay much better.

Are Retail Clinics a Good Thing?

Editorial
San Diego Physician
2007;94(11):6

My wife is a big fan of Martha Stewart. I often hear about something being a "good thing." Does this expression apply to retail clinics, those easy access modules popping up in Wal-Marts, Targets, and CVS pharmacies?

A time honored behavior in society is that when you get sick, maybe you should see a doctor. In the days when two thirds of physicians were in general practice, all you had to do was call or go right into your doctor's office, sign in, and be seen in a reasonably short period of time. Now, primary care works much differently. The appointment slots are guarded by a trained staff and filled in advance with scheduled visits. Good luck seeing a doctor the same day you get sick and want to. If "they" will fit you in, it is when "they" want, not necessarily when it is convenient for you. And, if you do not have insurance, you get that dreaded "self pay" label, immediate suspicion of being a deadbeat.

Retail clinics are popping up because of a real or perceived need for ready access to simple primary care. Nurse practitioners are replacing physicians as lower-cost providers. The care will be so convenient that you can even shop while you wait. Given the shortage today of primary care physicians and the large number of uninsured people with cash to spend for basic healthcare, retail clinics seem like a sure winner.

I consider retail clinics an unfortunate sign of a breakdown in office practice. Separate care delivered by a nurse practitioner in one of these clinics further fragments the healthcare of a patient. The retail clinic becomes another place where important medical record information is kept. Without a unified system of care, a person's medical record is scattered over a community, creating a high-risk situation for errors in diagnosis and treatment.

Will retail clinics reduce healthcare costs? Will they save money for the patient? Not likely. When a person is seen by a stranger, more tests get done than when a person gets care from someone who knows them and where their health information is readily available. Even though nurse practitioners have lower wages than physicians, they may drive up the overall cost of care through more testing and referrals. A recent meta-analysis showed that while patients are satisfied with care from nurse practitioners, the costs are higher because of more testing and referrals.[1] Nurse practitioners have an important place in providing quality and efficient healthcare, but this comes from working with physicians, not instead of them.

My hope and prediction is that retail clinics will have some initial success and then flop. Their emergence is a wake-up call for office practice. Ready access to common, acute primary care is important to people, and physician offices must provide that. Having a physician or nurse practitioner dedicated to same-day, acute visits are important. Patients should be able to walk in and not always have to call for an appointment.

Some medical groups and hospital systems are opening acute care clinics in places where people shop. In the past, it was considered unprofessional to have a "storefront office." In today's society, convenience trumps the fancy separate building where you might even have to pay to park. Electronic health records allow a medical group to have the patient's medical record available in multiple places.

Online access to communication and care makes much of what retail clinics do unnecessary. Most common acute illnesses, like upper respiratory infections, do not need an office visit. If a person at home could go online with their physician's office and share information and receive care as appropriate, why would the person even consider paying $50 at a retail clinic? Pay $25 for an E-visit from home versus driving to a Wal-Mart? Think of the reduced sharing of cold viruses! I'm not sure I want to be in a Wal-Mart, Target, or CVS pharmacy with a bunch of sick people walking around.

These are dynamic times for healthcare. Retail clinics, online care, and electronic health records in the patient's possession are all disruptive to traditional office practice. Being in a successful practice today means being responsive to changing societal wants and needs … and new technologies. The delivery of healthcare will be much different in the coming decades.

Physicians in general are not keen on changing how they work. But in today's world, change is a necessity for continued success. Rather than let a retail clinic steal some of your business, think about how you might put them out of business by providing better service.

Reference

1. Carter AJ, Chochinov AH. A systematic review of the impact of nurse practitioners on cost, quality of care, satisfaction, and wait times in the emergency department. CJEM. 2007;9:286-295.

Practicing Excellence

Editorial
San Diego Physician
2008;95(3):6-7

Excellence is a habit, not a single act. We are what we do repeatedly. — Aristotle

Excellence in medical practice today goes beyond the comparison with pornography: I know it when I see it. Sure, a great patient visit or disease outcome gives the impression of excellence. But repeated and consistent excellence in medical practice is rare, even among the best physicians.

What constitutes practice excellence? There are at least three dimensions. First, the patient must feel as if they received excellent care. The patient satisfaction score is all the way to the top. Secondly, what was done for the patient matches the highest current standards of care. Current best practice was delivered. Thirdly, the outcome of the care was optimal, given all realistic possibilities. Best outcomes are derived from consistently repeated best practice.

How do we achieve such an ideal in medical practice? Is excellence a realistic goal and a consistently achievable outcome? Yes, according to Steve Beeson, Sharp-Rees Stealy physician leader of the Sharp Experience and author of Practicing Excellence: A Physician's Manual to Exceptional Health Care.[1] His article in this issue tells the story of the Sharp Experience from the physician perspective. Steve Beeson does not just talk the talk of excellence. He walks the walk, both for himself in full-time practice and for his group.

Steve Beeson's book is a wonderful read, and I recommend it highly to all physicians, regardless of specialty. After making the case for excellence, everything from improving patient compliance, building patient loyalty to reducing malpractice risk, he dissects the clinical encounter into detail most of us have never thought about. Did you know there are eight parts to each visit? They are:

1. The First Impression
2. Exam Room Preparedness
3. Techniques in History Taking

4.   The Physician Exam
5.   Providing Patient Information
6.   Patient/Physician Collaboration
7.   Patient Follow-up
8.   Effective Appointment Closure

Each of these has room for error or inadequate performance. Beeson gives pointers for excellence with each of these steps. He then provides pointers for difficult patient situations.

The book then goes beyond the individual physician and staff to the medical group. How does an entire group achieve excellence? Beeson provides nine steps that were used at Sharp Rees-Stealy to accomplish their amazing turnaround.

Steve Beeson was the keynote speaker at the Sharp Primary Care Conference in Hawaii. Fifteen of his colleagues were present. I enjoyed listening to the early skeptics, for example, the urgent care and occupational medicine physicians, who felt that they were doing as well as they could under difficult circumstances. They are now doing incredibly better and look back on their past performance as an earlier time of substandard practice.

Converting to consistent excellent practice is not easy. Physician coaching is often necessary, not something we in a traditionally autonomous profession are inclined to admit that we need. Finding and developing coaches is an important and challenging process, but one that is necessary for group-wide excellence. Other companies known for consistent excellent service, like Nordstrom or Starbucks, use coaching and development continuously. We need to also, and not just for our office staff.

Steve Beeson's keynote presentation highlighted nine essential elements of practice excellence. Everyone must be present for a group to sustain excellence. I find a list of nine things intimidating, and I quickly wondered how realistic that could be. They are: Vision, Leadership, Passion, Relentlessness, Ownership, Recognition, Accountability, Measurement, and Execution. I could not think of any one of these to remove and still have excellence.

It has been five years since I became the director of the San Diego Center for Patient Safety, an organization that is no longer active due to lack of funding. Benchmarks of quality of care in San Diego County revealed lots of gaps. One study on several common conditions even put us in the bottom 25 percent of major metropolitan areas! A lot has happened here since that time. I am convinced that San Diego County is now in the top 25 percent nationally. Every major hospital and medical group has had dedicated efforts to improve quality, as this issue of San Diego Physician describes. Sharp's recent Malcolm Baldridge Award is a crowning achievement. Steven Beeson has emerged as a major champion of physician excellence. We would all do well by following his teachings and example.

Reference

1. Beeson SC. Practicing Excellence: A Physician's Manual to Exceptional Health Care. Gulf Breeze, FL: Fire Starter Publishing (Studer Group), 2006.

Patient Portals

Editorial
San Diego Physician
2008;94(4):6-7

Electronic Health Records (EHRs) are the most visible tool for modernizing the process of patient care. 20th-century healthcare was marked by scattered paper charts and handwriting by doctors and nurses. 21st-century healthcare has digital patient information in one place, portable to wherever the patient is cared for. While the EHR symbolizes modern care, it is the applications within EHRs that transform the process of care.

Two EHR applications that are basic for improving patient care are registries and electronic prescribing. The registry function allows for the planning and evaluation of care to a population of patients. All patients with a certain disease, such as diabetes, are gathered together with proactive disease management efforts and continuous evaluation of the quality of care. The registry function is necessary for efficient participation in pay for performance programs. Electronic prescribing adds great convenience to patient prescriptions and reduces the risk of medication errors.

A higher order function within EHRs is knowledge management

for clinical decision support (CDS). Most early EHRs have drug-drug interaction information at the point of care and reminders for preventive services. More advanced EHRs have imbedded clinical guidelines to help the care team provide consistent best practice to patients. CDS applications make an EHR intelligent and providers are not limited to what they can think of at the moment, or have to break away from care to look something up.

The EHR application that I believe will truly transform the process of care is the patient portal. The patient portal is a secure communication function built into the EHR. Two-way communications between the patient and care team happen within the medical record, with the communication automatically captured as part of the care.

Early applications of a patient portal look more like convenience than transforming care. I visited a practice recently that just launched its patient portal, and it is being used for the patient to request appointments, refills, and to ask questions that would have been done over the telephone. The care team will use the patient portal for appointment reminders and to share information with the patient such as lab and other test results. Nothing revolutionary there.

Whether you realize it or not, the patient portal is a gateway to two major transformations of patient care. The first is that patients have direct access to their own medical record. 20th-century healthcare was paternalistic, with providers owning the medical records and patients had difficulty even getting copies. With EHRs containing patient portals, patients share in the ownership of their records. This is patient-centered care in which patients becomes active coordinators of their care. The shift to patient coordination of care is big, just like people being able to manage their own financial accounts, travel, and other services. Soon, patients will be arranging for their own preventive services, such as lab work and mammograms. They will be filling out their own checklists for the management of chronic health problems, such as diabetes. Patient responsibility for their own care increases. Through patient portals and the evolution to personalized medical home pages, patient centered care in the 21st-century will blossom.

The second transformation is that through patient portals, care does not depend on patient visits. Patients and the care team communicate in a continuous way rather than depend of getting everything done during hurried patient visits. The first rule of redesign in the IOM report, Crossing the Quality Chasm (2001), is that care is based on continuous healing relationships. Patient portals make access to care continuous, at mutual convenience, and become the new first platform of care. Face-to-face visits, group sessions, and telephone communication will increasingly be driven by communication which starts through the patient portal.

What looks like a simple new convenience for patient communication becomes a transformative tool for patient care. I think the patient portal is the most exciting and powerful application of an EHR. Methods of making patient portals financially viable are available. Like online banking, health care online will be remembered as the major transformation of care in the early 21st century.

How to Save Medicare (and America)

Editorial
San Diego Physician
2008;95(7):6-7

The conservative, market-oriented chairman of the Federal Reserve Bank, Alan Greenspan, stated on his retirement that his greatest fear for America was the cost of the Medicare program. With 78 million baby boomers becoming over 65, twice the number as today, the unfunded Medicare mandate for this generation is estimated at $67 trillion! What is a trillion dollars? To put that into perspective, one million seconds ago was last week. One billion seconds ago was the early 1970s when Nixon left the White House. One trillion seconds ago was 30,000 BCE! The current federal deficit is approaching $10 trillion. A doubling of the Medicare population, and business as usual, will certainly bankrupt America for our children.

Medicare is already in crisis. Current estimates show that Medicare will run out of money in 2019, just 11 years from now. Reimbursement cuts are being proposed, a mindless method of reducing costs that will certainly be counterproductive. Most hospitals are already losing money on patients that only have Medicare. Physicians are in the same situation and are fleeing from taking Medicare patients. Further reimbursement cuts will make this access even worse as emergency rooms, not equipped to manage the chronic diseases of seniors, face further overcrowding.

Healthcare researchers estimate that medical waste makes up 30-35 percent of healthcare costs. Price Waterhouse Coopers recently estimated this at 50 percent! Medical waste is expenditures that provide no benefit to the patient. Even using the lower 30 percent figure, for the $500 billion Medicare program, the waste is $150 billion! Add the $300 billion Medicaid program, and we have about $250 billion of taxpayer-funded medical waste in this country. Saving the Medicare program should begin with reducing medical waste. How much money will we keep borrowing to pay for unnecessary and overpriced tests, procedures, and medications?

Medical care is a dance among people, the medical profession, and the overall healthcare system. This dance has become overly expensive as we have medicalized normal parts of living, such as aging and death, and have made common health problems overly expensive. When a third party pays the bills, what happens in the patient-physician relationship becomes unrestrained. Restraint must come before we bankrupt America and leave a problem for our children that is beyond solution.

In 1981 when Ronald Reagan took office, he appointed the 34-year-old David Stockman as federal budget director. Stockman's job was to apply "tough love" to the federal budget and reduce spending by 30 percent. The government should only pay for socially necessary programs. No frills, no fat, and no payment to compensate for poor human behavior. Stockman did just that, although what finally passed Congress were lesser savings. Unfortunately, Medicare was considered untouchable during the Reagan years, and the escalation in costs rivaled the rate of today and the federal deficit tripled.

Will Durant in his 11-volume Story of Civilization states that one factor in the decline of ancient Egypt was that healthcare became "overspecialized." The Greek and Roman civilizations declined in part due to slothful human behavior and a sense of entitlement to its maintenance. America is already the most overweight developed country in the world, and Medicare is planning for three million bariatric surgeries a year! I know about the cost effectiveness data supporting bariatric surgery, but come on, would entitlement to this procedure using taxpayer dollars pass a voter referendum?

It is time to apply "tough love" to Medicare. If we provided only healthcare that was evidence-based, cost effective and necessary for health, we would save hundreds of billions of dollars. We could provide that for everyone, the foundation of a healthcare system, and let people pay for or buy supplemental insurance for everything else they want.

None of the candidates for president is expressing anything close to this bold vision for fixing Medicare. They only want to tweak our current failing system. Cut reimbursement but still provide for almost everything under the sun. How stupid. This is a recipe for continued social decline. The richest country in the world with the best medical schools and higher education can do better. We can provide necessary healthcare for all Americans, not just the seniors and disabled, be affordable, and have the best healthcare in the world. Right now we need to focus primarily on reducing the waste in the system and a lot of tough love.

The Secret Sauce of Office Practice Redesign

Editorial
San Diego Physician
2009;96(4):6-7

Making the Process of Care Continuous Rather Than Episodic – Being Proactive With Care Rather Than Reactive – Activating Patients for Greater Self-Management

This issue marks the third year for devoting an issue to health information technology (HIT). Computer applications have already changed front office procedures, and their clinical applications are spreading to change the face of medical practice. The computer with an EHR is becoming the "third person" in the exam room. Increasingly, that computer contains not just the patient's health record but rapid access to all medical knowledge.

2009 may go down in history as the year of healthcare reform in America. If not, it certainly will be the start of major change. The current wasteful and inefficient non-systems of care are not sustainable. We need methods that are better, faster, and cheaper — the dream of any redesign engineer.

The imperative of healthcare redesign for today is to achieve a combination of cost reduction, quality improvement, and service improvement. All that is possible today with HIT applications and new methods of care. Major change has happened in most other service industries and will happen to us in medical office practice. Secure online communication with patients, even automatic communications for things like making appointments and refilling some prescriptions, is just one of the many efficiencies that HIT will bring to office practice to improve service and lower costs.

Besides using Internet communications, how do we improve the quality of outcomes and improve service while lowering the cost of care? Current office practice is reactive, episodic, and physician dependent. Our workday has us reacting to whatever is on our schedule and whatever urgencies arise. Our care is delivered episodically during office visits. As physicians, we carry the major responsibility of providing the totality of medical care to our patients. We are in charge of ensuring that our patients get all the preventive services, chronic illness care, and acute care they need. As medical knowledge grows, this responsibility becomes overwhelming. New methods of care are needed.

Despite our best efforts, traditional office practice results in only about 25 percent of our patients getting all their recommended services or having their outcomes of chronic illness care at the target levels. It is easy for us to say that the responsibility for these gaps is on the patient. If they just came in regularly and complied with all our care, many more would be at target. While this is true, there are emerging models of care that are achieving much better outcomes.

Demonstration projects of chronic illness care have shown that working differently may result in improved quality of care at lower cost. There is a "secret sauce" of care strategies that when put together have a major impact on the outcomes of care to a population of patients. The three "ingredients" to this secret sauce are: making the process of care continuous rather than episodic; being proactive with care rather than reactive; and activating patients for greater self-management. While these three strategies can be done without HIT, using HIT makes them much more efficient and begins to move healthcare into modern processes much like other service industries today (banking, travel, accounting, etc.).

An online platform of communication and care services makes the access to care continuous for patients. They may log into their personal medical home anytime and have access to their medical record and participate in whatever care services that are available. The online platform allows both sides of the care equation — the physician team and the patient — to communicate around care at any time asynchronously at mutual convenience.

Once a practice has a registry of all its patients and is able to stratify patients by age, sex, preventive services, and any given disease, proactive strategies of care may follow. If you want to know how your diabetics are doing, turn on the computer application and look. Rather than spending the day reacting to the patients that are on your schedule, you and your care team may embark on productive interactions with patients to improve their care. With better information systems, care to a population of patients may become strategic. Of course the finances must support this proactive care and reward better outcomes. That is where pay-for-performance, or, better stated, payment for results, replaces payment for just doing care.

Once patients get their medical records and are linked into us as their providers of care, why not let them take a greater role in their own care? We know what preventive services we want our patients to have; why not let them obtain them directly? The experience over the past decade of studying patient self-management shows that the more the patients are involved in their own care, the better the outcomes. Conversely, the more the patients remain totally dependent on the physician to provide all the care, the worse the outcomes.

The tools of HIT do not improve healthcare without the right applications. HIT is not the answer. People using HIT wisely have the potential to redesign care for the better. HIT creates new processes of care that offer the potential to greatly improve the outcomes of care. The financing of care is moving toward improved outcomes to a population of care. All physicians may begin to apply the "secret sauce" concepts to improve quality and service at lower costs. What an exciting time to be in medical practice.

How Obama Could Slash Health Care Costs

Editorial
San Diego Physician
2009;96(5):6-7

It looks as if major healthcare reform is going to happen this time. The March 11, 2009, USA Today proclaimed that healthcare costs are the biggest problem facing the United States. In the worst economic crisis since the Great Depression, the United States can no longer afford to spend more than $8,000 a year per person on healthcare. The pressure to make major changes is mounting, and we have a charismatic and practical president and a Congress of the same party, both determined to act this year.

When you ask the leaders just what the future U.S. healthcare system will look like, their eyes seem to glaze over. They look like a deer in headlights. The single-payer advocates know what they want, but the majority in the United States is not inclined to have the government run the whole system. Most agree that healthcare in the United States should be a partnership between public agencies and private enterprise. We have that now in a patchwork non-system of care that leaves out 15 percent (and growing) of the population. We must do something to reform healthcare in the United States, but what? Many books out there offer different solutions, and none seems palatable to a majority of stakeholders.

I'd like to offer five things that President Obama could do right now that would slash healthcare costs with our system of public and private health plans covering care delivered by largely private providers. By reducing costs and expanding coverage, everyone would have access to care, not just in the emergency room but also in a medical home.

1. Stop Unnecessary Care

Many analysts tell us that 30–35 percent of care currently being delivered is of no benefit to the patient. As a primary care physician, I see it every day. MRIs hum day and night imaging degenerative disease of the spine with no neurologic deficit to justify the expense. Fibromyalgia patients bounce among specialists getting big workups for no benefit. As I watch medical students and residents order what they do, I get the impression that we train physicians to waste money.

We need a "green movement" in healthcare. We need to look at healthcare spending like a precious resource not to be wasted. I have this fantasy of being a healthcare czar and proclaiming that everyone please stop wasting money. We all know the waste around us. There would be an immediate 10 percent reduction in cost. Penalize rather than reward those regions of the country that are notorious for wasteful healthcare spending.

2. Provide Liability Protection for Appropriate Care

Defensive medicine, especially in emergency departments, is wasteful yet done to avoid liability exposure just in case there is a bad outcome. The public needs to be reminded that we all will die, and we all will die of something. Bad things happen with disease, despite our best efforts. Whenever there is a question of liability, an impartial review panel should look to see if the care was appropriate, and, if so, there would be no litigation. When current clinical guidelines are followed, there is immunity from litigation. All of the United States should have the tort reform of California's MICRA. Obama was a community organizer, not a trial attorney, and we can no longer afford the wasteful spending that comes from liability risk.

3. Reduce Administrative Waste

We spend an enormous amount of healthcare dollars for work that has nothing to do with clinical care. Just like how the Obama administration is going line by line in the federal budget to eliminate programs that are not working, there should be a line-by-line review of all administrative spending in healthcare. A massive simplification effort could save many billions of dollars.

Today we can buy a ticket on the Internet and fly across the country for less money than ever before in commercial aviation. Part of that is because we never have to interact with anyone from the airline company until we arrive at the gate to board the plane. Personal banking is now done for pennies compared with the high cost of teller transactions. How many automated applications in healthcare are out there ready to be discovered if we had the cost-reduction imperative to simplify the process of care?

4. Use Patient Visits Only When Necessary • Use Other Methods for Communication and Care

Our visit-based system of care is highly wasteful when less-expensive methods of communication and care are available. Redesigned practices such as Greenfield Health in Portland, Oregon, show that 40–60 percent of healthcare can be delivered well online or with planned telephone encounters. The new medical home projects are paying physicians for care coordination separate from visits. When the impact of the Internet is fully appreciated in healthcare, most Americans will have a web-based personal medical home and be able to coordinate much of their own care with their chosen providers. Modernize the process of healthcare delivery like other service industries have, and many billions of dollars are to be saved. That is the type reimbursement reform and practice transformation that Obama should support, and not simply throw money at HIT in practices that continue the wasteful dependence on visits as the only means of care.

5. Lower the Cost of Brand-name Drugs

Drug pricing in the United States is a scandal that we can no longer afford. There is no market competition when the person getting the drug is not paying the true price and the person ordering the drug has no stake in the costs. For complex reasons, U.S. drug companies charge what the market will bear for drugs in the United States while other countries regulate prices. I am all for the continued development of new drugs, and that is expensive, but it is time to reckon with wasteful spending by drug companies in marketing and pricing medications. Coca Cola and Pepsi have suppressed the generic sodas by pricing their products competitively and being affordable to everyone. Today's drug companies price their brand products such that most of the people who need them cannot afford the cost. Obama should ask for cost reductions in exchange for support in developing promising new drugs. He could just mention price controls and send shivers down the spine of drug companies. If these companies are good corporate citizens, they will become part of the solution and not part of the problem in healthcare costs.

While we wait and wait for some new model to emerge (which may never happen), we can act to drastically reduce our healthcare spending without changing the system. We can offer affordable healthcare coverage through employer programs, individual purchasing, and government programs for those who need them. To get everyone under the health coverage tent, we will need legislation, but it should not be into a wasteful system of care. The solutions offered here are oversimplified because space only allows a short mention of what are certainly complex problems.

In this time of economic crisis, wasteful healthcare spending is especially egregious. The time is now for the Obama administration to get smart in waste reduction, and the good news is that we do not have to radically change the public.

Thomas Friedman continued to be a major influence on my thinking and I used his ending to The World is Flat to call for a new generative of progressive change agents for family medicine. Having come of age in the 1960s where we did not trust anyone over 35, it seemed strange that the voices for change in family medicine were coming from those of us over age 50.

Family Medicine Needs a Generation of Dreamers

Family Medicine
2006;38:548-549

Does your society have more memories than dreams or more dreams than memories?

Thomas L. Friedman, The World Is Flat.[1]

Thomas L. Friedman addresses this question to societies such as the United States today and to corporations. We might ask the same question of family medicine.

He follows the question with the observation, "When memories exceed dreams, the end is near."[1]

The generation of pioneers that founded and established our specialty between 1965 and 1975 were definitely dreamers. They focused much more on a new specialty of family medicine than on the preservation of general practice. The first residency-trained generation of family physicians were also dreamers. They focused on making family medicine a legitimate academic specialty and one that was exciting for medical students and residents.[2]

Today, the pioneer generation is older and understandably nostalgic. The first residency-trained generation, to which I belong, also seems nostalgic and is wondering what happened to family medicine. Fewer than half the US medical students who chose the specialty a decade ago are doing so today. Family physicians are struggling to get through their work days and feel powerless to change their work environment.

The future of family medicine rests with a new generation of family physicians, training now, during an era that has little contact and identification with the pioneers and first generation of residency-trained family physicians. They grew up during the dawn of the information age and the new globalization. If relationship-centered care and the commitment of being a comprehensive personal physician are to survive in family medicine, this new generation will have to invent a 21st-century application of these principles.

Previously, I have described the redesign imperative in family medicine,[3] an imperative because the complexity of the work in primary care and family medicine no longer fits the traditional brief visit care model. We are now expected to provide comprehensive prevention and the continuous management of chronic illness, along with treating whatever acute problems our patients may have. A review of our records or a survey of the populations we serve show that we do not do this well.[4] It is not our fault; rather, our care model is faulty. We need a new model of care that matches our work requirements. This model should be rich in information management and provide "on demand" access to services.

Who will come up with new models of family medicine and implement them in our education programs and clinical practice? Will the dreamers come from the medical directors who worry about the next month's productivity report? Will they be the residency directors who prepare for the next Residency Review Committee accreditation visits and worry about how to keep the budget going? Will the dreamers be the experienced family physicians who have spent a career learning how to squeeze an hour of caring into 10 minutes of face-to-face time with patients?

No, I don't think it will be any of these. Just like the young pioneers of family medicine 30–40 years ago and the first generation they trained, the dreamers need to come from the young who readily see the limitations of how family medicine has been practiced and how it could and should be different. This new generation grew up with the Internet, handheld devices that store and present hundreds of hours of entertainment, and cell phones that allow connectivity from virtually anywhere.

The Future of Family Medicine report has been written and is a start of the reform process.[5] Like the prior Millis and Willard reports,[6,7] the change generation may not read the report but will capture the need and vision for change in the new social context of information exchange, communication methods, and caring interactions.

Today, medical students look at how family medicine is delivered, and they run the other way. That is not how they want to spend their careers. The idea of being a personal physician to a community of patients is appealing but not while running on a hamster wheel of brief encounters. Today's residents are as tired as ever, and the excitement of clinical practice in the clinic is rarely felt. Do they have the vision and energy to dream of a better way?

The biggest challenge facing family medicine today is to develop a new generation of dreamers who will change the specialty into new care models that fit the emerging social context of communication, caring, and service. No doubt health care in general is embarking on a major process of change, with interactive Web sites and embedded secure communication, electronic health records shared with patients from their home, and a public with complete access to all health information on the Internet. Who will reinvent family medicine to fit into new health systems? Will nursing and other health professionals become the new first tier of health service online while primary care physicians remain relegated to the back rooms of medical office buildings seeing those patients who still benefit from brief visits? Who will want to enter that line of work except physicians who want a simple work schedule and a low-stress clinical setting?

At the end of The World Is Flat, Friedman calls for a:

. . . generation of strategic optimists, a generation with more dreams than memories, ... a generation that wakes up each morning and not only imagines that things can be better but also acts on that imagination every day.[1]

How do we create this new generation in family medicine? Current leaders in family medicine must do the hard work of initiating the change process based on a new vision for family medicine. The Future of Family Medicine report is a great beginning. Translating that report into action may come from the New Partners Initiative embarked on by the leadership of the Society of Teachers of Family Medicine[8] and TransforMED, a new initiative developed by the American Academy of Family Physicians.[9] We need to create a spirit of change and revolution in family medicine that sweeps into all of primary care. That requires discussion and efforts at the grassroots in all family medicine settings. Let us get on with it!

References

1. Friedman TL. The world is flat: a brief history of the twenty-first century. New York: Farrar, Straus and Giroux, 2005.
2. Scherger JE. Phase three of academic family medicine. Fam Med 1997;29(6):439-40.
3. Scherger JE. The end of the beginning: the redesign imperative in family medicine. Fam Med 2005;37(7):513-6.
4. Institute of Medicine. Crossing the quality chasm: a new health system for the 21st century. Washington, DC: National Academy Press, 2001.
5. Future of Family Medicine Project Leadership Committee. The future of family medicine: a collaborative project of the family medicine community. Ann Fam Med 2004;2(Suppl 1):S3-S32.
6. Citizens Commission on Graduate Medical Education. The graduate education of physicians. Chicago: American Medical Association, 1966. (Millis Report)
7. Meeting the challenge of family practice: the Report of the Ad

Hoc Committee on Education for Family Practice of the Council on Medical Education. Chicago: American Medical Association, 1966. (Willard Report)

8. Mygdal WK. Our medical and medical education crisis—a bursting point? Fam Med 2005;37(9):615-6.

9. American Academy of Family Physicians. TransforMED. www.aafp.org/x40604.xml.

The Future of Family Medicine Report (2004;2:S3-S32) set the change for rethinking family medicine residency programs. Larry Green invited me to prepare one of the papers for the Preparing Practicing Physicians for Practice (P4) project, and encouraged me to let my reasoning run wild in his words.

Preparing Personal Physicians for Practice: Essential Skills for New Family Physicians and How Residency Programs May Provide Them

Journal of the American Board of Family Medicine
2007;20:348-355

Abstract: Family Medicine residency programs must change substantially to prepare for new family physicians a model of practice for the 21st century. This article describes 10 essential skills that are part of a new model of family medicine and the educational changes and resources needed to obtain them. These skills include management of a population of patients, patient-centered care, personal medical home, best knowledge at the point of care, continuous access to multimodal communication, a new platform of are, time intensive visits, group visits, teamwork and interpersonal skills, and financial practice management. (J Am Board Fam Med 2007;20:348-355.)

There is an imperative for change in the process of how Family Medicine is delivered. A New Model of Family Medicine[1] is ready for experimentation, application and education for a new generation of family physicians. Now comes the hard part in changing practices and residency programs to achieve much higher levels of both service and outcome quality. The tools of Health Information Technology are available and are rapidly improving. Quality improvement methods from many industries demonstrate how service processes can be delivered with great safety and consistent best practice. All of medicine is on verge of a major process transformation,[2,3] and the challenge for Family Medicine is to be a leading specialty for change rather than a vestige of the past.

TransforMED was formed by the American Academy of Family Physicians to be a catalyst for the New Model of Family Medicine. The first National Demonstration Project (NDP) of TransforMED consists of 36 practices throughout the U.S. randomized equally to an intervention group with professional facilitation and a self-directed group. The second NDP is for residency programs to embrace the transformation process. This paper describes the essential skills that new family physicians must have to succeed in the transformed practice setting, and what residency programs must do (read change) to provide their residents these skills. A portrait is presented with the professional life of the new personal family physician, and a new weekly schedule for residents.

Family Medicine is moving into uncharted territory in this transformation process. The skills described here are a best estimate of what will be important. Through this evolutionary process of change, new skills and priorities are likely to emerge. New technologies will emerge to automate, customize and personalize high quality patient care. What is described here for residency programs is a starting point on this journey into the future. New methods of training residents will emerge to better prepare graduates for a practice environment that is part of this new century of progress in medicine.

Ten skills are highlighted here with suggestions as to how residency programs can provide them. These skills and educational methods form a framework for the TransforMED NPD for Family Medicine residency programs. The portrait of the new personal family physician provides an exciting challenge for residency programs to create a new context for education. Family Medicine for the resident must return as the centerpiece of the residency experience, rather than as a part time duty as residents focus on a series of block rotations. The visionary efforts behind this project are similar in historical impact as the original requirements for Family Medicine residency training developed almost 40 years ago.

Skill 1. Management of a Population of Patients

Family Physicians serve as personal physicians to a population of patients. Residents are given a patient population to care for at the start of residency, usually about 200 patients or about 50 families. This number increases during the residency to about 800 patients or about 200 families. Residents take primary responsibility in managing these patients, similar to what they will do in later practice with a panel of about 1500-2000 patients. For the past 35 years, residents have been in their clinics for limited hours each week and care for their patients' one at a time with breaks in continuity of care more the norm than the exception. Care occurred only during visits, except for the occasional telephone call following up on some test. This visit dependent model of primary care results in marginal health care outcomes from a population analysis.[2,4,5]

The new model of family medicine calls for family physicians to manage both the population of patients as a whole and the individual patient. New family physicians are proactive in reaching out to patients to achieve high levels of preventive services and chronic illness management. They have the tools to provide this care in a continuous way. They are incentivized through pay for performance reimbursement based on achieving high levels of successful care to populations of patients.

What Residency Programs Can Do To Achieve This Skill: All residents are electronically connected to a list of their patients at the start of residency with ready access to their health records and an ability to audit the records for targeted care outcomes. This resident patient panel is updated as the practice grows. Residents are expected to maintain their "In Box" of patient care needs both in and out of clinic time and while on various block rotations. Residents receive regular reports of their performance in caring for their population of patients, and have the ability to self-audit their practices. All productive interactions with patients are measured (visits, telephone contact and online communication) as a reflection of resident productivity. Group visits and group online communication is available.

Resources Needed: Electronic health records with a registry function, accessible from any computer in the health system and elsewhere. The residency program has continuity of care and patient management policies that support population management.

Skill 2. Patient Centered Care

The traditional paternalistic model of the patient-physician relationship is replaced with patient centered care in which patients are taking an active role in their health and health care. With patient centered care, physicians serve their patients with continuous respect for the patient's autonomy and self-control. Personal family physicians are advisors and caregivers on the patient's terms whenever possible. There are times when a physician must step in and assertively provide patient care, such as in medical emergencies and with major illnesses, but this is always done with the utmost respect for the patient's needs and desires. The practice has a patient centered, relationship oriented culture that emphasizes the importance of meeting patients' needs, reaffirming that the fundamental basis for health care is "people taking care of people".[1]

What Residency Programs Can Do To Achieve This Skill: A statement of practice philosophy for the program embodies patient centered care. This statement is highly visible in all materials relating to the residency practice. Most importantly, this philosophy of patient centered care is practiced by all faculty, residents and staff. Patient care discussion groups, such as Balint groups, are held regularly to facilitate discussion, learning and growth in patient centered care. Patient input is regularly obtained, and patients have continuous access to their records and communication with the practice, ensuring that their needs are being addressed. All patients receive care that is culturally and linguistically appropriate.

Resources needed: Policies which support patient centered care. Open access to communication between patients and their personal physicians and care team. Training for faculty, residents and staff in a service model of culturally competent patient centered care. Recognition for excellence in providing patient centered care.

Skill 3. Personal Medical Home

The residency practice serves as a personal medical home for each patient, ensuring access to comprehensive, integrated care through an ongoing relationship.[1] A traditional concept of the personal family physician is one of being a member of the patient's extended family. This substantive role deteriorates with breaks in continuity of care. New online communication methods allow for a continuous connection between the family and a resident physician (Skill 5). The basket of services provided by the program becomes a home for health care to the population being served. Patients feel connected and have a sense of ownership of all the resources available for their care. The personal family physician is the steward for the patient and family in this medical home.

Home implies a place, and the medical office is designed to be a personal medical home for patients. However, for many patients, the office is not their primary medical home. Their own home and their workplace are where they live their health and illness every day. The personal medical home reaches out electronically to patients wherever they are as a virtual medical home. Patients have a "home page" electronically connected with the medical practice that is able to provide many of their health care needs. This electronic connection is rich with services as described in Skill 6.

What Residency Programs Can Do To Achieve This Skill: Redesign patient care settings to become a personal medical home. The waiting room is replaced by a "medical home resource room" where patients may update their personal information and obtain guided access to medical information. Preserving what is necessary for good clinical care, the office has an atmosphere which makes patients feel at home. More importantly, the practice has an advanced information system which allows for patients to be connected with their personal health records and to the virtual medical home of the practice. Residents as personal physicians interact with their patients continuously through this electronic platform of care.

Resources Needed: Office redesign using the principles of patient centered care and a personal medical home. Advanced information systems with a virtual medical home for all patients.

Policies which have the residents continuously active in the virtual medical home with their patients.

Skill 4. Best Knowledge at the Point of Care

Family physicians should use the best scientific knowledge in the care of patients. Family physicians are committed to evidence-based medicine and have the skills to evaluate the quality of medical information. Residents develop this evidence-based philosophy of care from the very beginning of the program, taking advantage of the low patient volume both in clinic schedules and in the overall population of patients served. Since the complexity of modern medicine exceeds the inherent limitation of an unaided human mind, knowledge management and clinical decision support tools are used routinely at the point of care. Patients consistently receive the best available clinical care. Currently, access to the best knowledge at the point of care is the goal. Soon, best knowledge will be imbedded into the electronic record and will help guide patient care. Increasingly, some routine care will be automated for the patient to receive best practice upon request.

What Residency Programs Can Do To Achieve Skill[2]: All residency programs have a commitment to a culture of evidence-based clinical practice, and all providers demonstrate this. Faculty supervisors ensure that residents practice evidence-based medicine at all times, supported by advanced information resources available at the point of care. Decision making "off the top of the head" is discouraged.

Resources Needed: Clinical decision support tools which promote evidence-based practice are available at the point of care. Increasingly, clinical decision support is imbedded into the electronic health record to guide excellence in patient care. A relationship with an IT vendor committed to this level of clinical decision support is essential.

Skill 5. Continuous Access to Multimodal Communication

Quality of care is achieved through a continuous healing relationship.[1,2] This requires that patients and providers have access to secure communication at all times. The care team in family medicine handles patient messages in a timely manner, and important health information is proactively given to patients. Residents participate as family physicians continuously in responding to their patient's messages and proactively communicating with patients through a secure online portal, by telephone and by arranged patient visits.

What Residency Programs Can Do To Achieve This Skill: Provide secure online communication methods for all the providers, staff and patients. Policies are developed for these communications which include appropriate use, timeliness, and how messages are triaged. Residents are expected to maintain their patient and staff communication "In Box" at all times, both in and out of clinic scheduled time. All patient related communications are captured in the patient's health record.

Resources Needed: A secure online communication portal based in the electronic health record and/or in the practice website. Communication policies are developed and regularly updated to cover online messaging, telephone and visits. Residents have greater flexibility in scheduling patient visits.

Skill 6. A New Platform of Care

The convergence of these skills provides a new platform of care which makes the previous model of family medicine obsolete. The new platform of care offers an electronic health record available from any computer including by the patient in their home (their personal health record). This record has imbedded evidence-based knowledge management to guide clinical decisions. Secure online communication is imbedded in the electronic record, allowing for access to all patient information with online or telephone communication. This is the new platform of care is being rolled out by advanced health care systems such as Kaiser Permanente.[3] Residents are trained to provide care using this new platform, even if one or more of the electronic tools are still separate applications.

What Residency Programs Can Do To Achieve This Skill: Purchase and implement advanced information systems which support the new platform of care. All residents and faculty interact with patients using these tools in a continuous manner.

Resources Needed: An advanced information system as described above. Policies are developed to support its use on a continuous basis.

Skill 7. Time Intensive Visits

With family physicians having productive interactions with patients online and by telephone, fewer office visits are needed in caring for a population of patients. Office visits in the new model are scheduled selectively and time intensively based on patient needs.[6] Brief visit office schedules are replaced by flexible and time intensive schedules. Residents are encouraged and supported to spend from 30 minutes to more than an hour in the care of complex patients. The number of office visits is reduced, but the overall number of productive interactions with patients increases from the traditional brief visit model of care. Time intensive office visits reflect a thorough provision of care using a biopsychosocial model.

What Residency Programs Can Do To Achieve This Skill: Eliminate the visit requirements for residents and replace it with measurements of all productive interactions in the care of a population of patients. Give residents more control in scheduling the patients to be seen and the time requested for the appointment, all derived from the new platform of communication. Residents are trained in effective time intensive visits through methods such as video monitoring and role playing.

Resources Needed: Flexible scheduling of patient appointments. An ability to capture all resident interactions with patients.

Skill 8. Group Visits

Family physicians use group visits to consolidate care with patients having similar conditions, such as obesity and diabetes, and to create a dynamic where patients help each other. Residents are trained to provide group visits as part of their clinic experience. When organized well using the entire care team, with appropriate coding and billing for services, group visits become an important part of a modern family medicine practice.7 Technology applications allow for a virtual presence of some members of the group, or possibly an entire virtual group visit.

What Residency Programs Can Do To Achieve This Skill: Make Group Visits a regular part of the office practice. Residents participate in group visits for their patients on a regular and rotating basis, especially through the resident's identification of appropriate patients among their population. The office staff and faculty are proficient in successful Group Visits and provide training for the residents.

Resources Needed: Group Visit training and policies. Use of an appropriate room which will maintain confidentiality of the group visit discussion. Technology for virtual connection of patients for group visits.

Skill 9. Teamwork and Interpersonal Skills

The new model of Family Medicine requires a high level of teamwork and interpersonal skills for the family physician. Traditional practice was a physician "craft" with office staff as ancillary. Successful wellness care and chronic illness management requires that the entire office staff be engaged in the care of patients.[8,9] The family physician not only communicates well with patients, but also with the entire staff in a collaborative care manner. Everyone knows their responsibilities and the responsibilities of others, and the team "huddles" at the start of every patient care session. Residents learn to model teamwork in their practice and are measured on the quality of their interpersonal skills with patients and staff.

What Residency Programs Can Do To Achieve This Skill: Train residents in team practice and interpersonal skills. Model team practice in the clinic through training of all the office staff. Collaborative care with shared patient responsibility is the norm. Everyone on the care team as access to the electronic health records with an "In Box" for messaging. Residents, along with faculty and staff, are measured in teamwork and interpersonal skills at least once a year using a 360 degree evaluation.

Resources Needed: Training and modeling of team practice and collaborative care. Communication training regularly occurs for effective interpersonal skills. Advanced information systems are available to all team members.

Skill 10. Financial Practice Management

The new model of Family Medicine must be financially successful.

Residents should realize the financial aspects of all the care activities they provide. The new platform of care requires financial contracts and policies which support it. Residents are trained in coding and billing for all the services they provide. Prepaid services such as for online care should be considered as part of the contracts with patients and insurers. A first step in a financial analysis of the new model of family medicine was provided by Task Force 6 in the Future of Family Medicine project.[10] While there are new delivery methods in the new model such as online communication with patients and group visits, there is much efficiency created which should allow for the new model to enhance revenues. In the words of design engineers, it should be "better, faster and cheaper". While education is primary in residency training and should not be shorted to enhance revenue, residency programs exist in a real world of patient care and should be financially viable. Better yet, they should be models of smart financing of care. The residents should have a detailed understanding of the finances which support the entire family medicine care model.

What Residency Programs Can Do To Achieve This Skill: Develop financial relationships with patients and payers to support the new model of care. Online communication with patients can be delivered as fees for "e-visits" or through prepaid arrangements such as a monthly or annual service charge. Practice management education with a full understanding of the organization and finances of the practice are built into the resident's experience. Residents are responsible providers of care from a financial perspective throughout the residency experience through accurate and complete coding of services.

Resources Needed: Financial contracts which support the model of care. A coherent financial model for the overall practice. Resident education to include financial practice management.

Portrait of the New Family Medicine Resident and Physician

The new model family physician cares for a population of patients with robust information systems and continuous healing relationships. The care team takes pride in achieving high levels of patient satisfaction and excellent clinical outcomes whenever possible. Patients are actively involved in their care. Face to face visits occur selectively, time intensively and include family and group visits. A continuous platform of care, secure and web based, is the dominant means of coordinating patient care needs and communication among patients and caregivers. Residents participate as personal family physicians to a population of patients using this model while simultaneously participating in targeted learning activities.

New model family physicians and residents do not spend most of their time on keyboards. Keyboards are very early 21st century. Like Dr. Bones in Star Trek, new model family physicians listen, observe, think and speak. All thinking is technologically enhanced. Soon, finger print or retinal scan identification and voice recognition will replace keyboards as access to patient data and medical knowledge. New model family physicians will balance their time between functioning through an electronic system of care and being face to face with patients and families.

As population based providers of care, new model family physicians play a unique role in the communities they serve. The primary care teams across a health care delivery system have knowledge about the health and heath needs of a community which were never before realized. Pooled patient information allows for a regional health information network which is able to respond to community needs in prevention and chronic illness care. Planned care to populations of patients will be rich with information and options for providing care. New model family physicians will be drawn into activated community care roles.

A Week in the Life of a Resident

Sally is a second year family medicine resident on her maternity care rotation. Her family medicine patient population has recently expanded from 200 to 400 patients with the graduation of a residency class. She is on labor and delivery with some free time waiting for her patient to progress. She logs on to her family medicine "In Box" for messages and lab results. She also studies her new patients and is able to sort them by age, sex and illness, curious as to how her practice has expanded. She looks for priorities to address in the health of her patients, diabetics who are poorly controlled, asthmatics who have had frequent acute visits, seniors who have not had their recommended screenings. She sends personalized information messages to her new patients, all individually addressed but for Sally these are group messages. She encourages her new patients to come and meet her either through individual or group visits.

Sally now has 3 half days in the Family Medicine center. She is able to see her upcoming schedules in advance, and is able to schedule the appointments of many of her patients. She has the flexibility of scheduling her patients for a standard 30 or 60 minute visit, or even longer for a family conference or group visit. She is also able to schedule a brief 15 minute visit to quickly look at a patient with a rash or possible ear infection. She communicated with her office staff team to schedule new patients to come and meet her. The Family Medicine center has the flexibility to allow her to see one of her patients anytime the office is open, and after hours. Sally sees 4-6 patients, couples and families in a usual clinic session, 2-3 such visits scheduled at other times during the week. She has a weekly group visit with her patients. She has about 50 patient interactions each week electronically and by telephone, and reviews a similar number of faculty and staff messages and lab results.

Sally attends educational sessions and meetings with her Family Medicine program in person and virtually depending on her location and other responsibilities. She has adjusted to the dual continuous roles of a family medicine resident, which are focusing on a block rotation while maintaining the continuity of a clinical practice as a personal family physician. The advanced information system provides a platform of care which facilitates this duality of purpose and learning.

Sally also enjoys a rich personal life with her spouse and two children. She is often able to leave early to attend a function of one of her children, and finish her messages and documentation from home when her children are in bed. Most of Sally's communication with patients is done asynchronously at the mutual convenience of her and her patients.

Fortunately, her residency program has a philosophy of patient centered care balanced with a spirit of vitality for the physicians and staff. Turnaround times for nonemergency patient messages are 24 hours during the week and none required over the weekend. She is happy not to be part of a program which gives a Blackberry to all the residents and expects rapid responses to almost everything.

Discussion

In many ways, the essential skills and portrait described here are back to the future. The original model of family medicine residency training emphasized a continuity of care experience with a panel of patients. Residents would be "model" family physicians caring for patients in a "model family medicine center". While block rotations would be necessary to obtain advanced education and skills, the residents would not be separated from their longitudinal patient responsibility. Some programs in the 1970s developed pairing systems for residents on block rotations so that the continuity of care in the family medicine center could be maintained. Even non-rotational programs were developed so that the home base and identification with the family medicine center was maintained. There has been considerable entropy with the original concept of the longitudinal residency experience, and resident identification with their panel of patients has been reduced in many programs.

The new model of family medicine calls for a renewed and intensified identification with a population of patients. The tools of health information technology (HIT) allow for data access to patients never before available. Residents and faculty family physicians may provide care for their patients outside of clinic schedules. HIT and a renewed commitment to ongoing patient responsibility provide a new opportunity for residents to manifest continuity of care and achieve health outcomes for their patients never before experienced.

The first rule in Crossing the Quality Chasm is that care is based on continuous healing relationships.[2] The first concept in the Future of Family Medicine is the personal medical home.[1] If residency programs make a firm commitment to these as the primary applications of the resident experience, they will have joined in the redesign of family medicine and will be preparing their residents for a new and exciting future.

References

1. Future of Family Medicine Project Leadership Committee. The future of family medicine: A collaborative project of the family medicine community. Ann Fam Med 2004;2(Suppl 1):S3-S32.

2. Institute of Medicine. Crossing the Quality Chasm: A New Health System for the 21st Century. Washington, DC: National Academy Press. 2001.

3. Kilo CM, Leavitt M. Transforming Care Using Information Technology. Chicago: Health Information Management and Systems Society (HIMSS). 2005.

4. Meissner I, Whisnant JP, Sheps SG, Schwartz GL, O'Fallon WM, Covalt JL, Sicks JD, Bailey KR, Wiebers DO. Detection and control of high blood pressure in the community: Do we need a wake-up call? Hypertension. 1999;34:466-71.

5. McGlynn EA, Asch SM, Adams J, et al. The quality of health care delivered to adults in the United States. New Engl J Med. 2003;348:2635-2645.

6. Ludmerer KM. Time to Heal: American Medical Education from the Turn of the Century to the Era of Managed Care. New York: Oxford University Press. 1999.

7. Jaber R, Braksmajer A, Trilling J. Group Visits for Chronic Illness Care: Models, Benefits and Challenges. Fam Pract Man. 2006;13(1): 37-40.

8. Robert Wood Johnson Foundation. Improving Chronic Illness Care. www.improvingchroniccare.org

9. Lawrence D. From Chaos to Care: The Promise of Team-Based Medicine. Cambridge, MA: Perseus Publishing. 2002.

10. Spann SJ, Task Force 6 and Executive Editorial Team. Report on financing the new model of family medicine. Ann Fam Med. 2004 Dec 2;2 Suppl 3:S1-S21.

My closest friend in family medicine was Jack Rodnick and his untimely death was very sad. I was honored to be asked by STFM to write this tribute:

A Tribute to Jack Rodnick

Family Medicine.
2008;40:158-159

Family medicine lost one its most likeable, dedicated, and energetic leaders on January 26, 2008. Jonathan (Jack) Rodnick, MD, died suddenly while running on the beach in paradise—the island of Kauai. Born on the 4th of July, Jack was 65. His death came as a shock to all who knew him because he always seemed so alive.

Jack graduated from medical school at the University of California, Los Angeles in 1968, did his internship at San Francisco General Hospital, and worked in rural Alaska before completing his family medicine residency at the University of Vermont. Later, Jack served as chair of the Department of Family and Community Medicine at the University of California, San Francisco (UCSF) for 14 years, building it from a small faculty to one of the top departments in the county.

Jack's early academic career began in Santa Rosa, California, where he taught in the family medicine residency program, serving as the tuberculosis medical officer for Sonoma County, working in community clinics. I will never forget going with Jack to a community clinic in Guerneville during my student rotation in 1974. Jack introduced me to what real community medicine was about. He introduced me to the "Common Health Club," a group of activated people taking charge of their own health, 1970s style. Naturally, the group sought out Jack as their medical advisor. I am blessed that I had a continuous friendship with Jack for 34 years. To a degree I will never fully comprehend, he molded me into the family physician and person that I am.

Jack was the 15th president of STFM (1987–1988), and promoting high-quality research in family medicine was his primary focus. His commitment and service to STFM never stopped, and right up to his death he edited the "International Family Medicine Education" column in Family Medicine. He was also the editor of a special issue of Family Medicine, published in 2007 as part of an international effort on global health that involved more than 235 medical journals around the world.

Jack's work in international health led STFM to select him as STFM's representative to the World Organization of Family Doctors (Wonca) in 2007, and his strong interest in family medicine in developing countries will be greatly missed. Working closely with the American Academy of Family Physicians (AAFP) on its international activities, he recently made a trip to Albania. In the 1980s, Jack helped Japan develop postgraduate programs in family medicine and did the same in China during the 1990s. This decade, his work extended to other countries in Asia and Africa.

Jack was an outstanding clinician scholar. He loved to write important articles and dedicated himself to writing at least two every year. His article on HIV testing in the November 2007 American Family Physician is a great example.1 His articles on international issues in family medicine gave us insights into the world. Jack was often ahead of the timely issues of the day, writing about computers and electronic health records in the 1980s and how to make managed care work for family medicine in the early 1990s. He would also write about the clinical articles that changed his practice. At the time of his death, Jack had just begun a term as the chair of the AAFP Commission on Science. And through all of this, he never stopped caring for patients.

Jack's personal life was every bit as rich as his professional one. A devoted husband and father, Jack's wife Judy would often light up a room with him. I will never forget Jack's 65th birthday party last July 4 in San Francisco at a hotel with a band, friends from all over, and hours of expressions of love and admiration.

Jack was a legendary outdoorsman, taking multiple hikes and backpack trips every year. For more than 30 years, Jack would lead a 7–8 day trip in the high Sierra Nevada with a group of old friends from Santa Rosa and professional colleagues. Every year was a new adventure, meticulously planned for many months. I had the pleasure of going on about 10 of these trips, and for me and my sons, they are a highlight of our lives.

There is a lesson in Jack's death for all of us in medicine. Knowing Jack as a consummate teacher, I believe he would want me to share this. Jack had a congenital bicuspid aortic valve. Over the years, he developed aortic stenosis, and his valve was being closely monitored. There was a growing recommendation that Jack have his aortic valve replaced, and restrictions were being put on him, such as the altitude at which he should backpack. Jack put off having the surgery. Jack's wife related to Roger Sherwood that he did not want to go on warfarin (Coumadin) for the rest of his life, fearing the risk of bleeding. Unfortunately, aortic stenosis is notorious for causing sudden death during exercise, and patients should be urged to have valve replacement surgery when the time is right. Most likely, Jack's aortic valve caused his untimely death.

Jack, maybe this is the way you wanted it—a sudden and painless end while running in paradise.

We all miss you enormously, and for so many of your friends and colleagues, our lives have a vacancy without your friendship, your leadership, and your warmth and support. You are the greatest role model in so many ways and one of the nicest people we will ever know.

Reference

1. Rodnick JE. The CDC and USPSTF recommendations for HIV testing. Am Fam Physician 2007;76:1456, 1459

Blogs emerged on the scene as a rapid way to get material into print on the internet. No more waiting for publication. My first efforts at writing blogs were as the men's health blogger for a patient website, Revolution Health. After that site went too commercial, I was invited to be the primary care blogger for <u>modernmedicine.com</u>. A selected number of these blogs relating to new models of practice are reprinted here:

Do You Accept Emails From Your Patients?

Blog
Modern Medicine
Posted November 2008

Email is now the most common form of communication in society. Email has the convenience of being asynchronous, done at the mutual convenience of both parties. It would seem ideal for the many communications between patients and a medical practice. Yet, few medical practices take advantage of email communication with patients.

I started giving my email to my patients in 1997. It is one of the best things I have ever done in patient care. Now, more than half of my patient communications occur over email. It saves me and my patients considerable time and inconvenience.

I'd like to share some myths about email with patients:

Myth #1:   Hackers could read my patient's confidential messages.

That could happen, but it is more unlikely than your phone being tapped or your mail being intercepted. As long as patients accept this level of privacy (part of your HIPAA security policy), email is safe and security compliant. Most physicians are moving onto secure patient portals for email with patients, the more professional way to handle such communications.

Myth #2: It will take more time from my day, and I will not get reimbursed for it.

If done right, email with patients should save you time. An email can be handled in 2-3 minutes, even with attachments of web links, while telephone communication is more time-consuming and often requires multiple calls, with no structured documentation. The daily demand on you is rather fixed, and email allows you to handle that demand most efficiently. You may now charge for e-visits with patients, and some practices have an increased revenue stream through this method of payment or through monthly email access charges.

Myth #3: If I allow my patient to email me, I will receive a flood of email messages.

That has not been the experience of physicians sharing email with patients. We all get fewer emails than we expect. The comfort of this access does not drive up use. Sure, most emails come from a small percentage of patients, but email is a more efficient way to handle high demand patients than being stuck on the telephone or in frequent office visits.

Myth #4: Patients will ramble.

Typed email seems to limit the length of messages. You can read a long message quickly and offer a brief response in most cases. When email becomes video, we need to have time limitations.

Myth #5: I may get sued, and a lawyer will discover my email messages.

Sure, email is part of your care. Do not do anything over email that requires a visit. Be careful in your communications, and always offer follow-up instructions. Email should lower liability risk by improving communications, improving record keeping, and by bringing physicians and patients closer in a caring relationship.

I believe that online communication with patients will be a standard part of medical practice soon. Try it; I think you will like it.

Medical Home Model Gaining Steam

Blog
Modern Medicine
Posted January 2009

The Medical Home Model is gaining steam and looks to be the means for renewal in primary care. This year, Medicare is embarking on a program for paying primary care practices for the coordination of care of patients with certain chronic illness. Other health insurers are preparing to follow suit. The National Committee for Quality Assurance (NCQA) has established the official criteria for a Patient-Centered Medical Home and is the source for measurement that will lead to payment. The NCQA is the home of HEDIS measures and, as a non-profit organization, is considered the standard for quality measurement in health care.

Medicare's Medical Home demonstration project will launch this year in 8 states and will run for 3 years. Primary care practices will be paid between $40 and $52 each month per patient depending on their Medical Home score established by the NCQA. Since $50 per month for 600 patients is $360,000 per year, just for care coordination, this is really important for primary care. All practices that want to succeed in the future should prepare now to become Medical Homes.

The official NCQA definition of a Patient-Centered Medical Home is "... a model of care provided by physician practices that seeks to strengthen the physician-patient relationship by replacing episodic care based of illnesses and patient complaints with coordinated care and a long-term healing relationship." The scorecard used by NCQA to measure a Medical Home becomes vital for establishing whether care coordination payment will come and how much. This scorecard measures:

- Access and Communication
- Patient Tracking and Registry Functions
- Care Management
- Patient Self-Management Support
- Electronic Prescribing
- Test and Referral Tracking
- Performance Reporting and Improvement
- Advanced Electronic Communications

Every primary care practice should study carefully the Patient-Centered Medical Home criteria available at www.ncqa.org. Succeeding with these measures requires an advanced electronic health record and other information systems. There needs to be a redesign of practice style from reactive—just responding to those patients that come in for appointments—to proactive—reaching out to patients with chronic health problems. This is a tall order, but it is what will be required not only for success in primary care in the near future, but also for survival in the long run.

Inventing a New Primary Care Practice Today

Blog
Modern Medicine
Posted April 2009

I have been given a wonderful opportunity: Effective May 4, 2009, I am Vice President for Primary Care at Eisenhower Medical Center in the Palm Springs area of California. One of my assignments is to start a new primary care practice. If you had this opportunity in 2009, what would you do?

My superiors who are supporting this effort to not want a traditional brief-visit productivity practice model. They want personalized and efficient care. This is the model we are going to use.

Membership in the practice will cost a dollar a day, or $365 dollars a year. For that fee, patients get open access to online and telephone communication. The panels for the primary care physician will be capped at 1000 patients. This gives a base gross income for the physician of $365,000 per year.

Visits will be done as needed and will be charged separately and billed to insurance or Medicare. We will also do house calls, both virtual and real. It is estimated that each physician will see 8 to 10 patients a day in the office, spend about 1.5 to 2 hours a day in online or telephone communication, and do 1 to 2 house calls, hospital visits, or nursing home visits a day.

The practice will have an EHR with all important functions like patient registries and ePrescribing. The overhead will run 60%, so the physician's income will be 40% of gross revenues. Estimating

$200,000 each year in billed revenues on top of the membership fee, the total gross income generated by the physician is $565,000 a year, with 40% or a $226,000 net income for the physician.

How does this practice model and base income sound to you? Would you not agree that this model is affordable to almost everyone? Would you not agree that seeing 8 to 10 patients a day in the office in unhurried visits is a much more professional way of working? I believe that this describes the new primary care. Let me know what you think.

Practicing Ideal Primary Care

Blog
Modern Medicine
Posted December 16, 2009

Eight months ago I posted a blog here titled "Inventing a New Primary Care Practice Today." Here is an update. Our group is now providing ideal primary care, no joke.

At Eisenhower Medical Center in Rancho Mirage, California, every patient gets 5-star treatment. This not-for-profit health system makes its margin on donations, not from medical practice, where it loses money every year on Medicare, its dominant payer. With substantial reserves, Eisenhower is able to invest in whatever care it wants. After 35 years of investing in specialty service lines, the system is now investing in primary care. Not ordinary, brief visit, always-in-a-hurry, patients-wait-longer-than-they-see-the-physician primary care. Ideal primary care.

So what is ideal primary care? We borrow the slogan from the Institute for Healthcare Improvement (IHI) in Boston: We give you the care you want and need, how, when and where you want and need it. Patients get all the time they need with 30 and 60 minute appointments, longer if necessary. Our group of 6 physicians (and growing) sees 5 to 6 patients each half day session. Once the relationship is established, the access to dialogue with the patients is continuous on a secure communication platform, Relay Health.

Ideal primary care is not only great service, it is also the best quality of care, based on current clinical evidence. Our records are fully electronic, using a McKesson system, and linked with the hospital and specialists. We have robust and growing Clinical Decision Support to guide our care. We have transparency so that we can see at any time how we are doing with our patients. Rather than practicing episodic, reactive care that depends on the physician doing everything, our care is continuous, strategically proactive and empowers patients for greater self-management. We are not perfect in all these areas yet, but we are getting there.

So what does all this cost and who pays for it? While Eisenhower is fronting the money, we have a sustainable business model. In my previous blog, I indicated a fee of $365 a year paid for by the patients for all the non-visit communication and care. That works only if all physicians are instantly full with 1000 patients. Since we are a growing practice and it takes 1 to 2 years for each physician to get a full panel, our annual fee is $595 a year with a $40 discount for couples and families. We use the patient centered medical home hybrid payment model of billing for office visits taking Medicare and other insurance. We are an advanced Patient Centered Medical Home, the bright future for primary care.

Because half of our patients are seniors who require more time, we are capping our panel size at 900 patients per FTE physician. With that we are able to have physician salaries start in the $200k plus range and that will grow based on the hybrid revenues. We bonus physicians based on quality of care and patient satisfaction.

It is so much fun to practice ideal primary care. I was getting to dread the frustrating challenge of seeing 12 patients each session, knowing that I was always in a hurry and shortchanging people's care. Being able to sit back and get the entire patient story is such a reward. The patient's regularly tell us they have never had doctors like us. This is primary care the way it should be, and it is sustainable. Do it!

The Medical Home Gains Momentum

Blog
Modern Medicine
Posted March 1, 2010

Real health care reform is happening in the trenches. While Washington struggles to do something meaningful, improved and redesigned primary care practices are springing up all over the country.

I am attending the second National Medical Home Summit in Philadelphia this week. Last year there were 21 medical home demonstration projects going on in 18 states. Now the number is too numerous to count, and almost every state is involved. The use of EHRs and HIT as tools for the modernization of medical practice is rising exponentially, at least by medical practice standards, which ordinarily change at glacial speed.

So what is this Medical Home thing if you are still in a traditional paper-based, appointment-based practice seeing 30 or more patients a day? The Medical Home means that you strategize the care of your patients individually and as a population. You have a registry function that allows you to see which of your patients have received their recommended preventive services and which have not. Your office staff are calling women who have not have a mammogram in the past 2 years, and all patients over 50 that have not had colon cancer screening. You know which of your diabetic patients are in control and who have their last A1c over 7.5. You are starting to see the patients you really need to see in order to improve your overall outcomes and set yourself up for any pay for performance incentives.

I do not have time to see all these patients, you might say. Work with them over the telephone or over secure e-mail. That is more efficient. The additional payment of the Medical Home model is for care coordination by your team outside of visits. Our population outcomes will advance if we can provide care that does not depend on visits.

This is the real health care reform, and the methods of care in the information age. It is time for all medical practices to get on this bus. Go to www.pcpcc.net and read all about it and join a demonstration project near you, or start one.

Reinventing Primary Care

Blog
Modern Medicine
Posted May 28, 2010

Health Affairs is the leading health policy journal in America. It is read by the people who make big decisions in how health care should be delivered, not clinically, but the organization and finance. In May this year, an entire issue is devoted to Reinventing Primary Care - 47 articles! For those interested in the future of primary care in America, this issue is a collector's item to be read and used in discussion.

The issue begins with an editorial about how primary care is too important to fail. Primary care is the foundation of the health system. Primary care improves the health of a population more than specialty care does and keeps it efficient and affordable. Yet, only 1 in 14 medical students in the United States is planning to go in to primary care. That must change!

The history of primary care is well described here before going into future models. There are a number of historic transitions underway. One is the movement from the individual physician doing everything to team care. Led by a primary care physician, a team is able to achieve much greater control over the chronic diseases that contribute to 80% of health care costs, such as diabetes, asthma, and heart failure.

A second transition is moving primary care into the information age. Instead of paper records that cannot be searched, electronic records with registry function allow for an analysis of the population being served. Care moves from reacting just to those patients who make an appointment to strategic proactive care coordination to the entire population of patients.

My favorite transition is the moving away from a busy office schedule of 15-minute appointments to seeing just 10 to 12 patients a day, giving them more time, and spending 1 to 2 hours in online or telephone communication with patients.

There is truly a paradigm shift in how primary care is being delivered, and with that comes a change in how it is paid for. Medical home care coordination payments become a major source of revenue for the practice. As Medicare and other insurance companies are actively exploring this payment, with savings overall through better primary care, many practices are not waiting for that and are charging patients the fee to receive better primary care.

This is truly an exciting time to be in primary care. We are in an historic time of transition that only comes once in a career. I hope the medical students get the message and get on board. We need to spread the word that a new and exciting primary care is coming. We all need to take steps to make it happen today.

Ideal Practice Update

Blog
Modern Medicine
Posted July 4, 2010

On February 8, 2010, the Eisenhower Primary Care 365 practice was launched in La Quinta, Calif. I wrote about my opportunity to idealize primary care at Eisenhower in two previous blogs (Inventing a New Primary Care Practice Today, April 2009[1] and Practicing Ideal Primary Care, December 2009.[2] I am here to report that the success of this practice has exceeded expectations.

Our business plan stated that 1075 patients would join this practice by June 30, 2010, by paying a fee of $595 per year ($555 for each member of a couple, no charge for children if the parents joined). By June 30, we exceeded this number by 163 patients and more than 25 patients continue to join each week. Overall, our patients believe that this fee is very reasonable, especially compared with most concierge medicine. It gives them open access to online communication 24/7/365 with a same-day (within 24 hours) turnaround, longer visits, and a smaller panel size per physician (up to 900). It is gratifying to learn that many patients are willing to pay for a better primary care experience. I get 3-6 online messages each day, and about half of them are thank you notes!

On June 30, I did a national audio conference on Creating Ideal Primary Care. More than 100 people subscribed, the largest number that the sponsor has ever had. The interest in improving primary care is intense right now, as reflected in my last blog discussing the May, 2010, issue of Health Affairs with 47 articles on Reinventing Primary

Care. Eisenhower Medical Center in Rancho Mirage, California, has the Annenberg Center for the Health Sciences and we are planning a conference on Optimizing Primary Care sometime the fall.

Real change in how primary care is practiced is definitely happening, and I believe that future recruitment of new primary care physicians will depend on new models of care. Of course all this change requires financial sustainability, and the payers such as Medicare, Medicaid, and private insurance companies must follow through on plans to support primary care beyond visit-based reimbursement. Growing evidence of better outcomes and lower overall costs will drive these changes. Better preventive care and management of chronic diseases keeps people out of the hospital, and this is where the money is saved.

I urge all involved in primary care practice to become part of the Patient Centered Medical Home movement and help to optimize primary care practice. You too can have a practice like that at Eisenhower. The future of primary care depends on that.

References

1. http://community.modernmedicine.com/_Inventing-a-New-Primary-Care-Practice-Today/blog/249876/33379.html
2. http://community.modernmedicine.com/_Practicing-Ideal-Primary-Care/blog/1617837/33379.html).

Is Obamacare the Real Health Care Reform?

Blog
Modern Medicine
Posted February 6, 2011

It seems that everyone is talking about Obamacare. Whether you hate it or like it, the name is associated with health care reform today. Whether repealed or not, so called Obamacare is not the real health care reform going on today. The real revolution is happening, under the radar of media and politics.

Let's put this in perspective. Obamacare is about health insurance reform, and an individual mandate that everyone have health insurance. The latter is the most controversial. Remember that the individual mandate is the plan promoted by the mostly Republican American Medical Association, and was started in Massachusetts by then Republican governor, Mitt Romney. It is a personal responsibility plan using a philosophy usually associated with Conservatives. I guess it is the mandate part that bothers some people. If so, I suggest those people be taxed to pay for the uninsured when they show up in the Emergency Department. I do not want to pay for them anymore like I am paying now with higher health insurance premiums. Health care is not an option when you are sick or injured, and that happens to all of us eventually.

But what is real health care reform today? I suggest that it is the revolution being caused by the internet and health information technology. How we have given and received health care for the past 40 years has been driven by the automobile and the telephone. People call for appointments and then drive to a doctor visit. Before that doctors made house calls and there were no appointments. My general practitioner from the 1950s did not even have a sign-in sheet. The nurse went to the waiting room and called next. You had better be sure you figured out who came in before and after you.

Now this telephone and automobile process is getting outdated too. Smart phones and applications (Apps) on the smart "pad" are connecting us to an increasing amount of our health care. People will communicate with their doctor's office using new technology and face to face visits will only be done when necessary. Membership payments or care coordination reimbursements are coming into practice creating a new hybrid reimbursement model.

While this might be the decade of Obamacare, it will be the decade when the process of giving and receiving health care will change radically. I'm excited about that. How about you?

Online Communication with Patient is Ready for Primetime

Blog
Modern Medicine
Posted March 5, 2011

After more than a decade of some physicians communicating with patients online, it is time for this platform to become mainstream. A new survey from Intuit Health indicates that Americans "expect their physicians to be easily accessible online." The poll found that 73% of Americans surveyed "would use a secure online communication solution to make it easier to get lab results, request appointments, pay medical bills, and communicate with their doctor's office." Steve Malik, president and general manager of Intuit Health, said "patient anxiety is rising…they want some measure of control, convenience and better communication with their doctor."[1]

I started giving my email to my patients back in 1997. Soon I was doing more email communication than phone calls and face-to-face visits. Communication and care became continuously accessible rather than episodic based on visits. Fewer important things "fell through the cracks" between visits. Now we have available secure online patient portals that allow for secure and professional communication, often within the electronic medical record. Medical care has finally entered the information age.

It is important to be paid for online communication and care. Fee-for-service for e-visits is one option, but most online communication would not qualify as a true e-visit. The practice where I work has a membership fee that covers all out-of-office communications, $30 to $50 a month, depending on age. Patients like this so much we have trouble keeping up with the growth of our practice. Continuously accessible online communication takes away most of the frustrations people have with their medical practice. It is rare for this communication to be abused, and some training of patients is occasionally necessary.

Our incomes are significantly higher because we are now paid for all communication and care coordination activities. Online messages with patients usually take no more than 1-3 minutes, a very efficient way to take care of questions and provide basic services. If you are not doing this, I suggest you get on board before you have to just to compete in your community.

Reference:

1. http://www.ihealthbeat.org/articles/2011/3/7/survey-most-patients-want-online-access-to-their-physicians-office.aspx

How Many Patients Should We Take Care Of?

Blog
Modern Medicine
Posted May 7, 2011

An interesting thing is happening in the world of concierge medicine.

MDVIP is now owned by Proctor and Gamble. The business model is based on the concierge physician taking care of 600 patients, but many of the physicians are calling for a halt in new patients after 400-450.

Why?

When all of a physician's patients have direct access to them via cell phone, the physician's life becomes too disrupted after 400-450 patients, even though they would make more money if they went to 600. When you give all patients your cell phone number, the "sweet spot" for panel size seems to be in the range of 200-450. The lower numbers apply if your patients are older. It seems amazing to primary care physicians used to panel sizes of 2000 or more that such a low number of patients can keep you that busy.

At Eisenhower Primary Care 365 (EPC 365), our business model is based on each physician caring for 900 patients. Instead of giving patients our cell phone numbers, patients have direct access to their personal physician via secure e-mail. A promise of a reply within 24 hours, 7 days a week, is given. The group shares emergency calls on the phone. Since online communication is done at mutual convenience, the theory is that the physician could care for more patients than with concierge practice.

In addition to providing 7 days a week online direct access to their physician, we strive to optimize the primary care of patients through longer visits (30 and 60 min routine appointments) and coordinating the care of patients with referrals. That is, we strive to do primary care right for every patient. We work as a team with our staff. In a population when half our patients are 65 and older, and almost 75% are over age 55, we are finding that a panel size of 600 keeps a full time physician very busy with a full appointment schedule.

Practicing this way, we realize what a sloppy job we do when we try and care for 2000 or more patients. Many things fall through the cracks and do not get done, like good explanations of lab results, and communication among physicians caring for the patient. The work of primary care is much more complicated than the days when patients only came in when they were sick. Comprehensive preventive care and management of chronic illness takes time, with the need for frequent communication. We need to rethink the number of patients that primary care physicians should take care of in order to do a good job.

I know that makes our shortage even worse, but unless we do primary care right, who would want to go into it? Also, the financial model needs to change to allow for a good income caring for a smaller panel of patients. Concierge medicine does that, but it is very expensive. We use a hybrid model with a membership/access fee of $30 to $50 a month depending on age, and then we will bill for visits. That does work well for us even with a panel size of 600 patients. It is time to make smaller panel sizes for primary care physicians as active topic of discussion and research in order to move forward with success. What do you think?

Social Rounds Are Not Social

Blog
Modern Medicine
Posted August 2011

We are all familiar with "social rounds" on our hospitalized patients. This is when we take the time to go and see the patient, talk with the family, and not bill for our services. Only one primary care physician can bill on hospitalized patients daily, and when a hospitalist is managing our patients, our rounds become "social rounds".

I know that for me, and for many of you, this term is insulting and not reflective of the real value these rounds provide. Usually we are the ones explaining to the patient and family what is going on with their care, and what the future holds. We often speak to the various physicians involved with our patients and provide an important care coordination function. We know our patients well, while hospitalists and specialists are only involved with their care temporarily.

With the health care cost crisis, I do not see us getting paid for these rounds anytime soon. Maybe if there were a global care coordination payment we received for patient continuity of care, these rounds would be part of that. Regardless, I'd like to see a better term for this work than "social rounds".

Does anyone have any suggestions?

Are You Practicing in the 21st Century?

Blog
Modern Medicine
Posted September 20, 2011

Is your practice using 21st century methods of communication and care or are you still in the 20th century? The 21st century is a time of internet applications, the ability to communicate anytime from anywhere, and to receive services remotely from a smart phone or tablet computer. Computer workstations, considered mini-computers 25 years ago now, now seem big and cumbersome. The world of communication and providing services has changed dramatically, yet medical care has lagged behind slowly clunking its way into the information age. The tipping point is past and by the end of this decade, your office needs to be an App on your patient's smart phone.

The 20th century had three phases of methods for medical communication and care. Early in the 20th century people had to fetch the doctor. There were few telephones and the doctor arrived by horse and buggy staying as long as necessary. Only the poor went to most hospitals and the outcomes were not pretty. By the mid-20th century most people had telephones and automobiles and fetching the doctor was easier. Most physicians has "surgeries" in an office, often attached to their home, and spent about half the day seeing patients there (the $2 office visit was born) and the other half making house calls. There were few appointments and patients came and signed in to be seen, waiting their turn. During the last decades of the 20th century, with advances in communication and transportation, the "make an appointment and come and get it" mode of health care developed. Physicians were most efficient staying in their offices, now in larger office buildings, seeing many patients each day. Same day services became less common replaced by waiting for next available appointments. Urgent care centers were developed to make up for the fact that most physician waiting rooms were full of patient coming for recheck visits or physical exams.

By 21st century methods, all the modes of care in the 20th century care seem archaic. Most medical practices are still in the late 20th century because change is difficult and "fee-for-visit" reimbursement and productivity measurement still dominate. The new communication methods are better, faster and cheaper, the dream of any redesign engineer, yet they are coming into application slowly.

I am fortunate to practice primary care in a fully 21st century mode of practice. About 75% of all communications with our patients occur over a secure online platform. Patients pay between $30 and $50 a month depending on their age for unlimited use of online services and care coordination outside of visits. Face-to-face visits start the care process and then are used as needed. We bill insurance for all visit related services. We care for a large number of patients yet our office is calm, quiet and all patients who are seen are heard fully in lengthy, unhurried visits. Our patient satisfaction scores are at the top of the chart, and our physicians enjoy their work every day because the intensity of the relationships with patients is so satisfying. The sweet spot of productivity seems to be seeing about 10-12 patients every day and communicating with about 30 patients in non-visit care. All our staff helps with communication and care coordination so we can optimize the delivery of primary care. The specialists we refer to love the level of service we give them and our patients.

More information about the online platform of communication and care is presented in a longer version of this article in one of the October issues of Medical Economics.[1]

Reference

1. Medical Economics. Interactions for the 21st century. October 25, 2011.

10-12 Visits a Day, 50-60 a Week

Blog
Modern Medicine
Posted October 2011

The October 10, 2011 issue of Medical Economics[1] has an article discussing the number of visits per week for the primary care specialties of FPs/GPs, internists, OB/GYNs and pediatricians.

While in 2010 the number of visits per week fell slightly, about 5% for each specialty, almost all are still doing more than 90 visits per week (OB/GYN was at 89). The summary point was that primary care physicians saw 93 patients per week in 2010. No mention is made of online or telephone visits, although it was mentioned that patients are less willing to come in for office visits to discuss test results.

The survey shows that in 2010, the dominant form of primary care is still the visit dependent 20th century model. Most primary care reimbursement is still fee-for-visit. As I have discussed in this Blog, new models of primary care have fewer visits and more communication and care provided online and over the telephone. Reimbursement must change to support these more efficient methods of communication.

Two very large prepaid health plan providers, Kaiser Permanente and Group Health Cooperative in Washington State, have their primary care physicians seeing only 10-14 patients per day. The physicians spend one hour or more doing "desktop medicine", communicating with patients and other team members online. Group Health is the most advanced in this and the physicians average 10-12 visits per day. Even in high-demand practices with lots of patients, physicians can limit their visit volumes, and spend more time with patients, through the use of PAs or NPs and with everyone practicing to the limit of their license in the care of patients.

As I have said repeatedly, the work of primary care, with comprehensive prevention, chronic illness management and the biopsychosocial model, is too complex for hurried brief visits. The quality expectations today require enough time to complete everything expected in care. The Medical Home models uses care coordinators, powered by information systems, to provide care outside of patient visits.

I look forward to one of the annual Autumn issues of Medical Economics finally showing that the practice of primary care has changed dramatically. For many of us, it already has.

Reference

1. Hertz BT. Patient visits down slightly, but not workload. Medical Economics. 2011

The work of Kate Lorig at Stanford and David Sobel at Northern California Kaiser Permanente pointed the way toward greater patient self-management as an important change in primary care. I tried to capture this phenomenon in this article for Family Medicine:

Future Vision: Is Family Medicine Ready for Patient-Directed Care?

Family Medicine
2009;41(4):278-281

A growing number of Americans will soon have a Web-based personal medical home with connectedness to their chosen providers of care. The personal health record will become integrated with the electronic health record. Like other services on the Internet, patients will be able to direct much of their health care using clinical guidelines, such as prevention, chronic illness care, behavior change, and arrangement for minor acute care. Physician control and autonomy will give way to greater patient control over their care, a major culture change in medicine away from paternalism. While the personal family physician will continue as a primary caregiver, there will be a shift toward greater patient involvement in the coordination of care. Family medicine educators should begin now to educate medical students and residents for this new model of care. Fam Med 2009;41(4):285-8.

In 2012, what will an average American be able to do when they log into their Web-based personal medical home? Will the Internet fulfill the dream of patient self-management? What will become of the personal family physician? How should we train family physicians when more and more patients begin directing their own care?

Is the Medical Home Model Really Patient Centered?

The Medical Home Model has captured the hopes of primary care physicians who are yearning for a better day. After a prolonged period of decline, primary care is poised for a comeback if better reimbursement and greater medical student interest can be accomplished. A rational and affordable health care system depends on a healthy foundation of primary care. The Medical Home Model, with its patient-centered coordination of care, seems to be just the right concept on which to pin the hopes of primary care.

Primary care enjoyed a period of rapid growth in the 1990s, riding the wave of managed care. It was a period of cost reduction based on primary care physicians serving as gatekeepers. The gatekeeper model was doomed to fail, however, among an American public that demands choice over where it gets health care. As the popularity of managed care waned, so went primary care. In cynical terms, one might say that today's medical home model is the gatekeeper over again with nicer words. They share the strategy of asking patients to have their comprehensive care coordinated in a single primary care environment, though recent innovations in primary care coupled with the changing demographics of an aging population offer hope that the medical home will not suffer the fate of gatekeepers. Coordinated chronic illness care, team approaches, and health information technology all combine to offer new processes of care not understood or available 15 years ago.

In 2007, the major primary care organizations agreed on a set of guiding principles for the patient-centered medical home.[1] These describe the innovations necessary in primary care to achieve improved coordination of care and better outcomes. All the principles are progressive except one that sticks out as a commitment to the past -- physician-directed care. Apparently, the crafters of these principles did not want physicians to lose any control over patient care.

Is this Medical Home Model care, with its commitment to physician-directed care, really patient centered? It depends on what you mean by patient-centered care. To some, being patient centered means that you focus on the patient, not just the disease. Another view of being patient centered is to put the patient on the care team, even at the center of the team.[2] In the Institute of Medicine report Crossing the Quality Chasm, patient centered is one of the six aims for quality health care, and the report defines it as care that "encompasses qualities of compassion, empathy, and responsiveness to the needs, values, and expressed preferences of the individual patient.[3] Shared decision making has emerged as a care model, especially when the evidence is not completely clear about what tests and treatments are preferred, such as with breast or prostate cancer screening and treatment. These concepts allow for patient centeredness while preserving the traditional physician control over medical practice. That may change, even radically, as more health care moves onto the Internet.

The Internet Releases the Power of Patient Self-Management

The Internet makes it possible to give patients more control over their care and challenges the concept of physician-directed care. When patients have their personal health records connected to their chosen providers of care through Web-based personal medical homes, what is to stop them from coordinating some of their own care? Physicians who think they will direct patient care in the future might reflect on what has happened to personal bankers, stockbrokers, and travel agents. Health care has had a delayed reaction to this revolution in consumer control—a degree of control that would have been unimaginable a few decades ago.

Of course, some health care will always be physician directed. Physicians will always be in charge of providing care for trauma, surgical emergencies, and major acute medical problems. When patients become acutely ill, whether with a myocardial infarction or acute appendicitis, they need and desire a physician to take charge. Indeed, for some complex medical and surgical problems, even arrogance on the part of physicians has its place.[4] In complex health and illness matters, an objective professional physician is a source of comfort and care, and for many patients, having a personal family physician is desirable even if they are able to coordinate much of the care. Other patients, especially those with limited education or inadequate literacy, may always need to rely on a physician and health care team to direct their care.

Outside of the aforementioned exceptions (acute care of major illnesses, trauma, and emergencies and patients incapable of coordinating their own care), there is a question about whether the physician should still be in charge. Ed Wagner developed the chronic care model based on informed and activated patients interacting with a prepared and proactive medical team.[5] The relationship is symmetric, with the control of care equally shared. Patients are asked to become experts themselves, to develop an understanding of their chronic illnesses that matches or perhaps exceeds
that of their physician. With the Internet, all knowledge becomes available for free, and learning happens rapidly. Patients, supported by their families and friends, only have their own problems to learn about.

This type of patient self-management has been studied for more than a decade, and the evidence for better control of chronic illnesses is impressive.[6-10] David Sobel, medical director at Kaiser Permanente Northern California, has found that the greater the degree of patient self- management, the better the outcomes. Conversely, dependence on the physician is detrimental to the management of chronic illness.[11] Indeed, Kaiser has launched a Web platform where its members may directly access recommended care services. Why should a physician stand in the way of a patient getting recommended preventive services or tests for the monitoring of their chronic illness? If what should be done is known, why require a visit to a physician? As patients become knowledgeable and have the power to direct aspects of their care, the primary care physician becomes an unnecessary "middleman." Rather, the primary care physician should become a resource for the patient—a consultant or coach—rather than a gatekeeper through which the patient must go to receive routine preventive and chronic illness care.

Patient-directed care does not, of course, mean that the care team backs off and leaves the patient unattended. Patients should not be alone making sure that they get their recommended services. For quality outcomes to occur in patient-directed care, the care team is proactive in communicating with the patient about services with the patient and works hard to ensure that timely optimal care is received.

What Care Will Be Physician Directed?

If patients will be orchestrating much of their own care, what care will be directed by physicians? The answer is seen in the stratification of primary care services currently being undertaken by large health care systems like Kaiser, which is organizing health care around five distinct areas: prevention, chronic illness care, maternal and infant care, trauma and major acute care, and minor acute care.[12] If those are in different places in the health care delivery system, where is primary care and family medicine? Primary care becomes the integration of ongoing care—prevention, chronic illness, minor acute illness—all best done from a biopsychosocial perspective. Family medicine also provides pregnancy care and early infant care. Rural physicians continue to provide trauma and major acute care. But, the specific role of family physicians in this new delivery system is not the same as family medicine of today.

What Care Will Be Patient Directed?

What about the patient? What services will the informed and activated patient, armed with a Web-based medical home, be capable of obtaining directly? The obvious ones are recommended preventive services; self-management of common chronic illnesses such as diabetes, hypertension, and asthma; behavior change such as smoking cessation and weight loss; and arranging for minor acute care. The family physician becomes a resource serving many roles desired by the patient—provider and coordinator of care, coach, or consultant—helping with tough decisions like what to do for colon, breast, and prostate cancer screening and treatment. Even the prenatal care schedule could be managed by activated patients.

This is not about putting patients in charge of what they do not want to do or of what they are unable to do. Rather, it is about patients being enabled to play an active role in their care as they access all the resources available to them and seek care within recommended clinical guidelines. Who will want to sit in a crowded waiting room to have a brief encounter with a physician when they can find out on their own what needs to be done? When visits become selective encounters for issues about which patients can't find answers, rather than the sole source of care, visits should all happen on time in unhurried and less crowded environments.

Major steps in the direction of patient-directed care have already been made by Kaiser's Health Connect platform and Geisinger's Personal Health Navigator.[13] Microsoft with HealthVault and Google Health are partnering with major groups such as Mayo Clinic and Cleveland Clinic, and these organizations have the vision of revolutionizing health care around patient-directed services. Dossia has been formed by a consortium of major employers, and even Wal-Mart employees have their personal health records and will soon be directing their care with willing providers.

Does this mean that patients will get any care they want? Of course not, especially care for which they do not directly pay. Patient-directed care would operate under recognized clinical guidelines and represent care the provider and payer would want the patient to have. Everything else would come through communication to agree on appropriate services.

Training Family Physicians for Patient-Directed Care

The service model of most industries has changed radically in the age of the Internet. That is now happening in health care, too. The change process is still early, but the horse is out of the barn. Physicians and other caregivers need to adjust to patients having more control over their care. This is a culture change for a health care system that is currently very paternalistic. Physician control and autonomy arose during the 19th and 20th centuries, but this approach will have to change.[14] Health care has had its social transformations before and will have one again in the 21st century.

Unfortunately, most clinical settings in medical education are also highly paternalistic. From the day of the white coat ceremony, medical students becoming physicians are taught to respect and "take care" of the patient. Professional respect in medicine is fine, but the message of control begins early. The boundary between health care professionals and the public forms and becomes two distinct worlds, and patients have limited access to communicating about their own care. While this separation may persist in major acute hospitals, it will erode in chronic care and prevention. Health caregivers, including physicians, will need to learn to serve patients who have much greater control over their care.

Patient-directed care will be a culture change for medicine. It will not happen overnight, and strata of the population will move to it at different rates. There will always be a segment of the population that does not want to be bothered with or is afraid of their health care decisions and that is happy to have physicians direct the care. There will always be people who want to be taken care of and who desire paternalism or maternalism from physicians. There will always be tensions between what patients want and their evidence-based needs and tensions among payers, providers, and recipients of care. Health care is messy, which is one reason why it has been slow to change its processes. But, the need for family physicians to be chameleons, able to change styles to adapt to the patient, is everlasting.

The Role of Family Medicine

Family medicine, with its emphasis on patient-centered communication, is well positioned for this transition. However, loss of control of patient care will be threatening to many family physicians. The personality of our specialty may undergo a shift much like it did in the transition of general practice to family medicine.

That shift needs to be driven by medical education. Family medicine educators should prepare new scripts for role modeling and additional training for simulated patients. Paternalistic tendencies will need to be exposed and addressed in both teachers and learners. Physician-directed electronic health records should be integrated with patient-directed personal health records through secure portals that become new communication platforms for care coordination. Are we prepared for a single shared health record controlled largely by the patient? Are we reducing the toxicity of dependence and releasing the power of patient self-management? We all strive to be healers, and our healing skills are shifting more to what we always strived to do, helping patients take care of themselves.

The Future of Family Medicine project along with TransforMED has sought to define the personal physician for future practice. Green et al, in a commentary on preparing the personal physician for practice (P4) papers evokes the time-honored perspective of the personal physician by T.F. Fox in the 1960s (apologies for the male gender):[15]

The doctor we have in mind . . . is looking after people as people and not as problems. He is what our grandfathers called 'my medical attendant' or 'my personal physician;' and his function is to meet what is really the primary medical need. A person in difficulties wants in the first place the help of another person on whom he can rely as a friend—someone with knowledge of what is feasible but also with good judgment on what is desirable in the particular circumstances, and an understanding of what the circumstances are. The more complex medicine becomes, the stronger are the reasons why everyone should have a personal doctor who will take continuous responsibility for him, and, knowing how he lives, will keep things in proportion—protecting him, if need be, from the zealous specialist....[16]

Dr. Fox could not have imagined patients with Web-based personal medical homes directing much of their care. He would argue for the continuation of the personal family physician. A great class discussion would be an analysis of the truth versus paternalism in this statement and the delicate navigation in store for family medicine.

References

1. American Academy of Family Physicians, American Academy of Pediatrics, American College of Physicians, American Osteopathic Association. Joint principles of the patient-centered medical home. February 2007. http://www.aafp.org/online/etc/medialib/aafp_org/docume nts/policy/fed/jointprinciplespcmh0207.Par.0001.File.tmp/02 2107medicalhome.pdf. Accessed October 12, 2008.

2. Berenson RA, Hammons T, Gans DN, et al. A house is not a home: keeping patients at the center of practice redesign. Health Aff 2008;27:1219-30.

3. Institute of Medicine. Committee on the Quality of Health Care in America. Crossing the quality chasm: a new health

system for the 21st century. Washington, DC: National Academy Press, 2001.

4. Inglefinger FJ. Arrogance. N Engl J Med 1980;303:1507-11.

5. Improving chronic illness care. www.improvingchroniccare. org. Accessed October 12, 2008.

6. Lorig K, Mazonson P, Holman H. Evidence suggesting that health education for self-management in patients with chronic arthritis has sustained health benefits while reducing health care costs. Arthritis Rheum 1993;36:439-46.

7. Lorig KR, Ritter P, Stewart AL, et al. Chronic disease self-management program: 2-year health status and health care utilization outcomes. Med Care 2001;39:1217-23.

8. Barlow JH, Wright CC, Turner AP, Bancroft GV. A 12-month follow-up study of self-management training for people with chronic disease: are changes maintained over time? Br J Clin Psychol 2005;10:589-99.

9. Lorig KR, Ritter PL, Jacquez A. Outcomes of border health Spanish/English chronic disease self-management programs. The Diabetes Educator 2005;31:401-9.

10. Sobel DS, Lorig KR, Hobbs M. Chronic disease self-management program: from development to dissemination. The Permanente Journal 2002;6(2):15-22.

11. Sobel DS. Patient self-management and activation. Presentation to the California Clinical Quality Improvement "Right Care" Initiative, RAND Corporation, Santa Monica, Calif, September 29, 2008.

12. David M. Lawrence, former CEO of Kaiser, personal communication, 2008.

13. Paulus RA, Davis K, Steele GD. Continuous innovations in health care: implications of the Geisinger experience. Health Aff 2008;27:1235-45.

14. Starr P. The social transformation of American medicine. New York: Basic Books, 1982.

15. Green LA, Pugno P, Fetter G, Jones SM. Preparing personal physicians for practice (P4): a national program testing innovations in family medicine residencies. J Am Board Fam Med 2007;20:329-31.

16. Fox TF. The personal doctor and his relation to the hospital. Lancet 1960;1:743-60.

The California Academy of Family Physicians asked me to write this article as part of a "toolkit" monograph to members about the redesign of their practice.

New World of Family Medicine
Family Medicine is Leading the Redesign of Medical Care

Family Medicine Toolkit
California Academy of Family Physicians
February 2009;2:4-5

Family physicians continue to provide an incredible variety of front line medical care - from preventive, acute and chronic care to people of all ages. A family physician can enter any community in the world and immediately care for everyone there. As health information technology (HIT) and new quality methods bring new models of care, family medicine remains on the cutting edge of patient care. The Patient Centered Medical Home (PCMH) is the unifying concept for primary care in the 21st Century, and family medicine is leading the way in its development and implementation.

In 2007, the American Academy of Family Physicians (AAFP) partnered with other primary care organizations to develop the guiding principles of the PCMH.[1] Among the principles are:

• Personal physician - Each patient has an ongoing relationship with a personal physician trained to provide first contact, continuous, and comprehensive care.

• Physician-directed medical practice - The personal physician leads a team of individuals at the practice level who collectively take responsibility for the ongoing care of patients.

• Whole person orientation - The personal physician is responsible for providing for all the patients' health care needs or taking responsibility for appropriately arranging care with other qualified professionals. This includes care for all stages of life - acute care, chronic care, preventive services, and end of life care.

• Care is coordinated and/or integrated across all elements of the complex health care system (e.g., sub-specialty care, hospitals, home health agencies, nursing homes) and the patients' communities (e.g., family, public, and private community based services). Care is facilitated by registries, information technology, health information exchange and other means to assure that patients get the indicated care when and where they need and want it in a culturally and linguistically appropriate manner.

• Quality and safety are hallmarks of the medical home. These include patient-centered outcomes defined by a care planning process, evidence-based medicine, clinical decision support tools, and voluntary participation in performance measurement and improvement. Patients actively participate in decision making, and feedback is sought to ensure patients' expectations are met. HIT is utilized appropriately to support optimal patient care, performance measurement, patient education, and enhanced communication.

• Enhanced access to care is available through systems such as open scheduling, expanded hours, and new options for communication between patients, their personal physician, and practice staff.

• Payment appropriately recognizes the added value provided to patients who have a patient-centered medical home.

What is so exciting about this new concept for family medicine? The new tools and methods of the PCMH promise to make family physicians more effective than ever before. Previously, in the traditional model of care, family physicians evaluated and treated patients based on what they could personally find out about a patient. Call this "off the top of the head" medicine. Most family physicians are quite skilled at this, but patients do not reliably receive the best that medicine has to offer. As David Eddy has said, "the complexity of modern medicine exceeds the inherent limitations of an unaided human mind."[2] HIT provides the tools that combine all important patient information to guide the best treatment. Family physicians in the 21st Century will continue to have meaningful personal relationships while helping patients and families, but the readily available world of medical knowledge will be shared and harnessed with highly informed and activated patients playing a greater role in their own care.

The practice of family medicine is in a period of rapid change. More patients are using web-based personal health records (PHRs) through vendors such as Google™ and Microsoft®. They expect their family physician to be able to download the PHR in the practice's electronic health record (EHR). Leading EHR companies are developing these systems through secure patient portals so that there is one medical record shared between the patient and the PCMH. A secure online platform of communication and care is emerging that promises to be the new "front door" of a PCMH practice. Payment methods for the PCMH are emerging to pay physicians for non-visit care such as e-visits and scheduled telephone visits. The proposed care management fees paid to family physicians for patients with chronic illness will provide a much greater financial base for primary care than in the past.

Relationship-centered care delivered by family physicians has an emerging care model that will make the traditional "make an appointment, come and get it" model of care obsolete. Patients will have advanced access to timely communication and care with their family physicians, and the outcomes will be far superior than before.

This is such an exciting time to be starting a career in family medicine! We are on the cusp of a great transition in how care is delivered both to populations and individuals. The information age is a boon for family medicine. As personal physicians caring for entire families and communities, family physicians will benefit most from the new knowledge management tools. The economic picture looks bright for family physicians since the PCMH requires less overhead, delivers improved quality and service to patients, and enhances provider satisfaction.[3] The mission, vision, and values of family medicine will not change, but will be enhanced by the emerging model of practice. Now is the time to become a 21st Century family physician. The communities of America and around the world need us, and serving them will be the best it has ever been.

References

1. American Academy of Family Physicians, American Academy of Pediatrics, American College of Physicians, American Osteopathic Association. Joint principles of the patient-centered medical home. 24 October 2007. www.medicalhomeinfo.org/Joint%20Statement.pdf.
2. Millenson, M.L. Demanding Medical Excellence: Doctors and Accountability in the Information Age. Chicago: University of Chicago Press, 1997. p.75.
3. Report on Financing the New Model of Family Medicine. Annals of Family Medicine. 2004 2: S1-S21. www.annfammed.org.

By 2010 it appeared that family medicine was on the rebound in the match after 5 years of decline, helped by the growing re-awareness of the importance of primary care.

What Does the Match Mean for the Growth and Development of Family Medicine?

Editorial
Family Medicine
2010;42(8):538-9

Over the past 4 decades, the number of medical students matching in family medicine has followed a sinusoidal curve. The 1960s were a period of major decline in graduating medical students entering general practice, reflecting the post-World War II "age of specialization" (I remember reading about that as a child in the World Book Encyclopedia update circa 1960). The growth of family medicine residency programs and medical students matching in the new specialty in the 1970s are upswing curves we are all familiar with (at least those of us with some grey hair).

The 1980s was a decade of rapid cost inflation in health care, and incomes for procedurally oriented specialists rose as fast as major league baseball players' incomes. I was a predoctoral director in the

1980s and commented that going into family medicine was like being a missionary. The Match in 1988 was known as "black Tuesday" with precipitous declines for both family medicine and internal medicine.

Family medicine made a comeback in the 1990s riding the wave of managed care. There were all-time highs in students matching into family medicine in 1997. The backlash against managed care and other factors resulted in steady declines since then. Now, in 2010, family medicine and primary care are poised for a comeback with expanded access to health insurance coming and the need for accountable care organizations wanting a foundation of primary care using a Patient-centered Medical Home model. The 2010 Match with US seniors is showing the first signs of recovery.[1] The early signs are that here we go back in favor again.

What does this up and down in the Match mean to the growth and development of family medicine as a specialty and to family medicine education? The practice of family medicine during these same 4 decades has been much more stable. The number of residency programs and residency positions peaked in the late 1990s but only declined modestly during the past decade. New residency programs are springing up again as the need for primary care has become more acute.

International medical graduates have populated our residency programs over the past decade in large numbers providing substantial diversity. The quality of students entering family medicine remains strong. I serve on the Board of Directors of the Pisacano Leadership Foundation, and the number and quality of applicants for Pisacano Scholarships over the past decade have remained steady and incredibly impressive. I served on the Board of Directors of the American Board of Family Medicine, and the graduating resident board scores have remained strong as the number of diplomats continues to grow. Despite the downturns, family medicine remains the second largest specialty behind internal medicine and the largest if you consider that most internists subspecialize.

As reflected in this issue of Family Medicine, the evolution of scholarship in family medicine has been steady and impressive. Opinion pieces have given way to more rigorous analytical and quantitative research. The articles by Myerholtz et al, on a communication assessment tool, and Bloom et al, on an evaluation of an electronic medical record implementation are both sophisticated scholarship.[2,3]

Family medicine has stayed the course despite the ups and downs of medical student interest and selection of the specialty. Family medicine is a "high road" specialty and central to the solution of what ails health care in America. Pride in being a family physician or a family medicine educator remains consistent and strong. My observation is that general surgeons seem to be in a funk these days but not family physicians.

What will be required to support and sustain an upswing in family medicine? Not the same style of practice that characterized the last decades of the 20th century. We are now in a new information age, and the population no longer needs us for medical information; it is everywhere. People want control over their own health care, and they will soon have the tools to manage much of their own care.[4] The interpersonal advising, coaching, and healing skills of the family physician become primary, a trend that the founders of the specialty would smile about.

Riding a positive wave of medical students matching into family medicine is a lot of fun, and I'm glad to get another ride with that before I retire. If we seize the information age and develop new models of education and practice that keep family physicians and others on the team central to the health of populations, this upswing might just last longer than a decade and achieve a new level of stability. Family medicine is also an eternally optimistic specialty.

References

1. McGaha AL, Schmittling GT, DeVilbiss Bieck AD, Crosley PW, Pugno PA. Entry of US medical school graduates into family medicine residencies: 2009–2010 and 3-year summary. Fam Med 2010;42(8):540-51.
2. Myerholtz L, Simons L, Felix S, Nguyen T, Brennan J, Rivera-Tovar A, Martin P, Hepworth J, Makoul G. Using the communication assessment tool in family medicine residency programs. Fam Med 2010;42(8):567-73.
3. Bloom MV, Huntington MK. Faculty, resident, and clinic staff's evaluation of the effects of EHR implementation. Fam Med 2010;42(8):562-6.
4. Scherger JE. Future vision: is family medicine ready for

patient-directed care? Fam Med 2009;41(4):285-8.

In 2007, four primary care organizations, AAFP, ACP, AAP and the AOA, developed joint principles for the patient-centered medical home (PCMH). It became clear that the future of primary care depended on an improved model of care, with recognition and reimbursement for the care coordination activities essential to a quality practice. Lots of long lists and accreditation requirements created confusion as to what a PCMH actually was. In 2009 I joined the editorial advisory board of Medical Home News and tried to provide clarity with this article:

The Essence of the Medical Home

Medical Home News
2010;2(5):2

The Medical Home means different things to different people. Position papers and articles go on at length describing the principles and applications of the Medical Home model, often called the Patient-Centered Medical Home. After reading such pieces I often wonder just how the Medical Home is different than good traditional medical office practice. Too often the trees are being described without first making clear what the new forest is all about.

The essence of the Medical Home model can be described in eight words: care coordination by a team independent of visits. If you only use two words, they are care coordination. Traditional office practice reacts to those patients who make appointments. Information systems that allow for strategic proactive care to a population are missing. In a Medical Home, the population cared for becomes clear, and efforts are made by the care team to reach out proactively to achieve better outcomes.

The additional payment in the Medical Home model is for the care coordination outside of visits. There are two payment methods emerging. I will call them low payment and higher payment. The low payment method, such as $2-$4 per member per month, is common in Medicaid applications of the Medical Home. This amount of money gives a practice the funds to hire a care coordinator as part of the team. This person or persons reaches out to patients, usually by telephone, to get patients back into the care system. Outcomes improve, and visits to the emergency department and even hospitalizations may decline. The rest of the team, including the physician, continues to practice in the same way with a busy office schedule of mostly brief visits.

The higher payment method, such as $30-$50 per member per month, allows for a redesign of the care model away from a dependence on office visits. This payment allows the entire care team, including the physician, to communicate with patients on a new platform, such as online and the telephone. Visits are done selectively and more time intensively to establish care relationships and provide essential visit based care. Interactions with patients occur outside of visits each day, and these are more efficient than intermittent face-to-face encounters. A new care model emerges with physicians seeing about 10-12 patients per day in longer appointments and spending 1-2 hours per day in care coordination activities. This new model of primary care has the potential of attracting more medical students to primary care and avoiding burn-out among providers. It is the new primary care for the information age.

With all of the issues surrounding the Medical Home movement and the call for redesigning primary care, remember the essence that is supported by data as being cost effective and improving outcomes. Proactive care coordination by a team supported by information systems is the new care model. As it becomes the new primary care, such care coordination will migrate into specialty care as those office practices also should use care coordination by a team independent of visits to provide higher quality continuity of care to patients.

New jargon and a distrust of the government often get in the way of appreciating real progress. Meaningful use of HIT was thought by many to be an onerous regulation more than an improvement in the quality of care. The following article gives a positive perspective on meaningful use of HIT:

Meaningful Use of HIT Saves Lives

Editorial
Medical Economics
May 2010

Since the meaningful use criteria came out, many providers of healthcare have been crying out, "Not so fast!" You have got to be kidding. I have no sympathy for them. Meaningful use of health information technology (HIT) saves lives, and it is inappropriate, if not unethical, for us to delay its use any longer.

Electronic health records (EHRs) came on the scene in the 1970s. Yes, the 1970s. The family medicine department at the Medical University of South Carolina and other daring practices implemented them. The computer age had begun.

In the 1980s, networking with personal computers won the battle over the big machines, and more EHR options became available. Microsoft's dominance in business was in full swing, and MS-DOS was a great operating system for EHRs. More innovative practices came on board.

The 1994–1995 time period was the official start of the information age, writes Tom Friedman in The World is Flat. The first Web browsers went public, and a second generation of EHRs, Web-enabled products such as Logician, became available. The writing was on the wall for the universal adoption of EHRs, yet most medical practices continued to suffer from "mural dyslexia" (difficulty reading the writing on the wall).

In 2004, Department of Health and Human Services (HHS) Secretary Michael Leavitt and the first HIT "czar," David Brailer, MD, PhD, declared the 2000s the decade of HIT. They stated a goal of universal penetration of EHRs by 2014. In 2009, President Obama reiterated this goal for 2014 and provided $19 billion in funding via the Health Information Technology for Economic and Clinical Health Act as part of American Recovery and Reinvestment Act of 2009.

More than 10 years ago, the Institute of Medicine released its groundbreaking report "To Err is Human" and called for the end of physician and nurse handwriting within five years to reduce errors and save lives. Politicians across the political spectrum, from the liberal Patrick Kennedy to the conservative Newt Gingrich, declared that "paper kills" and have called for universal adoption of EHRs.

Now, in 2010, a large number of private practices have yet to implement EHRs, and the government is getting tough. After all, most of the modern world is way ahead of us. In Europe and New Zealand, more than 90 percent of physician practices have had EHRs for years. If there were an Olympics for the use of HIT, the United States would be far down the list of medal winners.

The meaningful use criteria were written by physicians for physicians. David Blumenthal, MD, MPP, the federal government's second and current HIT czar (his HHS title is national coordinator for HIT), and Paul Tang, MD, MS, chairman of the federal HIT Policy Committee's Meaningful Use Work Group, which advises HHS, are both experienced primary care physicians. They know how certain applications of HIT will avoid medical errors and save lives. It is time for all of medicine in America to follow their lead.

Significant medication errors happen in seven percent of all hospitalizations, and such errors are even more common in office practice. A leader in the retail pharmacy industry told me that more than 30 percent of all handwritten prescriptions need some correction at the pharmacy. The pharmacies cannot catch all the mistakes. Successful lawsuits have been brought against physicians because of harm caused by poor handwriting.

It is impossible for humans—and physicians are human—to remember all significant drug interactions. More than 50 commonly used drugs cause prolongation of the QT interval of the heart and if used together in an at-risk patient may cause sudden death. The list of drug interactions with warfarin in both directions of anti-coagulation effect is too long for anyone to remember.

Rocket scientists need computer support to do their jobs correctly, and we physicians do, too. It is time for us to give up "medicine by the seat of our pants" and work with HIT to provide safe and consistently effective care. The standard of care now requires that, and you know what that means in legal terms.

EHRs and other HIT applications are expensive, and the quality of the software has been a problem, but the time for excuses is over. We do not tolerate a lack of safety in industries such as air travel and automobile manufacturing. The number of people dying in the United States from medical errors could fill two jumbo jets every day. The meaningful use of EHRs and other HIT such as clinical decision support software will go a long way in making medicine safer.

Members of the public and their elected representatives are lowering the boom on us, and it is time for us to respond en masse. Welcome meaningful use of HIT and get a certified EHR system application for use in your office.

In 2009 I was hired by Eisenhower Medical Center in Rancho Mirage, CA to develop the best possible primary care practice. The leadership at Eisenhower believed that in fulfilling the mission of excellence in patient service and quality of care, margins would follow. I was forbidden by the CEO to develop a productivity model of primary care, but rather to develop the best primary care the patients have ever experienced. The wisdom here was to improve market share in the area led by outstanding primary care. Using new tools of HIT and the internet, and the quality methods of the PCMH, we strived to develop ideal primary care in our setting. Looking at the innovations in primary care emerging around the U.S., two very different models seemed to be emerging based on the needs of the populations served. These articles describe idealizing primary care practice and describe both the relationship centered models and the organized team models of care:

Creating Ideal Primary Care

Medical Home News
2010;2(7):1,5

Hospitals and health systems have been setting up "Centers of Excellence" for many years. Cardiovascular disease, cancer, orthopedics, and neuroscience are common targets for idealizing care. Why not primary care? That may sound far-fetched with the current state of primary care practice and its hurried office visits, crowded waiting rooms, and frustrated patients, providers and staff. But creating ideal primary care is just what I was asked to do at Eisenhower Medical Center in the Coachella Valley (Palm Springs area) of California.

Another way to describe ideal primary care is to say that it meets the following criteria:

- Patients receive all the time they need and want for care with great service
- Patients receive the best care
- Physicians and staff enjoy their work and sustain high level professional satisfaction
- Medical errors are minimized
- Physicians are supported by a team and care for the right number of patients

This article describes two models of idealizing primary care. The first is an organized team model capable of care for a large population per physician. The second is a relationship-centered model focusing on a limited panel of patients per physician. These models are not mutually exclusive, and any given health system or practice may want to have elements of both.

In the organized team model, the physician focuses on the sicker or more complex patients requiring the extensive medical training of a specialist in primary care. Routine preventive care and treatment of common acute and chronic conditions are handled by a nurse practitioner or physician assistant. The care team includes other resource providers such as a counselor, nutritionist, pharmacist, diabetes educator, and fitness expert such as a physical therapist. Each of these providers is "right sized" to match the population being served, and everyone works to the limit of their license. A care coordinator, such as a nurse, makes sure that all patients are receiving the care they want and need. A shared information system allows for strategic proactive care and evaluation of patient satisfaction and outcomes. Depending on the size of the population being served, team members may be located together or close by. The organized team model fits an organization caring for a large population with limited resources, such as a community clinic or a staff or group model HMO such as Kaiser Permanente. As conceived by Tom Bodenheimer, a single physician may be responsible for as many as 4000 patients in this model.[1]

In the relationship-centered model, all patients have a personalized connection with their chosen primary care physician. This physician knows all the patients well and focuses on optimizing their health. A new platform of online communication and care makes the physician continuously available to the patient. Most clinical communications go directly to the physician and may be triaged to an activated medical assistant or other team member. Given the smaller panel size, such as 1000 patients or less depending on the number of seniors, the practice team is small and may include just an assistant who is trained by the physician as a care coordinator. Other resource providers are readily available in a "neighborhood" of care provided by an integrated delivery system. A shared information system again allows for strategic proactive care and evaluation of patient satisfaction and outcomes.

The relationship-centered model of care resembles the service of concierge medicine, although most concierge practices simply provide cell phone access with the physician and do not have advanced information systems. Gordon Moore of Rochester, NY started the "ideal micropractice" model in 2002, and this has been refined by him and many "member" practices into the Ideal Medical Practice model.[2] Charles Kilo and colleagues started an idealized primary care practice that has grown to two offices and nine physicians in Portland, OR called Greenfield Health.[3] Eisenhower Primary Care 365 is modeled after Greenfield Health but had to modify the structure since more than 50% of the practice is composed of seniors.[4]

It is not clear if the primary care physician's workday changes in the organized team model of care. One would hope that by focusing on the more complex patients, the physician would have more time with patients and see fewer each day. The busy office schedule with many brief visits has been described as running on a "hamster wheel" and is a major reason for dissatisfaction among primary care physicians.[5] In the relationship-centered model, the smaller panel size allows the physician to spend more time with patients and have fewer visits daily, as low as 8-12 patient visits per day.[2,6] Online and telephone communication with patients, and meeting with team members to discuss care coordination, become an important part of the physician's workday in ideal models of primary care.

The financial viability of any ideal model of primary care requires payment reform. There must be reimbursement to support the care coordination and communication with patients outside of visits. Prepaid models of care support this when the overall expenses are reduced through efficiency and a reduction of office visits. In the more dominant fee-for-service model based on office visits, a care coordination or "medical home" payment is required to support the work done outside of visits. Pay for performance revenue would then reward any ideal model of practice for improved outcomes.

Primary care is the foundation of any rational health care system. Quality primary care adds tremendous value to the overall health care enterprise, reducing costs and enhancing quality population outcomes. As specialty care in the U.S. has enjoyed a long period of idealized development, it is high time to optimize primary care practice. Doing so might save U.S. health care from a financial implosion as millions more people have access to health insurance in the coming years as a result of health reform.

References

1. Margolius D, Bodenheimer T. Transforming Primary Care: From Past Practice to the Practice of the Future. Health Affairs. 2010;29:779-784.
2. Moore GL, Wasson JH. The Ideal Medical Practice Model: Improving Efficiency, Quality and the Doctor-Patient Relationship. Fam Pract Manag. 2007 Sep;14(8):20-24.
3. www.greenfieldhealth.com
4. www.eisenhower365.emc.org
5. Morrison I, Smith R. Hamster Health Care. BMJ. 2000;321:1541-1542.
6. Casalino LP. A Martian's Perspective for Primary Care: Overhaul the Physician's Workday. Health Affairs. 2010;29:785-790.

It's Time to Optimize Primary Care For a Healthier Population

Editorial
Medical Economics
2010;87(23):86-88

What specialty in medicine compromises the quality of its work based on its model of care? While I do not suggest that all specialties provide optimal care, only in primary care do I see that the model of care actually limits the quality of the work. The complexity of primary care today includes preventive services, common acute problems, the management of 1 or more chronic illnesses, and attention to the psychosocial determinants of health. That work cannot be done well in 15-minute appointments and an office schedule based on seeing 4 to 6 patients an hour.

We know that primary care is important to the health of any population. We know that a rational healthcare system has a strong foundation of primary care. We know that primary care done well provides value by controlling healthcare costs while delivering services focused on the whole patient.

The current primary care practice model of a busy office schedule and fee-for-service visits is a recipe for burn-out and only a small percentage of new medical school graduates are choosing this line of work. I do not blame them. It is time to reinvent the work model of primary care. It is time to optimize the experience of primary care for the patient, the physician, and the staff and achieve a healthier population. New models exist to show that primary care can be radically changed to achieve these goals in a successful business model. I call this optimal primary care for the information age.

WHAT IS OPTIMAL PRIMARY CARE?

Optimal primary care would mean:

• Patients receive great care: easy access to communication and care services, all the time needed to handle their health needs, and great outcomes for both wellness and the management of the medical problems.

• The providers enjoy the work by having enough time with patients to provide comprehensive care without the need for rushing and interrupting patients due to time demands. The provider sees the right number of patients each day and has time to communicate with patients outside of visits and time to do care coordination with other team members to improve the health of the population being served.

• State-of-the-art information systems are in place to provide easy access to patient records, registry functions to search the outcomes and care needs of the patient population, electronic prescribing for medication safety and convenience, clinical decision support systems imbedded in the record system to help guide evidence-based care at the point of service, and a secure communication portal imbedded in the record system so all interactions with patients and among caregivers are captured in 1 place.

• The patient population being served is attaining the highest known outcomes in all the areas of primary care.

I know this scenario may sound pie-in-the-sky to most primary care physicians. But optimal primary care—or something close to it—already is happening in many progressive healthcare settings in the United States, by intentional design and by keeping an eye on continual improvement. Optimal primary care is being developed in large health systems like Group Health Cooperative in the Pacific Northwest, in medium-sized practices like GreenField Health in Portland, and where I work at Eisenhower Medical Center in Southern California, and in small practices such as the Ideal Medical Practice network developed by L. Gordon Moore, MD, from Rochester, New York. There's no running on the treadmill in constant hurry mode for these primary care physicians.

The May 2010 issue of Health Affairs devoted 47 articles to the theme of reinventing primary care. The focus was on the need for major change in primary care to save it and improve the health of Americans. Detail on many of the practices I mention above is there. From this effort, I see 2 general models emerging for optimizing primary care that I will discuss in this article. These are not mutually exclusive and many practices will have elements of both.

The Patient-Centered Medical Home (PCMH) has emerged as a general descriptor for improved primary care. The essence of PCMH is providing care coordination by a team that goes beyond patient visits to improve outcomes. I strongly support the PCMH movement but believe that optimizing primary care goes beyond the current descriptions of PCMH. Most PCMH models have added care coordinators, information systems, and teamwork for improved care, but many do not address the overall work model for the primary care physician who is still trying to see too many patients.

Two emerging models for optimizing primary care are what I call the Relationship-Centered Model and the Organized Team Model.

They are best used for different populations and with different available resources.

RELATIONSHIP-CENTERED MODEL

The Relationship-Centered Model of care focuses on a close personal relationship between the patient and his or her chosen primary care physician. Patients have direct access to their physician at essentially all times. Concierge medicine has emerged out of a desire for this model and many people are paying lots of money to have it. However, direct access to the physician does not have to be expensive. Rather than give every patient the physician's cell phone number, online communication done at mutual convenience connects the doctor and patient 24/7/365 without untimely disruptions.

The Ideal Medical Practice network, formerly called Ideal Micropractices, started by Dr. Moore in Rochester exemplifies this approach with very low overhead and personalized care (see http://www.idealmedicalpractice.com). The physician may have only 1 employee and often meets the patient in the waiting room and does the vital signs.

GreenField Health in Portland, Oregon, started in 2001, developed this approach on a larger scale and now has 2 offices and 9 primary care physicians (see http://www.greenfieldhealth.com). Building off this model, I helped start in 2009 Eisenhower Primary Care 365 and after proving the model in 1 practice site, we are opening it in 4 locations this year (see http://www.eisenhower365.emc.org).

Relationship-centered practices have reduced panel sizes in order for the physician to provide continuous personalized care. Concierge practices typically have 200 to 600 patients. Eisenhower is in the process of growing from 5 to 10 EPC 365 doctors and will have 600 to 900 patients at each practice site with a high percentage of seniors; GreenField Health along with the Ideal Medical Practices generally go up to 1,000 patients per physician. Some physicians will work in co-practice with a nurse practitioner (NP) or physician assistant (PA). All train their staff to assist in the care coordination with patients. Typically, no more than 12 patients are seen by the physician each day in visits that are usually 30 minutes or longer, and much care is provided online and on the telephone. Information systems are required to optimize the care to the population being served.

The finances of relationship-centered care require adequate funding for non-visit services. This could be the medical home payment in PCMH models being proposed for Medicare by the Centers for Medicare and Medicaid (CMS) and by private insurers. Current models with these numbers of patients do not require concierge prices, but rather $30 to $50 per month is adequate to support the non-visit communication and care and the smaller panel size. Visits are still paid fee-for-service. Some physicians use this model and bill patients for all time spent with them, whether online, on the telephone, or face-to-face. Most of these Relationship-Centered Models are way ahead of insurance payers and require cash payments by the patients who join the practice.

Patient and physician satisfaction scores are typically very high in Relationship-Centered Models, with a general belief by both that this is how healthcare should be. The trouble is that there are not nearly enough primary care physicians to provide this model of relationship-centered care to everyone.

ORGANIZED TEAM MODEL

Tom Bodenheimer, MD, MPH, at the University of California, San Francisco, and others are promoting an Organized Team Model of care to provide optimal services to a larger population of patients, even as many as 4,000 per physician. In such models, everyone works to the limit of his or her license and provides care. The primary care physician steps back from the front line of care and focuses on those patients who need a physician's level of service, such as patients with multiple or complex health problems. The physician would only see up to 12 patients a day, provide supervision to other providers such as NPs and PAs, and play a lead role in the overall coordination of care to the population being served.

Organized Team Models are ideal for community clinics, rural and inner city practices, and anywhere where the needs of the population are great compared with the number of physicians. At Eisenhower, we are starting an Organized Team Model at separate practice sites for patients unwilling or unable to pay for our Relationship-Centered Model. Organized Team Models benefit from payment for care coordination outside of visits. Some Medicaid models have been successful with as little as $4 per patient per month. These funds come from a reduction in the amount of hospital care needed by the patients both in the emergency department and admissions. The Patient Centered Primary Care Coalition has compiled ample evidence that investing in such models of care reduces costs and improves outcomes (see http://www.pcpcc.net).

New models of optimizing primary care are incredibly exciting. They are win-win for everyone involved: the patient, the physician, the staff, and the payer. They require a major process change and that is always difficult in medical practice. But the alternative—a gradual disappearance of primary care because few are willing to do it—is not tenable.

Plenty of health systems and physician practices are out there striving to optimize primary care. If you are not happy with your traditional practice, do something about it. The new primary care for the 21st century information age is within reach if you are willing to make major changes. Help is out there, such as TransforMED sponsored by the American Academy of Family Physicians (http://www.transformed.com) and Lumetra Health Solutions based in San Francisco (http://www.lumetrasolutions.com).

We expect our patients to change their lifestyles to be healthier; likewise, we should change our primary care practice for our health and well-being and for the better health of our patients.

Real Revolution in Healthcare Taking Place Under the Radar

Editorial
Medical Economics
2011;88(5):18

It seems that everyone is talking about healthcare reform. The current law, whether repealed or not, is not the real healthcare reform going on today. The real revolution is happening under the radar of media and politics.

Put in perspective, "Obamacare" (like it or not, that's the name associated with healthcare reform now) is about health insurance reform. The mandate that everyone have health insurance is its most controversial element. Remember, however, that that mandate is the part of the plan mostly promoted by the American Medical Association, and it was started in Massachusetts by then-Gov. Mitt Romney, a Republican. It reflects the philosophy of personal responsibility usually associated with conservatives.

Because physicians are required to treat everyone who comes to an emergency department (ED), mandating that people have health insurance means that we do not have to pick up the tab for this care through higher health insurance premiums. Healthcare is not an option when you are sick or injured, and all of us become sick or injured at some point. But the mandate part bothers some people.

But what is real healthcare reform today? I suggest that it is the revolution being caused by the Internet and health information technology.

The automobile and the telephone have driven how we have given and received healthcare for the past 40 years. People call for appointments and then drive to a doctor visit. Before that, doctors made house calls, and there were no appointments. My general practitioner from the 1950s did not even have a sign-in sheet. The nurse went to the waiting room and called "next." You had better be sure you figured out who came in before and after you.

Now this "telephone/automobile, make an appointment, and come and get it" process is becoming outdated, too. As with other service industries, more and more healthcare is being delivered online, and this practice will continue to grow in popularity. In my practice, I have an average of three online communications with patients for every one phone call or office visit. My patients pay a modest charge in advance—$30 to $50 a month—for this convenient and efficient service. Everybody wins, and money is saved because fewer patients need to visit urgent care centers or the ED. Wise insurance plans are starting to pay for this medical home-focused communication and care.

Soon, smartphones and applications on other portable devices will connect us to an increasing amount of our healthcare. People will communicate with doctors' offices using new technology, and face-to-face visits will occur only when necessary. New financial models to support all of this change will replace the traditional fee-for-service practice that requires in-person visits for revenue generation.

Although we may be in the decade of "Obamacare," it also will be the decade when the process of giving and receiving healthcare changes radically, driven by Internet technologies. I'm excited about that. How about you?

Is Your Office a Patient Centered Medical Home? Early 21st Century Medical Practice at Its Best

Editorial
San Diego Physician
2011;98(3):18-19

The patient-centered medical home means different things to different people. Position papers and articles go on at length describing the principles and applications of the medical home model. After reading such pieces, I often wonder just how the medical home is different from the good traditional medical office practice. Too often the trees are being described without first making clear what the new forest is all about.

The essence of the medical home model can be described in eight words: care coordination by a team independent of visits. If you only use two words, they are care coordination. Traditional office practice reacts to those patients who make appointments. Information systems that allow for strategic proactive care to a population are missing. In a medical home, the population cared for becomes clear, and efforts are made by the care team to reach out proactively to achieve better outcomes.

For example, a medical practice would know all its patients with diabetes. Those patients could be placed into three buckets: good control, fair control, and poor control. An analysis of who were coming into the office for care would probably show that those in good control were more likely to be coming in for regular appointments, and those in poor control were not. If the practice truly takes responsibility for the care of all its diabetic patients, the practice would reach out and contact the patients in fair and poor control and strive to improve their care proactively.

The additional payment in the medical home model is for the care coordination outside of visits. There are two payment methods emerging. I will call them low payment and higher payment. The low payment method, such as $2–4 per member per month, is common in Medicaid applications of the medical home. This amount of money gives a practice the funds to hire a care coordinator as part of the team. This person or persons reach out to patients, usually by telephone, to get patients back into the care system. Outcomes improve, and visits to the emergency department and even hospitalizations may decline. The rest of the team, including the physician, continues to practice in the same way with a busy office schedule of mostly brief visits.

The higher payment method, such as $30–50 per member per month, allows for a redesign of the care model away from a dependence on office visits. This payment allows the entire care team, including the physician, to communicate with patients on a new platform, such as online and the telephone. Visits are done selectively and more time intensively to establish care relationships and provide essential visit-based care. More productive interactions with patients occur outside of visits each day than face-to-face encounters. A new care model emerges with physicians seeing about 10–12 patients per day in longer appointments and spending one to two hours per day in care coordination activities. This new model of primary care has the potential of attracting more medical students to primary care and avoiding burnout among providers. It is the new primary care for the information age.

Proactive care coordination by a team supported by information systems is the new care model. As it becomes the new primary care, such care coordination will migrate into specialty care, as those office practices also should use care coordination by a team independent of visits to provide higher quality continuity of care to patients. The American College of Cardiology has placed the medical home as a high priority, and progressive cardiology practices are becoming proactive with patients with heart disease and related chronic conditions. Any practice caring for patients over time, such as a rheumatology practice with its arthritis patients or a neurology practice with its movement disorder patients, should apply the methods of proactive care. Even a surgical practice, such as in orthopedics with a joint replacement patient, should be a medical home for that patient from the day of the initial consultation to the rehabilitation after surgery.

Strategic, proactive care using the patient-centered medical home model achieves better outcomes in the many applications where it has been studied (see pcpcc.net for list of medical home applications and outcome studies). It is early 21st-century medical practice at its best. When our computers give us a snapshot of our practice population, a new dynamic of reach out care follows, especially if the payment system supports this activity beyond office visits.

Read more about: Managing Your Practice, March 2011 San Diego Physician, Patient-centered Medical Home, PCMH

Interactions for the 21st Century

Editorial
Medical Economics
2011;88(20):10-11

Is your practice using 21st-century methods of communication and care, or are you still in the 20th century? The 21st century is a time of Internet applications and the ability to communicate anytime from anywhere and to receive services remotely from a smartphone or tablet computer.

Computer workstations, considered mini-computers 25 years ago now, seem big and cumbersome. The world of communication and providing services has changed dramatically, yet medical care has lagged behind, slowly clunking its way into the information age. The tipping point is past, and by the end of this decade, your office needs to be an app on your patients' smartphones.

The 20th century had three phases of methods for medical communication and care. Early in the 20th century, people had to fetch the doctor. There were few telephones, and the doctor arrived by horse and buggy, staying as long as necessary. Only the poor went to most hospitals, and the outcomes were not pretty.

By the mid-20th century, most people had telephones and automobiles, and fetching the doctor was easier. Most physicians had "surgeries" in an office, often attached to a home, and spent about half the day seeing patients there (the $2 office visit was born) and the other half making house calls. There were few appointments, and patients came and signed in to be seen, waiting their turn.

During the last decades of the 20th century, with advances in communication and transportation, the "make an appointment and come and get it" mode of healthcare developed. Physicians were most efficient staying in their offices, now in larger office buildings, seeing many patients each day. Same-day services became less common, replaced by waiting for next-available appointments. Urgent care centers were developed to make up for the fact that most physician waiting rooms were full of patients coming for re-check visits or physical exams.

STILL IN THE 20TH CENTURY

By 21st-century methods, all the modes of care in the 20th century seem archaic. Most medical practices are still in the late 20th century because change is difficult and "fee-for-visit" reimbursement and productivity measurement still dominate. The new communication methods are better, faster, and cheaper, the dream of any redesign engineer, yet they are coming into application slowly.

I am fortunate to practice primary care in a fully 21st-century mode of practice. About 75% of all communications with our patients occur over a secure online platform. Patients pay between $30 and $50 a month, depending on their age, for unlimited use of online services and care coordination outside of visits. Face-to-face visits start the care process and then are used as needed. We bill insurance for all visit-related services.

We care for a large number of patients yet our office is calm and quiet, and all patients who are seen are heard fully in lengthy, unhurried visits. Our patient satisfaction scores are at the top of the chart, and our physicians enjoy their work every day because the intensity of the relationships with patients is so satisfying.

The sweet spot of productivity seems to be seeing about 10 to 12 patients every day and communicating with about 30 patients in non-visit care. All our staff members help with communication and care coordination so we can optimize the delivery of primary care. The specialists we refer to love the level of service we give them and our patients.

What transpires over the online platform of communication and care? Messages are evenly balanced between those initiated by patients and by the office. Obvious applications for the patient are requesting appointments and prescription refills. We encourage patients to report minor acute problems such as an upper respiratory infection to see whether an office visit is necessary. We like not having our waiting room filled with patients with colds spreading germs like a day care center.

Most commonly, we ask patients to report their progress with lifestyle changes such as quitting smoking, losing weight, or starting an exercise program. Patients also provide important chronic illness data such as blood pressures and blood glucose levels.

PRACTICE IS WELLNESS ORIENTED

Such communication makes our practice wellness-oriented. Messages we originate include reporting lab and imaging results to patients and making arrangement for specialty referrals or services such as physical therapy. We send group messages to our patients notifying them of services such as immunization clinics and patient education activities.

Telephone usage goes way down with online communication, a welcome advance because this asynchronous communication is self-documenting and you do not deal with voice mail problems of patient security.

Our practice, Eisenhower Primary Care 365 (http://eisenhower365. emc.org/), was started in early 2010 and was built off the Greenfield Health practice in Portland, Oregon (http://greenfieldhealth.com), which recently celebrated 10 years of successful service. Similar "advanced medical home" practices are springing up or maturing all over the country.

Insurance plans, seemingly always skeptical of the motives of physicians, realize in concept that what we are doing is better, faster, and less expensive, but they still are holding back in supporting this model of care, so patients continue to pay the fee for the online platform. Fully prepaid health plans such as Kaiser Permanente, Group Health Cooperative, and Geisinger have developed robust online platforms of care and are reaping the benefits.

Because other service industries such as banking, travel, shopping, money management, and education have developed robust online systems that now dominate, it is not difficult to vision a similar transformation in medicine. What could be more exciting?

Many patients are willing to "buy up" their primary care and are grateful that we are not as expensive as concierge medicine. We have trouble keeping up with our growth and will have more than 5,000 patients in the practice in less than 2 years.

The time to move into the 21st century is now. Learn from

modern practices or use a service such as TransforMED to get going. Change of this magnitude is difficult to do alone. The reward to primary care is enormous. Welcome to the 21st century.

Part of the patient safety and quality efforts triggered by the IOM reports was a change in resident work hours. The data on the impact of resident fatigue on the quality of patient care could no longer be ignored. In 2003 the ACGME limited resident work hours to 80 hours a week and dictated a number of days off. In 2011 the ACGME implemented much stricter regulations regarding how long residents could work at any one time. These new restrictions have been seen as negative by many program directors and the following article expresses my concerns:

Too Many Fences:
A Supporter's Criticism of Resident Work Restrictions

Commentary
Fam Med 2012;44(2):132-3.

"Any life truly lived is a risky business, and if one puts up too many fences against the risks one ends by shutting out life itself."
Kenneth S. Davis[1]

Ever since I was a medical student in the early 1970s, I have been in support of restrictions on resident work hours. Surgery was my first clinical rotation in my third year, and I was shocked by how long and hard the interns and residents worked. The chief resident on neurosurgery was on duty every day and night for 6 months! The residents were in a survival state of mind, and patients became burdens rather than people to be cared for. Empathy and compassion too often boiled over into resentment. I thought the residents had a multi-year prison sentence with a great lack of freedom over their lives. I did not like what this work experience did to them.

I wanted none of that. After choosing family medicine, I searched for programs where the work hours were "civilized," and learning was balanced with good patient care. Fortunately I matched in a program that used a pairing system on ward rotations in the first and second year so we could spend more time in the family medicine center caring for our continuity patients. Instead of being in the hospital every third night, we were there every sixth night, and we could read from home the nights our partners were admitting. I still got very good at starting IVs, even on children, and did lots of procedures, but I felt like I had escaped the prison sentence. I am not sure if I ever worked more than 80 hours a week. I suspect I did sometimes, especially when one of my patients had a 36- hour labor and delivery experience. These were draining but exhilarating. Other times I stayed at the bedside during a long dying experience, another profound and meaningful learning process. My work hours were generally 60 or more hours per week (that is still six 10-hour days), but I did learn that I could work the next day after staying up all night.

As research articles started to appear showing the patient safety problems from overworked residents, I cheered. Maybe something would be done about the barbaric process of residency training in America. Finally the evidence became overwhelming enough that the Accreditation Council for Graduate Medical Education had to act, first in 2003 and revised with much greater restrictions for 2011.[2] The 2011 standards were prompted by a major report in 2009 from the Institute of Medicine.[3] The evidence of danger to patients from sleep-deprived residents could no longer be denied.

Work shifts are now restricted to 16 hours for interns and 24 hours for second-year residents as long as there is "strategic napping" after 16 hours. Some do not think the new work restrictions go far enough and have called for 12–16 hour maximum shifts with 10 hours off duty between shifts.[4] These authors cite the data from the airline industry and call for residents, and all physicians, to have work restrictions similar to pilots.

All this is well and good looking only at patient safety and the cognitive and other abilities of a single caregiver. But physicians are more than "shift workers," and medical care is a team activity. Disease and illness are not scheduled like air travel. Patient experiences are often intense and last a long time. Residents and other physicians need to be capable of responding to patient needs in a variety of situations. If we train a generation of residents as shift workers, what will happen if we have a major disaster and physicians are called to work tirelessly for days? Will they be prepared for that? Training programs like Outward Bound show that we put far too many restrictions on our abilities based on limited experiences and when given the chance, we can perform in extraordinary ways.[5] Experience with that is important for survival in difficult conditions.

There is a balance between the patient safety literature and physician work hours. If a hardworking person experiences a decline in their abilities after 12–16 hours, patients should not have to suffer for that. A resident could remain involved in patient care while a fresh resident or faculty member becomes involved in primary decision making. As I experienced the 36-hour labor, I was happy to have help arrive. The same is true with the dying patient or the one in intensive care. But I would not want to be sent home unfulfilled by not seeing the experience through. I felt sorry for the nurses who were sent home when their shifts were done just as they were helping patients the most. Continuity of care is a core value in family medicine. Sending residents home away from the patients and families they care for is bound to be disruptive to the development of relationship-centered care. Family physicians are not shift workers.

It is hard to find rank and file residents and faculty who support the current resident work restrictions. I find myself holding my tongue and being embarrassed by my support of these. Why all the explicit restrictions when general rules would suffice? The ACGME has published a side-by-side comparison of the 2003 and 2011 standards.[2] The 2003 standards are more general and allow for some flexibility. The 2011 standards is an exhaustive list of restrictions, and most programs may not know when they are in violation. There are now too many fences around risk, and we are cutting out a major part of the residency training experience.

I am still in favor of resident work restrictions, but we should rethink these in the context of teamwork. Resident involvement with patient experiences is paramount to good training. Patient safety should never be compromised, and standards for that are important. Require a fresh physician every 12 hours, but do not force residents to leave the very experiences they will need to work in after training. Putting patients first means having the best care and continuity with a physician. Let's not create a generation of shift workers ill prepared for situations that are bound to arise, here and in other countries.

References

1. Famous quotes and authors. www.famous-quotesandauthors.com/topics/risks_quotes. html.
2. Accreditation Council for Graduate Medical Education. ACGME duty hours. Approved 2011 standards. www.acgme-2010standards. org/approved-standards.html.
3. Institute of Medicine. Resident duty hours: enhancing sleep, supervision and safety.2009.www.iom.edu/Reports/2008/Resident-Duty-Hours-Enhancing-Sleep-Supervision-and-Safe¬ty.aspx.
4. Blum AB, Shea S, Czeisler CA, Landrigan CP, Leape L. Implementing the 2009 Institute of Medicine recommendations on resident physician work hours, supervision and safety. Nature and Science of Sleep 2011;3:47-85.
5. Outward Bound Professional. www.outward¬bound.org/index.cfm/do/pro.index.

In 2012 STFM started a Blog and these are two of my contributions related to new models of care:

The Scope of Family Medicine Is Expanding

Blog
STFM News
Posted May 10, 2012

Many educators are lamenting today that the scope of family medicine is shrinking.

They refer to fewer family physicians working in hospitals and doing procedures. Warren Newton, MD, MPH, chair of the American Board of Family Medicine, recently sent out a letter expressing this concern. Such a grave outlook is dangerous to our specialty at a time when we are struggling to motivate medical students to go in to family medicine.

I think just the opposite. Family medicine today is more complex and expansive in some ways than ever before. Sure, fewer of us are delivering babies and doing hospital medicine, but family medicine is first and foremost a primary care specialty. Primary care is expanding and becoming far more complex in this new age of medical homes and the advanced use of information systems.

The Willard Report that set the stage for the transition from general practice to family medicine called for the creation of a new primary physician. That doctor would be the personal physician to individuals and their families. It is that personal physician role that is the essence of our specialty. New models of primary care, from concierge medicine to team-oriented medical homes to populations of patients, are deeply complex and expansive.

What do I mean? Prevention became part of primary care in the 1970s and continues to expand. Primary prevention includes all efforts to prevent disease, and since lifestyle causes 50% or more of disease, motivational counseling toward lifestyle change is a new and vital part of being a personal physician. Secondary prevention is the early detection of disease and knowing and applying all aspects of the US Preventive Services Task Force recommendations requires good information systems and skills. Tertiary prevention is the prevention of complications of chronic disease and is far more complex than when I finished residency 30 years ago.

Chronic illness drives about 75% of all health care costs so effective management of these problems is vital to our health care system. The routine visit of a type 2 diabetic patient is far more complex than before and requires much more time. Acute problems are still a major part of family medicine and if we are available to our patients online, we can manage or coordinate care much more efficiently. Relationship-centered care calls on us to know our patients well and provide the counseling services our patients need to deal with what life brings to them, attending to the biopsychosocial and spiritual dimensions of illness.

So, let's stop this talk about the scope of practice of family medicine shrinking. I am grateful to have more time to take a deep dive with my patients and be their personal physician with much greater complexity and effectiveness than ever before. Let's train our residents to do the same and show off this rewarding specialty to our students. What can be better than being a family physician

We Do Not Interrupt Our Patients

Blog
STFM News
Posted July 5, 2012

Ever notice a patient wince when interrupted describing his or her problem? It is well known that physicians interrupt their patients much of the time and usually within 30 seconds of the start of the visit. One study in Family Medicine1 showed that residents interrupted patients 12 seconds into a visit 25% of the time. We even teach interruptions as part of "controlling the conversation" and "limiting the agenda" for the visit.

In a practice where there is ample time for visits, there is rarely if ever a need to interrupt a patient. I'm now in such a setting after more than 30 years of brief office visits, and I had to train myself to not interrupt patients. What a great feeling that is! At our practice, we sit back and let every patient finish what he or she has to say. Patients notice this, too, saying they have never had a physician listen to them like we do. We learn things about patients they have not had the chance to share with physicians before.

Since we have an hour for every new patient visit, early in the encounter I ask the patient to tell me his or her story. The patient often asks, "Which story?" I say, "Where were you born and what happened after that?" It is amazing to me how most patients finish this story in about 5 minutes. As a matter of fact, I'm impressed with how brief most patients are when giving their narratives uninterrupted.

Our physicians are now demonstrating an uninterrupted communication style to medical students in their family medicine clerkships. By the time they arrive at our practice, they have already been taught to interrupt patients, so we teach them otherwise. Often, this helps them love family medicine. We look forward to training residents in uninterrupted narrative next year when our residency[1] program starts.

Interrupting patients is a part of the paternalistic culture of medicine where the physician's time is more important than the patient's, and the physician knows better than the patient what the problem is. Such paternalism is unprofessional and even dangerous and should not be a part of patient-centered care.

I admire professionals who let people have their say completely. Counselors are very good at this and so are good lawyers, realtors, designers, and many others. Interruptions seem to be mainly a physician behavior.

Visits with patient can be efficient without interruptions. When patients have been given the chance to say everything they want during the visit, they are more receptive to hearing our assessment and recommendations for managing their problems. After all, patients are in charge of their care. Our job is to serve them, respectfully and without interruption.

Reference

1. Rhoades DR, McFarland, KF, Finch WH, Johnson AO. Speaking and interruptions during primary care office visits. Fam Med 2001;33(7):528-32.

Collaborative family health care, having therapists integrated with primary care physicians to provide a true biopsychosocial model of care, is a concept that the new models of care emphasizing team practice finally encourage. I was asked by the Collaborative Family Healthcare Association to provide the following blog on the therapist role in value driven care:

Do Medical Family Therapists Bring Value to Health Care?

Blog
CFHA
Posted October 10, 2012

"The most important work of family therapists today is to make the case for being vital members of PCMH practice teams."

I suspect any family therapist reading this question would quickly say, "Yes, of course we add value to health care". From a health care policy perspective value is not a simple intuitive concept. Value is quality divided by cost, and today every health care system is focused on becoming value driven.

That the U.S. spends way too much money on health care is well known. Our health outcomes place us low in the world even though we spend twice as much or more on health care as other industrialized countries. Our spending is not sustainable, especially in Medicare with the influx of the Baby Boomer generation. We have to figure out how to spend less money.

A new IOM report indicates that we spend 700 billion dollars in health care every year that is of no benefit to patient care. These include unnecessary tests and procedures, overly expensive drugs when generics would do fine, and excessive treatment, especially at the end of life. Rather than just squeeze this money out of the system, the potential is here for transforming the system to provide value – actually improve the quality of care while we reduce costs.

Information technology makes much of value driven care possible. For the first time we can look at populations of patients in detail and make proactive strategic decisions to improve their health efficiently. Diabetic patients who are well controlled are much less expensive than ones who are out of control and develop complications. Through internet applications, we can communicate and care for patients at minimal costs compared with face-to-face visits.

So what role do family therapists play in this? We know that psychosocial problems are frequent in health care and usually are masked by physical complaints. Addressing the psychosocial problems early creates great efficiency rather than waiting until every physical evaluation has been done, only to show the patient is "simply" anxious or depressed. Yet this obvious situation remains hidden from the strategic planning to too many health systems.

Regional health systems committed to becoming value-driven are joining the Accountable Care Organization (ACO) movement. Developed by the Centers for Medicare and Medicaid Services (CMS), an ACO is committed to the Triple Aim:

1. Improving the individual experience of care

2. Improving the health of populations

3. Reducing the per capita costs of care for populations

Health systems know the future of health care financing will be directly tied to achieving these aims with their care, and information systems are able to measure it. At the patient care level, teams will operate in ACOs using the principles of the Patient Centered Medical Home (PCMH). PCMH practices have advanced information and communication technologies and are able to provide continuous access to strategic, proactive care rather than the tradition of simply reacting to patient appointments. Patients become activated to play an active role in the own care, ordering desired tests and treatments, according to accepted guidelines.

The most important work of family therapists today is to make the case for being vital members of PCMH practice teams. Working alongside physicians, nurse practitioners, pharmacists and others, family therapists will ensure that patients receive true biopsychosocial care from the beginning. Independent private practice is rapidly becoming a thing of the past. Organized and integrated health systems are the future. Family therapists are not automatically included in this discussion in most settings, so becoming knowledgeable about ACOs and PCMHs is critical today. Assertive inclusion of family therapists in demonstration projects around the country is needed to ensure the proper composition of team practice in the future.

Reference for more detail on ACOs, PCMHs and the Triple Aim:

Edwards TM, Patterson J, Vakili S, Scherger JE. Healthcare Policy in the United States: A Primer for Medical Family Therapists. Comtemp Fam Ther (2012) 34:217-227.

Many practices call themselves Patient Centered Medical Homes (PCMH)and are making incremental changes toward care coordination and use of information technology, but still provide episodic care based on brief visits. As called for in the IOM Report, Crossing the Quality Chasm (2001), 21st century health care needs to be continuous. In the following article I argue that this can only be done with practice transformation, highlighting the three changes described above in the "new model" articles.

PCHM: The Future Requires Practice Transformation

Medical Economics
2012;89(22):32-35

Goal is to improve patient population health, better manage chronic disease, and build a team to accomplish it

Care coordination are the two most important words related to the Patient-Centered Medical Home (PCMH).

It is important to note that this PCMH concept is taking on many forms, but the National Committee for Quality Assurance (NCQA) has identified six standards for a PCMH:

• Enhance access and continuity.
• Identify and manage patient populations.
• Plan and manage care.
• Provide self-care and community support.
• Track and coordinate care.
• Measure and improve performance.

To achieve the PCMH standards, the practice must have an information system to allow for the coordinated management of a population of patients.

Traditional practice is about caring for one patient at a time and reacting to those who made appointments. Population management means that you can look at your practice as a whole and see how you are doing with preventive measures such as mammograms in women aged more than 50 years, or with chronic disease management such as the overall control of diabetes, hypertension, or hyperlipidemia. Doing so requires having an electronic registry of all your patients, a function that many electronic health record (EHR) systems do not have currently.

Once you have an information system in place, your practice would hire or designate a patient care coordinator to focus on making the population of patients served by the practice healthier, that is, improve the quality metrics of the practice. Any one person cannot perform this function, so the care coordinator leads a team effort and all staff members and care providers in the office expand their roles to providing care coordination activities, during patient visits and outside of visits, using the telephone or online communication to achieve targeted outcomes.

Today, this function largely is being performed as an incremental change to a standard appointment-based office practice. The physicians are still running on the treadmill, seeing as many patients a day as they can. Patients may not notice much difference except that some are getting phone calls or e-mails reminding them to come for tests or to take their medications.

In the bigger picture, PCMHs are not about the incremental enhancement of office practice. As conceived by the 2001 Institute of Medicine report, Crossing the Quality Chasm, the process of quality healthcare in the 21st century requires practice transformation.

Traditional office-based practice uses the telephone to make appointments and the automobile or other transportation to get patients into the office. It is, by nature, episodic and reactive.

Information technology and the Internet have radically changed most service industries, and healthcare will not be the exception. Three transformational changes lie at the core of an advanced PCMH practice:

1. Care is continuous rather than episodic.

The practice has a new platform of communication and care using secure Internet applications. As with other modern service industries, patients may communicate with the office 24 hours a day, 7 days a week, and receive a timely response. The practice communicates with patients collectively and individually with efforts to improve their health. This online platform of communication and care becomes a new "front door" for the practice, and the power of asynchronous communication at mutual convenience makes the office practice much more efficient.

In the Eisenhower Primary Care 365 practice where I work, there are five times as many online communications with patients compared with face-to-face or via the telephone. A modest fee covers this service.

2. Care is strategically proactive rather than reactive.

Until now, without information systems that provide a snapshot of the practice and its quality metrics, all healthcare has been reacting to demand. Your workday and that of your staff has been dictated by who was on the schedule. With an improved information system, your practice may proactively reach out to patients and improve their care, in prevention and in chronic disease management.

Getting about 40% of your patients at the desired target for any preventive or chronic disease is a quality outcome most physicians can expect working in most traditional practices. Twenty-five percent or less at target is common for a traditional appointment-based practice.

Group Health Cooperative, Kaiser Permanente, and other advanced medical groups such as Geisinger in Pennsylvania and

Sharp in San Diego, California have achieved 80% control of diabetes, hypertension, and other chronic diseases, along with preventive services such as mammograms or colon cancer screening, through strategic proactive care by a team using their information systems. These improved quality outcomes save money far beyond the increased costs of providing these services. It will not be long before all payers require this level of quality.

3. Patients are able to self-manage much of their care rather than depend on getting all their care through healthcare providers.

Much of healthcare, particularly prevention and chronic disease management, is rules-based. When patients become knowledgeable about their own care needs, they can follow these rules as well as any provider. Activated patients truly become part of their healthcare team when they are not dependent on their care by others at all times.

In the self-management program at Kaiser Permanente, patients order their own mammograms and other preventive services through an online platform called HealthConnect. They play an active role in their own disease management by adjusting medications and getting scheduled tests under the watchful eye of a care team. Not surprisingly, self-managed patients see better outcomes and reduce the costs of care.

So what should your medical practice do now to begin a transformation to an advanced PCMH?

• Begin secure online communication with patients and promote applications back and forth about lab and other results, prescription refills, requests for appointments, handling minor acute complaints (ask whether a visit is necessary). Follow-up with information about chronic disease management, and coach for behavior change such as weight loss and smoking cessation.

• Get a patient and disease registry so you can have quality metrics for your practice and begin to contact patients proactively to improve those metrics. When quality outcomes is the new, finance and you will be paid more or less on how good a job you are doing, you will be happy you started this. PQRI and other incentives are already in place.

• Give up some of your control and activate patients to do more of their own care, such monitoring INR levels and adjusting warfarin according to protocol, and participating in diabetes and hypertension management. Think of your practice as a consultant or an adviser in a patient's wellness care rather than maintaining a paternalistic control over all things medical.

These three transformational changes, taken together, are a major departure from the "make an appointment, come and get it" care of the 20th century. Incremental change did not transform a Model T Ford into today's Mustang. Sometimes, a whole new model is needed.

My first article of 2013 is a rewrite of a 1995 article for Family Practice Management on working for an organization. In 2012, for the first time in the history of American medicine, the majority of physicians were employed by health systems rather being in private practice. This trend is likely to continue as integrated health systems functioning as Accountable Care Organizations compete in the new environment of President Obama's Affordable Care Act.

Leadership in a Health Care Organization: Not Like Private Practice

Family Practice Management
2013;20(1):17-20

A family physician shares what he learned about leadership when he was no longer captain of the ship.

Physicians have traditionally been an independent breed. A standard cliché among my generation is that you go to medical school partly to become your own boss. Private practice has allowed for such independent-spirited behavior, and many of us have been captains of our own ships.

All that is changing. Physicians are becoming part of large organizations, and many are taking positions that involve leadership responsibilities. Very few residency graduates are starting their own practices, and the number joining private practices is shrinking. Many are becoming salaried employees of large medical groups or health care organizations. This may say something about the lack of independent business spirit among the new generation of physicians, or it may say something about the changing landscape of health care in America. In any case, this new generation seems to be coping with the situation reasonably well. But what about the generation that has been in private practice for some time?

Many family physicians are adjusting to this new reality of working for a large organization. Those in positions of leadership or management face an especially challenging transition. In 1995 I wrote an editorial for Family Practice Management about what I had learned in this process.[1] Three years before, I had left behind 14 years of community practice in a small town to work for a large health care organization in a big city. Since then, I have worked for five large organizations, two not-for-profit community hospital systems, and three academic medical schools. I have learned much and have been well coached in leadership and management. I have also made some big mistakes along the way. Some of those mistakes came from the solo-practice mindset I brought with me. I hope my insights will be even more useful today than they were in 1995.

CULTURE EATS STRATEGY FOR LUNCH

Management guru Peter Drucker is credited with saying, "Culture eats strategy for breakfast." It can also chew up employees who underestimate its strength. Every organization has a culture, and adapting to that culture successfully is vital for anyone who wants to survive in the organization, let alone have any management or leadership success. If you are as self-confident as I was when I left private practice, you might think that you will change the culture of the organization you join. Although that might be true to some degree in the long run, thinking you can make that happen soon after you arrive is hopelessly naive, whether you come in as head of a department or head of the whole organization.

My first job coming out of private practice was to start a family medicine residency program in a community hospital that had never had graduate medical education. I informed the leadership of the leading medical groups what they would have to do to teach in the residency program. The idea of the residency was popular, but I had no idea how big a culture change I was asking for, and the resistance I faced was a shock. What I should have done was learn the culture first, and then learn how to work within it.

Eventually, I hired a management coach, and one of the first books he had me read was Organizational Culture and Leadership by Edgar Schein of the MIT Sloan School of Management.[2] It remains a classic work for understanding organizational culture and how to lead successfully in different organizational contexts.

BEWARD OF ASSUMPTIONS

Five years after Schein's book came out, another seminal management book emerged: The Fifth Discipline: The Art and Practice of the Learning Organization by Peter Senge.[3] Schein helps the reader understand organizations, and Senge focuses on how organizations should work. Senge's work has continued to inspire leaders and managers to this day. Senge describes three common assumptions that new and naive leaders like me make when coming to an organization. I'll put these in the context of my role and one that you may have.

I assumed it would be easy. Since primary care and family medicine are what health care organizations need most, I thought the organization would make it quick and easy to establish a new family medicine residency program. But my experience in small-group practice hadn't prepared me for the fact that any member of a large organization has to move at the speed of the whole organization and in paths the organizations has laid out. Large organizations are complex, their decision-making processes may be convoluted, and each has different information channels. And it isn't just that the decision-making process is slow, complicated, and unique to each organization: Simply learning how it works (and how to make it work) requires considerable time and effort.

In private practice, the clinical staff, the physicians, the operations staff, and the financial staff are all woven together as one system. In a large health organization, the clinical, operational, and financial are separate realms, each with its own language and processes. As a clinician, I thought good ideas based on sound reasoning would move quickly through those other realms, but that never happens. I'm dealing with one example of this now: My organization needs a memory assessment center, and one of the geriatricians is keen on leading it. From my perspective as a physician, setting it up seemed like a no-brainer. But that was before our financial staff questioned whether the geriatrician in charge would be as productive as he is now seeing patients on a normal schedule. That left me to figure out how to defend something that might not make financial sense to people whose sole concern is the financial well-being of the organization. Accounting pro formas are what matter to people working in the financial realm.

I assumed the organization would adjust to me. Every organization embodies a complex set of behavior patterns, values, and beliefs that tend to perpetuate themselves. Of course any organization must evolve to survive in the long-term, but while you may be an important part of this evolution, organizations change slowly. Ultimately you will be called upon to adjust to the organization rather than vice versa. We all think that we can bring our private practice savvy into the organization and make it more efficient. I and everyone I know who has moved from an efficient private practice into a complex health care organization is amazed by the difficulty and complexity of getting things done.

I assumed everyone would help me. Since family medicine is so clearly needed and my role has often been to develop and expand primary care, I used to assume that I would have all the support and assistance the organization could offer. But change or development in one area usually means de-emphasis in another. Some members in the organization will always be skeptical of or threatened by change, and they may act in ways intended to prove themselves right at the expense of your success. Moreover, even with general conceptual support for what you do, everyone is busy keeping his or her own house in order and may not have time to assist you. I have often felt that I would succeed despite the organization rather than because of it.

THE "LAWS" OF ORGANIZATIONS

Senge offers several "laws" of organizations. Five of them, in particular, strike me as applying directly to my experience and that of my colleagues who are trying to build something new within their organizations.

Every problem was once a solution (that someone was invested in). Before you go after perceived problems aggressively, think about who may be threatened by your actions – for example, key specialists in an environment of surplus or overpaid specialists. Your goal may be increased reimbursement for family physicians, and the additional income may have to come from monies now given to specialists. You will need a good relationship with key specialists in your organization to succeed.

The harder you push, the harder the system pushes back. Pushing your agenda or pushing for change is usually counterproductive. Learning the pace at which change takes place in an organization and the processes by which change proceeds is difficult and requires a great deal of patience.

Faster is slower. This follows directly from the above. If you try to accomplish something too fast and end up failing, you may not get another chance for quite a while. Slow and steady progress toward a goal will achieve the desired result in the quickest way. Don't try to make things happen too quickly. Help them fall into place.

Cause and effect are not closely related in time and space. For the quick, analytical mind, this may be frustrating. Taking a historical perspective is important. The managed care changes we went through in the '90s were a result of health care spending in the '70s and '80s, and not some 1990s' invention. The patient-centered medical home and accountable care organization movements of today, and related transitional models at the microsystem and macrosystem levels, are a result of our history of uncontrolled growth in costs without improvement in quality and of new health information technologies. Sometimes the right thing seems to happen for what seems to be the wrong reason.

There is no blame. Blaming someone in your organization for a bad situation doesn't improve the situation; on the contrary, it creates new problems. Assuming a victim mentality will compromise any chance of success you may have. Organizations are complex obstacle courses, even though almost everyone is simply trying to do the right thing. Blame just creates a new obstacle. Within an organization, any personal agenda takes a back seat to what the organization as a whole is doing or wants to do. Your job is to work within the organization to accomplish whatever the organization wishes or needs. However good they are, your ideas will seem bad if they are not in step with the organization's goals. If you push your ideas anyway, you will be seen as a problem, not a solver of problems.

DON'T LOOK BACK

Many family physicians are joining large organizations, and for many different reasons. It may make sense for your practice and community, or you may have leadership goals that can only be realized in a large organization. Regardless, understanding organizational behavior and culture will be critical to your success.

Leadership in a large health care organization can be very satisfying. Once you learn the culture and become a functional part of it, you come to enjoy the complexity and the relationships you form with a diversity of people. Being collegial with leaders in nursing, pharmacy, and even finance, as well as physicians, is both satisfying and educational. You'll find that it broadens your understanding.

If you work in a large organization where your primary role is patient care, and if your leadership efforts seem to be failing, concentrate on taking good care of your patients. After all, that is what you went to medical school for. By pouring your energies into patient care, you'll be able to avoid frustration with the pace of change. Keep your eyes and ears open for positive organizational developments, and you may get to seize opportunities to nudge things in the right direction.

It took me two years to get over the loss of my patients in private practice and feel comfortable in a large organization. Once I adjusted to the roles and relationships, I began to really like it. Now, I would not go back to a small practice. Not only will you learn much about any organization you join, you will learn much about yourself in the process.

References

1. Scherger JE. Working for an organization. Fam Pract Manag. 1995;2(8):10–11.
2. Schein E. Organizational Culture and Leadership. San

Francisco: Jossey-Bass, 1985.
3. Senge PM. The Fifth Discipline: The Art and Practice of the Learning Organization. New York: Doubleday, 1990.

For many, convenience trumps continuity for getting care for minor health problems and routine preventive services such as immunizations. Young, healthy people feel less need to have a personal physician and there is a growing market for low cost "retail clinics".

Is It OK if Our Residency Graduates Work for Walmart?

STFM
Posted on April 26, 2013

I attended a health care forecast conference recently and learned a sobering new reality. In the near future, Americans will be getting their primary care services in many different locations.

Walmart has announced that it soon will be offering comprehensive primary care in many of its stores. Walgreens, already the largest provider of immunizations outside the government, will expand its Take Care clinics and manage four common chronic diseases: diabetes, hypertension, hyperlipidemia, and asthma. A longtime colleague and family medicine educator recently went to work for Kroger's new clinic system, The Little Clinic. Large employers are setting up workplace clinics to provide common health services while keeping their employees on the job.

Discount department stores have already started to dominate certain areas of health care. The most convenient place to have hearing and vision testing and treatment in our area is at Costco. The pharmacies in Walmart, Target, and Costco are gaining market share rapidly over the traditional pharmacy providers. What is to stop these institutions from offering primary care?

All of these nontraditional primary care services are likely to be at lower cost than through traditional providers and be delivered in most cases by mid-level providers. How will a patient's medical record be kept whole? What is the future of the traditional family physicians' office? How many of our residency graduates will take positions as medical directors or providers in these nontraditional settings?

There has always been a distinction between a primary care physician and primary care services. The primary care physician, especially a family physician, provides continuity of care through a relationship. Primary care services include preventive services, common acute problems, and chronic disease management. Ever since the emergence of Urgent Care centers in the 1980s, primary care services have expanded beyond the primary care physicians' offices. Increasingly, the family physician has had to gather information from the patient about what and where they have received various services such as immunizations and procedures. The decentralization of receiving primary care services is likely to explode in the drive to deliver care faster and cheaper.

There are not many answers to this new reality of primary care. Only the patient will be able to keep an intact medical record. One thing that trumps care in a discount store is being available to patients online anytime from anywhere. Calling for the next available appointment will not suffice. The role of the family physician increasingly will be that of a health coach and advisor rather than the mandatory provider of primary care services.

Medical societies will fight against the expansion of primary care and other medical services to different providers, but it is likely that many new physicians will find that joining these convenience care teams is satisfying work. It may turn your stomach now, but your residency program may be giving out a Walmart award at a future graduation. How does family medicine education prepare us for this future?

While I support and practice evidence-based medicine, The U.S. Preventive Services Task Force has used evidence to create public policy. In an uncertain and changing world, this may be a mistake. I believe they were off target with their recommendations on PSA testing.

PSA screening: The USPSTF got it wrong

J Fam Pract.
2013;62(11):616, 618

Prostate cancer is an important disease. It is the second leading cause of cancer death in men who don't smoke, and in many cases it is detectable early and curable. The rates of both diagnosis and death from prostate cancer in men are similar to the rates of breast cancer in women.[1]

The current practical screening test for prostate cancer is the prostate specific antigen (PSA). Making routine use of it, as we know, however, is controversial. The false positive rate for PSA testing is high, for example, in men with chronic prostatitis and benign prostatic hypertrophy.[2] In addition, many prostate cancers are diagnosed that will never harm the patient. Treatment for prostate cancer may result in complications, such as incontinence and impotence. Because of these facts, the US Preventive Services Task Force (USPSTF) has recommended against routine screening.[2]

The PSA test itself never hurt anyone

It is just a lab value, a piece of information. What doctors do with the information is the issue. Physicians may cause more harm than good by being overly aggressive with elevated PSA levels and indolent or low-grade prostate cancer—and 75% of prostate cancer is considered indolent (Gleason score of 6 on biopsy).[3] Patients with such a finding can be watched, using active surveillance. The majority will never need treatment.[3]

The PSA test is just a piece of information. What doctors do with the information is the issue. Common sense tells us we must screen for prostate cancer. Not doing so on the basis of evidence-based medicine is not a defense when advanced cancer is diagnosed and screening was not offered to the patient.[4] Rather than using the data from past physician behavior and recommending against screening with PSA, the USPSTF should have criticized the response to PSA test results and recommended a better way. I see this change rapidly becoming current practice.

PSA testing saves lives

Since the early 1990s, when PSA testing became widespread, there has been a 40% decline in prostate cancer mortality.[5] A randomized trial in 7 countries in Europe clearly showed a survival benefit from screening for prostate cancer.[6] Clinical trials in the United States have been ambiguous.

Not screening for prostate cancer with PSA is unacceptable to many physicians and patients. Most physicians have seen preventable prostate cancer deaths. Two patients in my practice illustrate this point. The PSA of one of them—a 62-year-old man—went from 2.4 to 24 in 2 years. The PSA of another, age 56, went from 2.6 to 34 in one year. Both men had no symptoms, and their prostate cancer was found on routine screening. Both had a high Gleason score and locally invasive prostate cancer. Now, years after undergoing cancer treatment, both have undetectable PSA levels and full function. They think the USPSTF's recommendation not to screen is evidence of the government's attempt to save money, reinforcing the notion that the government cannot be trusted.

Patients are increasingly savvy

With all the controversy around prostate cancer screening and the adverse effects of treatment, patients are getting savvier. Shared decision making between doctor and patient is becoming the standard of care, and physicians can meet their professional obligations by offering screening and answering any questions the patient may have. I find that most men with low-grade disease are happy to avoid surgery and radiation if active surveillance is offered and explained.

The American Academy of Family Physicians adopted the recommendation of the USPSTF to advise against screening for prostate cancer.[7] The American College of Physicians recommends that men ages 50 to 69 be given the opportunity for informed decision making before screening.[8] The American Urological Association recently recommended that men ages 55 to 69 be offered screening, with a discussion about the risks and benefits;[9] and the American Cancer Society recommends screening starting at age 50, and earlier for high-risk men.[10]

Not satisfied that any of these organizations really knows what is best and aware that the data are confusing and evolving, I continue to follow my overall practice approach: Start routine cancer screening at age 50 in the general population and at age 40 for high-risk groups. This works for colon, breast, and prostate cancer, the big 3 that are common, sometimes fatal, and often curable with early detection. Recommending against screening for prostate cancer is not tenable.

Men in my practice are offered a PSA test starting at age 50, and every one to 2 years thereafter based on both patient preference and the results. Black men and those with a family history of prostate cancer before age 60 are offered screening starting at age 40. I suggest that screening be stopped at age 80, or earlier if the patient has a serious chronic illness with a life expectancy of less than 10 years.

Active surveillance for low-grade disease

What is done with elevated or rising PSA levels is most controversial, with lots of room for doing harm. Dramatic rises in PSA, like those of the patients I described earlier, are easy: Go right to biopsy and usually, treatment. Gleason 6 prostate cancer is likely to remain localized and indolent, and not threaten life. I work with urologists who are not aggressive and are willing to follow patients with PSA levels up to 10. Noninvasive options are available, such as fractionating the PSA (free and total) and imaging such as MRI. Genetic testing is available and can add to the evaluation of the patient's risk.

Active surveillance has become a standard of care in monitoring patients with low-grade disease. The outcomes for survival with active surveillance are as good as radical prostatectomy.[11] The goal is to be aggressive in treatment only with patients who have life-threatening disease. A collaboration among the patient, the primary care physician, and the urologist is crucial to optimizing patient outcomes.

Recommending against screening for prostate cancer is not tenable. The responsible approach is to continuously improve cancer detection and therapy to maximize good and minimize harm. This approach is available today.

References

1. Jemal A, Siegel R, Xu J, et al. Cancer statistics, 2010. CA Cancer J Clin. 2010;60:277-300.
2. US Preventive Services Task Force. Screening for prostate cancer: Ann Int Med. 2008;149:185-191.
3. Klotz L. Active surveillance: current and future directions. Curr Opin Urol. 2013;23:237-238.
4. Merenstein D. A piece of my mind: Winners and losers. JAMA. 2004;291:15-16.
5. Siegel R, DeSantis C, Virgo K, et al. Cancer treatment and survivorship statistics, 2012. CA Cancer J Clin. 2012;64:220-241.
6. Schroder FH, et al; ERSPC investigators. Screening and prostate cancer mortality in a randomized European study. N Engl J Med. 2009;360:1320-1328.
7. American Academy of Family Physicians Web site. Prostate cancer. Available at: www.aafp.org/patient-care/clinical-recommendations/all/prostate-cancer.html. Accessed October 16, 2013.
8. Qaseem A, Barry MJ, Denberg TD, et al. Screening for prostate cancer: a guideline statement from the clinical guidelines of the American College of Physicians. Ann Int Med. 2013;158:761-769.
9. Carter HB, Albertsen PC, Barry MJ, et al. Early detection of prostate cancer: AUA guideline. American Urological Association. 2013;1-28. Available at: www.auanet.org/common/pdf/education/clinical-guidance/Prostate-Cancer-Detection.pdf. Accessed October 16, 2013.
10. Wolf AM, Wender RC, Etzioni RB, et al. American Cancer Society guideline for the early detection of prostate cancer: update 2010. CA Cancer J Clin. 2010;60:70-98.
11. Wilt TJ, Brawer MK, Jones KM, et al. Radical prostatectomy versus observation for localized prostate cancer. N Engl J Med. 2012;367:203-213.

Ian McWhinney, who passed away in 2012, was a founder of family medicine in North America. As a social philosopher and a naturalist, he had a great influence on the development of family medicine It was a honor to write this tribute.

Remembering Ian McWhinney

Fam Med
2013;45(8):539-40

Back in 1974, as a third-year medical student, I made the counter-culture decision to go in to family medicine. My father wrote me a letter and said that I was not fulfilling my potential. I needed intellectual reinforcement. It came in an article in the New England Journal of Medicine, "Family Medicine in Perspective," by Ian McWhinney, MD.[1]

Having decided to devote my career to helping people rather than unlocking the secrets of medical science, McWhinney's opening hooked me in:

Family medicine is part of the process by which medicine adjusts to the changing needs of society. Family physicians have in common the fact that they obtain fulfillment from personal relations more than from the technical aspects of medicine.[1]

Ian McWhinney started his career as a general practitioner in England in 1954, practicing with his father. He became curious about the way patients presented and the thinking patterns in general practice. Following a rich tradition of observational scholars among British general practitioners (he had a special interest in the work of James MacKenzie), he wrote down his observations in his first book, The Early Signs of Illness: Observations in General Practice in 1964.[2] It is out of print, but I am grateful to Amazon.com for finding a used bookseller in England to get a copy.

McWhinney's career was also inspired by an article in the New England Journal of Medicine, this one by Robert Haggerty, describing postgraduate training in a new specialty of family practice.[3] He applied for and was given a Nuffield Traveling Fellowship to the United States, where he spent 8 weeks in a fellowship in family medicine with Robert Haggerty at Harvard, 1 year after Lynn Carmichael, the founder of the Society of Teachers of Family Medicine. He visited a variety of locations in the United States and Canada that were beginning postgraduate training in what was emerging as a new specialty.

The life-changing decision came as an offer to become the first chair of family medicine in Canada in 1968 at the University of Western Ontario. He was 40 and had a family that needed convincing to move to North America, and leaving his father was very difficult. His sense of mission to advancing family medicine won out.

From the beginning, McWhinney promoted clinical observation leading to clinical research. McWhinney referred to the natural history of disease as the basic science of medicine. He wrote about the naturalist tradition in general practice:

For me there have been two great satisfactions of medical practice. One has been the depth of human experience which, as physicians, we are privileged to have. The other has been the satisfaction of observing patients with illnesses of all kinds, in their own habitat, and over long periods of time. This is the satisfaction experienced by all naturalists.[4]

McWhinney's opus came in his single authored A Textbook of Family Medicine in 1981 with a second edition in 1997.[5] The book was an alternative to the textbooks that aimed to cover the field of knowledge in family medicine. McWhinney's aim was to define and conceptualize the field, which he did eloquently. Half of the book is devoted to the basic principles of family medicine, and the second half applies these principles to the treatment of common clinical problems.

Canadian family physicians revere Ian McWhinney as their Osler.[6] To the US founders of family medicine, he was a guiding light that both inspired and served as a kindred spirit.

McWhinney championed the exceptionalism of family medicine in a social context. The overlap between the writings of McWhinney and Gayle Stephens, MD, are not an accident; both served as the early social philosophers of the specialty. Ian McWhinney passed away 1 year ago this month, the occasion that prompted this editorial. His passing was not widely known in the United States last year, yet his influence lives on. John Frey, MD, and William Ventres, MD, interviewed McWhinney in 1991 and 1992, obtaining an oral history published in part in Family Medicine.[7] These are his words and are well worth reading again.

With managed care taking off in 1992, McWhinney realized that the old questions about general practice and family medicine need to be "reframed" since they are not answerable in the new framework. We are at such a time today with information systems and a new biology.

With the mapping of the human genome and the brain as an electrochemical grid, biomedical reductionists are having a heyday. Hence the controversy about whether the new Diagnostic and Statistical Manual of Mental Disorders, Fifth Edition (DSM-5) is scientific enough because it lacks a iochemical basis for mental disorders. The human spirit is not simply biology, and illness behavior is heavily influenced by experience.

Our chemicals are the often the effect rather than the causal basis of disease. We need more Ian McWhinneys to develop what he called the synthesis between science, technology, and art in medicine, not just family medicine but all of medicine.

References

1. McWhinney IR. Family medicine in perspective. N Engl J Med1975;293:176-81.

2. McWhinney IR. The early signs of illness: observations in general practice. London: Pittman, 1964.

3. Haggerty RJ. Training program for family practice. N Engl J Med 1963;26:160-1.

4. McWhinney IR. The naturalist tradition in general practice. J Fam Pract 1977;5:375-8.

5. McWhinney IR. A textbook of family medicine. New York: Oxford University Press, 1981 and 1997.

6. Pimlott N. Reflecting on Dr Ian McWhinney. Can Fam Physician 2012;58:1187.

7. Frey JJ, Ventres WB. Voices from family medicine:Ian McWhinney. Fam Med 1992;24:317-20.

It is fitting that this book end at a time of beginning. Family Medicine has finally entered a phase of transformation to a 21ˢᵗ century model of practice. I enjoy that now and look forward to a continued contribution to its fulfillment.

The Unfinished Story of Family Medicine Transformation

Fam Med
2014;46(1):5-6

1998 was a year of great change. How we communicate, bank, arrange travel and shop were being transformed by the new internet browsers that rose just three years earlier. Tom Friedman referred to 1995 as the beginning of the third phase of human civilization, the information age.[1] In 1998, the Institute of Medicine (IOM) convened the Committee on the Quality of Healthcare in America. The charge to the committee was to vision a 21ˢᵗ century health care system where the gap between the care most Americans received and what was available would be closed. What the committee found was not a gap, but a chasm, and a report was released in 2001 to cross that chasm by transforming how health care is delivered.[2]

Building on the IOM report, leaders in family medicine convened and released a Future of Family Medicine Report in 2004.[3] In order to meet the quality needs of the public, the process of delivering family medicine needed to change from brief episodic office visits on paper records to a continuous process of care using advanced information systems. Family medicine took the lead for all of primary care to bring about this transformation. Fewer medical school graduates were choosing to enter primary care making the need for transformation became an imperative.[4]

In 2007, the primary care organizations came together and released the principles for the patient-centered medical home (PCMH).[5] PCMH practices would offer continuous access to care through a team of caregivers all working to the level of their license. Care coordination outside of office visits became the hallmark of a PCMH practice. Multiple organizations are offering certification in

PCMH practice and this is becoming the new standard for primary care.

With the passage of the Affordable Care Act in 2010, many more Americans will have health insurance and access to care. The efficiencies of PCMH practice include greater teamwork, not relying on the physician to do everything, and nonvisit communication and care focused on delivering care to populations. Health systems are forming out of the cottage industry of independent private practice, and are being called upon to be accountable for the health of the population being served. Accountable care organizations (ACOs) are being challenging by financial incentives to follow the Triple Aim: improved health to populations, an improved experience of receiving care, and a reduction of wasteful healthcare spending.[6]

In his timely article in this issue to Family Medicine, Macaran Baird calls upon us not to be complacent with all that has been accomplished in the last 10-15 years.[7] PCMH practices are not the end of the transformation, but the beginning, and they need to become a new way of operating a practice, not a geographic location. Family Medicine should continue to lead all of primary care into a process of improving the health of populations, a complex task with multiple facets that must be addressed.

Pioneers in primary care have taught us much about how to make a difference in population health. Health is not just about receiving medical care, and the social determinants of health must be addressed to make a difference. Jeffrey Brenner in Camden, NJ has mobilized effective teams to bring health to some of the most challenging populations, including care to very high cost patients known as "hot spotters".[8] Baird has been among a group of leaders working to being mental health providers into primary care in a collaborative model that is gaining traction because it works to keep patients out of emergency rooms and hospitals, the standard for reducing wasteful health care spending.[9]

Innovations in primary care can be found at the Patient-Centered Primary Care Collaborative (www.pcpcc.org) and at the Center for Excellence in Primary led by Thomas Bodenheimer and Kevin Grumbach.[10] The complexity of advanced information systems, especially electronic health records and current coding practices, requires much greater teamwork and a changed role for the physician to be more efficient and effective.[11,12]

Nothing really changes until the financial incentives are in place. Internet based enterprises, such as Google, Cisco and Oracle, succeeded and became among the world's largest businesses by finding a path to financial success. If primary care continues to be paid on a visit-based productivity formula, that is what will dominate. Financial incentives for population health, and delivering care without visits, are growing and must continue to be supported to drive transformation. Financial disincentives for wasteful health care spending are working well in hospitals. For primary care, using internet communication and care offers great efficiency in reducing the need for expensive office visits for minor problems and ongoing communication about chronic illness care and preventive services. Prepayment for care coordination and rewards for successful performance will help drive this change.

Leaders in family medicine are convening again to provide a 2.0 version to the future of family medicine effort. Let's hope they head the words of Baird and not be complacent with the gains that have been made with PCMH so far. The transformation called for in the IOM report back in 2001 is still far from being realized, an unfinished story. Family medicine is still vulnerable to becoming an anachronism if it does not embrace the information age with internet based applications for communication and care. Primary care services can be provided by many different people in many different places, such as at Wal-Mart and the local pharmacy. Activated patients will increasingly be able to arrange their own care and even assemble their own medical homes. Through transformation, family medicine may remain the go to resource for providing health through personalized care.

References:

1. Friedman TL. The World is Flat. New York: Farrar, Straus & Giroux. 2005.
2. Institute of Medicine. Crossing the Quality Chasm: A New Health System for the 21st Century. Washington DC: Institute of Medicine. 2001.
3. Future of Family Medicine Project Leadership Committee. Future of Family Medicine: A Collaborative Project of the Family Medicine Community. Ann Fam Med. 2004;2:S3-32.

4. Scherger JE. The End of the Beginning: The Redesign Imperative in Family Medicine. Fam Med. 2005;37(7):513-516.
5. Kellerman R, Kirk L. Principles of the Patient-Centered Medical Home. Am Fam Physician. 2007;76(6):774-775.
6. Berwick DM, Nolan TW, Whittington J. The Triple Aim: Care, Health, and Cost. Health Affairs. 2008:27(3):759-769.
7. Baird MA. Primary Care in the Age of Reform – Not a Time for Complacency. Fam Med. Fam Med. 2014;46(1): 7-10.
8. Brenner J. Identifying "hot spots" of high health care costs and engaging patients. Keynote Address at the *Patient-Centered Primary Care Collaborative Stakeholder Conference.* April 23, 2012, Washington D. C.
9. Collaborative Family Healthcare Association. www.cfha.net.
10. http://familymedicine.medschool.ucsf.edu/cepc/
11. Bodenheimer TS, Smith MD. Primary Care: Proposed Solutions to the Physician Shortage Without Training More Physicians. Health Affairs. 2013;32(11):1881-1886.
12. Shipman SA, Sinsky CA. Expanding Primary Care Capacity by Reducing Waste and Improving the Efficiency of Care. Health Affairs. 2013;32(11):1990-1997.

POSTSCRIPT

My career in family medicine started in the infancy of the new specialty in the early 1970s and went through its early transformation in the information age. Family medicine is the modernization of general practice. A typical general practitioner in office practice would see 50-60 patients a day. In family medicine, more time was spent with patients with an expanded focus on the patient's biopsychosocial needs. Family physicians between 1970 and 2000 were trained to see 20-30 patients a day. With the internet, communication and care with patients become continuously accessible and seeing patients in the office is a selective activity rather than the primary way patients are cared for. The emergence of health information technology and the internet will radically change the delivery of health care, and in 2014 these changes are still in their infancy.

It has been a great honor and pleasure to participate in this 40 year history of family medicine. My health is good and I hope to be able to make many more contributions. Thank you for your interest in these articles and I hope they contribute to a richer understanding of a great specialty.

ABOUT THE AUTHOR

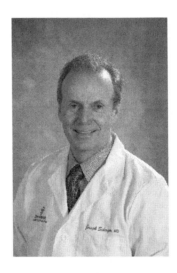

Joseph E. Scherger, M.D., M.P.H., is Vice President for Primary Care & Marie Pinizzotto, MD Chair of Academic Affairs at Eisenhower Medical Center in Rancho Mirage, California. Dr. Scherger is Clinical Professor of Family Medicine at the University of California, San Diego School of Medicine (UCSD), and at the Keck School of Medicine at the University of Southern California (USC). Dr. Scherger's main focus is on the redesign of office practice using the tools of information technology and quality improvement.

Originally from Delphos, Ohio, Dr. Scherger graduated from the University of Dayton in 1971, summa cum laude. He graduated from the UCLA School of Medicine in 1975, and was elected to Alpha Omega Alpha. He completed a Family Medicine Residency and a Masters in Public Health at the University of Washington in 1978. From 1978-80, he served in the National Health Service Corps in Dixon, California, as a migrant health physician. From 1981-92, Dr. Scherger divided his time between private practice in Dixon and teaching medical students and residents at UC Davis. From 1988-91, he was a Fellow in the Kellogg National Fellowship Program, focusing on health care reform and quality of life. From 1992-1996, he was Vice President for Family Practice and Primary Care

Education at Sharp HealthCare in San Diego. From 1996-2001, he was the Chair of the Department of Family Medicine and the Associate Dean for Primary Care at the University of California Irvine. From 2001-2003, Dr. Scherger served as founding dean of the Florida State University College of Medicine.

Dr. Scherger has received numerous awards, including being recognized as a "Top Doc" in San Diego for 6 consecutive years, 2004-2009. He was voted Outstanding Clinical Instructor at the University of California, Davis School of Medicine in 1984, 1989 and 1990. In 1989, he was Family Physician of the Year by the American Academy of Family Physicians and the California Academy of Family Physicians. In 1986, he was President of the Society of Teachers of Family Medicine. In 1992, Dr. Scherger was elected to the Institute of Medicine of the National Academy of Sciences. In 1994, he received the Thomas W. Johnson Award for Family Practice Education from the American Academy of Family Physicians. In 2000, he was selected by the UC Irvine medical students for the AAMC Humanism in Medicine Award. He received the Lynn and Joan Carmichael Recognition Award from the Society of Teachers of Family Medicine in 2012. He served on the Institute of Medicine Committee on the Quality of Health Care in America from 1998-2001. Dr. Scherger served on the Board of Directors of the American Academy of Family Physicians and the American Board of Family Medicine. From 2005-2010 he served as Consulting Medical Director for Quality and Informatics at Lumetra Healthcare Solutions.

Dr. Scherger serves on the editorial board of *Medical Economics* and is an Assistant Editor of *Family Medicine.* He was the Men's Health expert and a consultant for Revolution Health, 2006-09, and he has covered California for eDocAmerica since 2003. He was Editor-in-Chief of *Hippocrates,* published by the Massachusetts Medical Society, from 1999-2001. He was the first Medical Editor of *Family Practice Management.* He has authored more than 400 medical publications and has given over 1000 invited presentations.

Dr. Scherger enjoys an active family life with his wife, Carol, and two sons, Adrian and Gabriel. He has completed 30 marathons, eight 50K and three 50 mile ultramarathon trail runs.

Revised 06/14

Made in the USA
Columbia, SC
30 October 2017